Urological Surgery Handbook

Urological Surgery Handbook

Edited by Holly Penn

hayle
medical

New York

Hayle Medical,
750 Third Avenue, 9th Floor,
New York, NY 10017, USA

Visit us on the World Wide Web at:
www.haylemedical.com

ISBN: 978-1-63241-918-7

Cataloging-in-Publication Data

Urological surgery handbook / edited by Holly Penn.
    p. cm.
Includes bibliographical references and index.
ISBN 978-1-63241-918-7
1. Genitourinary organs--Surgery. 2. Genitourinary organs--Diseases--Treatment.
3. Urology. I. Penn, Holly.
RD571 .U76 2020
617.461--dc23

Table of Contents

Preface

This book has been an outcome of determined endeavour from a group of educationists in the field. The primary objective was to involve a broad spectrum of professionals from diverse cultural background involved in the field for developing new researches. The book not only targets students but also scholars pursuing higher research for further enhancement of the theoretical and practical applications of the subject.

The branch of medicine that is concerned with the surgical management of the diseases of the male and female urinary system and abnormalities of the male reproductive organs is called urology. The organs comprising the urinary system are closely linked with those of the reproductive tract. Therefore, any pathological condition affecting one is often seen to affect the other as well. This places several urological conditions under the spectrum of genitourinary disorders. Urological surgery is concerned with the management of bladder and prostate cancer, congenital abnormalities, stress incontinence, kidney stones and conditions arising due to traumatic injury. Transplant urology is an important area of urological surgery. This book discusses the fundamentals as well as modern approaches of urological surgery. The topics included herein on urological surgery are of utmost significance and bound to provide incredible insights to readers. A number of latest researches have been included to keep the readers up-to-date with the global concepts in this area of study.

It was an honour to edit such a profound book and also a challenging task to compile and examine all the relevant data for accuracy and originality. I wish to acknowledge the efforts of the contributors for submitting such brilliant and diverse chapters in the field and for endlessly working for the completion of the book. Last, but not the least; I thank my family for being a constant source of support in all my research endeavours.

Editor

1

Meta-analysis of female stress urinary incontinence treatments with adjustable single-incision mini-slings and transobturator tension-free vaginal tape surgeries

Peng Zhang[1], Bohan Fan[1], Peng Zhang[2*], Hu Han[3], Yue Xu[3], Biao Wang[2] and Xiaodong Zhang[2]

Abstract

Background: The study on SIMS and SMUS as a whole by Alyaa Mostafa et al showed that after excluding the TVT-S sling, there is no significant difference in patient-reported cure rate and objective cure rate between these two methods. In this paper, we systematically evaluate the relevant data on SIMS-Ajust and TVT-O/TOT and further confirm their safety and effectiveness, providing reliable clinical evidence.

Methods: By searching the Medline, Embase, Scopus, and Web of Science databases and the Cochrane Database of Systematic Reviews combined with manual searches, all reports on randomized controlled trials (RCTs) of single-incision mini-sling (SIMS-Ajust) and transobturator tension-free vaginal tape (TVT-O/TOT) surgeries were collected. Using RevMan 5.2 statistical software, the patient-reported cure rate, objective cure rate, operative time, postoperative pain, lower urinary tract injuries, groin pain, postoperative voiding difficulties, de novo urgency and/or worsening of preexisting surgery, vaginal tape erosion, repeated continence surgery, and other related data on both surgical methods were evaluated.

Results: A total of 154 relevant research reports were retrieved, and five randomized controlled trials were included in this study, involving a total of 678 patients. The meta-analysis results show no significant difference in the patient-reported cure rate and objective cure rate between SIMS-Ajust and TVT-O/TOT [$RR = 0.95$, 95 % CI (0.87 to 1.04), $P > 0.05$; $RR = 0.97$, 95 % CI (0.90–1.05), $P > 0.05$]. With respect to operation time and groin pain, SIMS-Ajust outperforms TVT-O/TOT [$MD = -1.61$, 95 % CI (-2.48 to 0.74), $P < 0.05$; $RR = 0.30$, 95 % CI (0.11 to 0.85), $P < 0.05$]. In terms of postoperative pain, lower urinary tract injuries, postoperative voiding difficulties, de novo urgency and/or worsening of preexisting surgery, vaginal tape erosion, and repetition of continence surgery, there is no significant difference between SIMS-Ajust and TVT-O/TOT [$RR = 0.50$, 95 % CI(0.18–1.43), $P > 0.05$; $RR = 2.82$, 95 % CI(0.14–57.76), $P > 0.05$; $RR = 0.64$, 95 % CI(0.28–1.45), $P > 0.05$; $RR = 1.06$, 95 % CI(0.66–1.71), $P > 0.05$; $RR = 1.04$, 95 % CI(0.24–4.45), $P > 0.05$; $RR = 1.64$, 95 % CI(0.41–6.61), $P > 0.05$].

Conclusions: SIMS-Ajust is safe and effective in the treatment of female stress urinary incontinence. Compared with TVT-O/TOT surgery, SIMS-Ajust surgery has the same high objective cure rate and patient-reported cure rate and low incidence of perioperative complications, in addition to its short operative time and low incidence of groin pain. Its long-term efficacy needs further observation.

Keywords: Single-incision mini-sling, Transobturator tension-free vaginal tape, Female stress urinary incontinence

* Correspondence: syfanbh@126.com
[2]Urology department, Beijing Chaoyang hospital Capital Medical University, 8 Gongren Tiyuchang NanluChaoyang District, Beijing 100020, China
Full list of author information is available at the end of the article

Background

The incidence rate of female stress urinary incontinence (SUI) in women in the United States is between 23 % and 67 % [1, 2]. Its risk factors include obesity and fertility, and studies have shown that when BMI increases by 5, the incidence rate of SUIrisk increases by 20 to 70 % [3]. Surgery has become a standard treatment for female stress urinary incontinence, and the surgical treatments can be roughly divided into six categories, namely, Marshall-Marchetti-Krantz operations (represented by the Burch operation), bladder neck suspension operations (represented by the Stamey and Raz operations), anterior vaginal wall repair operations, sling surgery, paraurethral injection, and artificial urinary sphincter [4]. As the operations are being improved and updated constantly, we are trying to find a treatment method that is not only effective, simple, easy to perform, with small trauma, and without long-term complications but also economical.

The SIMS-Ajust sling is a novel single-incision sling that appeared on the market in 2009 [5]. The patient-reported cure rate of SIMS-Ajust is between 73.9 % and 81.2 %, and its objective cure rate is between 76.8 % and 84.7 % [6–8]. The study on SIMS and SMUS as a whole by Alyaa Mostafa et al. [9] showed that after excluding the TVT-S sling, there is no significant difference in patient-reported cure rate and objective cure rate between these two methods. SIMS has an earlier and faster postoperative recovery. However, this report only performed an overall evaluation on single-incision mini-sling operations, including Mini-Arc, Ajust, Ophira, Needleless-Contasure, TFS, and Solyx, and did not include an individualized analysis on SIMS-Ajust. In particular, there is no report on the efficacy of SIMS-Ajust. Compared with the previous report, we have included two new randomized controlled trial literatures published in June and August 2013 [7, 10]. In this paper, we systematically evaluate the relevant data on SIMS-Ajust and TVT-O/TOT and further confirm their safety and effectiveness, providing reliable clinical evidence.

Methods

Data collection

Two urologists first extracted the relevant data and assessed their quality independently. The data were checked, and if there was a disagreement, experts were consulted to solve it. Computer searches were performed in the Medline, Embase, Scopus, and Web of Science databases and the Cochrane Database of Systematic Reviews. Manual searches were performed for meeting publications and abstracts of the International Continence Society (ICS), the International Urogynecological Association (IUGA), the American Urological Association (AUA), the European Association of Urology (EAU), and the Société

Internationale d'Urologie (SIU). SIMS-Ajust and TVT-O/TOT randomized controlled trials (RCTs) were included. The key words stress urinary incontinence, single incision mini-sling, and Ajust were used for the searches. All the reports were published in English. The searched literature begins in 2009 and ends in August 2014. RCT literature quality was assessed using the Jadad score [11]: (1) whether it is a randomized controlled trial; (2) whether it is a blind test; and (3) any treatment for loss to follow-up and withdrawal.

Inclusion criteria: (1) RCTs of studies on the efficacy of surgeries for female stress urinary incontinence; (2) prospective studies; (3) trials of studies on the comparison of Ajust methods versus the TVT-O method or versus the TOT method; (4) the characteristic baseline of surgical objects is roughly the same; (5) observed indicators include the cure rate and perioperative complications; (6) with or without allocation concealment or with blind treatment. Exclusion criteria: (1) design is rigorous, but sample data and intervention means are not clear; (2) statistical method is not appropriate; (3) loss to follow-up rate is too high; (3) assessment criteria are not uniform, and therefore, the efficacy values cannot be combined.

Statistical analysis

RevMan v.5.2 (Cochrane Collaboration, Oxford UK) was used to perform meta-analysis on the included papers. Figure 1 shows the literature search process. Clinical examination and related urodynamic examination results were used to determine whether diagnosed female stress urinary incontinence patients had complications of overactive bladder, urge incontinence, and pelvic organ prolapse. We collected information about cure rate, operation time, and postoperative complications, including postoperative pain, lower urinary tract injuries, groin pain, postoperative voiding difficulties, de novo urgency and or worsening of preexisting surgery, vaginal tape erosion, and repeated continence surgery, and we analyzed the effectiveness and safety on this basis. The mean difference (MD) for quantitative data and relative risk (RR) for qualitative data were used as statistical values for efficacy analysis; the interval estimation used 95 % as the confidence interval [12]. The Q test was used to test the heterogeneity of the included studies. When the heterogeneity difference of each test had no statistical significance ($P > 0.10$, $I^2 < 50$ %), a fixed effects model was used for meta-analysis; when the heterogeneity difference of a test had statistical significance ($P < 0.10$, $I^2 > 50$ %), the reasons for heterogeneity were analyzed, and subgroup analysis was performed. A forest plot was generated with the aid of software; if the included number of studies was too low ($n < 10$), a funnel plot was not drawn [12].

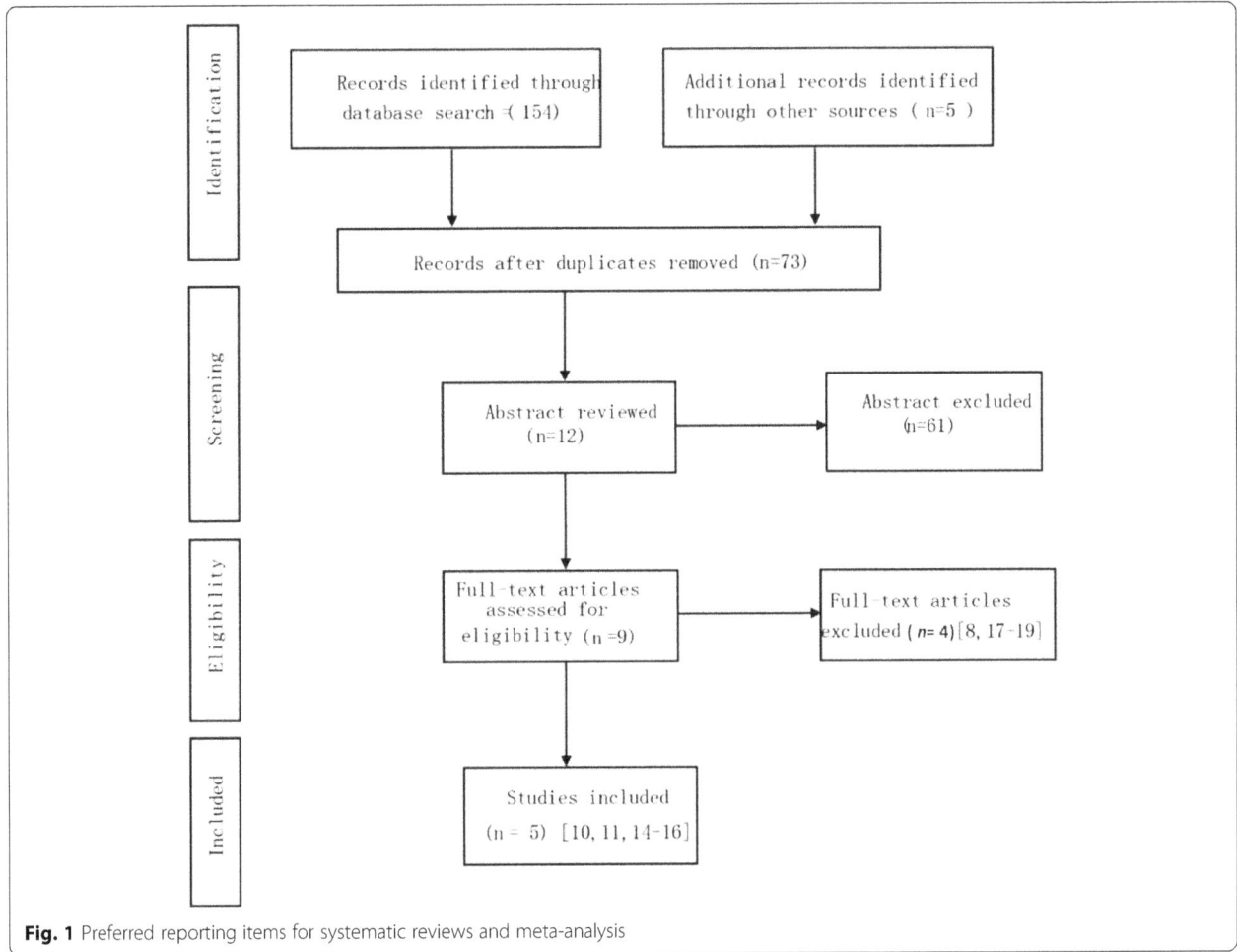

Fig. 1 Preferred reporting items for systematic reviews and meta-analysis

Results

A total of five RCT reports were selected, and the Jadad score for all five articles was three points (Table 1) [7,10,13,14,15] (SIMS-Ajust: $n = 361$, TVT-O/TOT: $n = 317$). A total of 13 people were lost to follow-up (SIMS-Ajust: $n = 3$, TVT-O/TOT: $n = 10$). The excluded papers and the reasons are listed in Table 2 [8,16-18].

Cure rate

A total of three studies were included to compare the objective cure rate of two sling surgeries: there are 235 cases in the SIMS-Ajust group, and the number of objective cure cases is 187; there are 200 cases in the TVT-O/TOT group, and the number of objective cure cases is 167. Heterogeneity test $I^2 = 0$ %, $P > 0.1$, and therefore, the included literature can be considered homogeneous, and a fixed model is used for the statistical analysis. The results show that the objective cure rate of the two groups has no significant difference [$RR = 0.95$, 95 % CI (0.87 to 1.04), $P > 0.05$] (see Fig. 2a). A total of four studies were included for the comparison of the patient-reported cure rate: 261 cases in the SIMS-Ajust group with 216 patient-reported cure cases; 261 cases in the TVT-O/TOT group with 222 patient-reported cure cases. The heterogeneity test $I^2 = 0$ %, $P > 0.1$, and therefore, the included reports can be considered homogeneous. A fixed model is

Table 1 Jadad score

	Randomized controlled	Blinding method	Loss to follow-up/ withdrawal	Total score
Dati 2012 [13]	2	0	1	3
Schweitzer 2012 [14]	2	0	1	3
Mostafa 2013 [10]	2	0	1	3
Grigoriadis 2013 [7]	2	0	1	3
Masata 2013 [15]	2	0	1	3

Table 2 Excluded literature

Boyers 2013 [8]	The same study as Mostafa 2013 [10]
Mostafa 2012 [16]	The same study as Mostafa 2013 [10]
Martan 2013 [17]	Two SIMS comparison randomized controlled trials
Palomba 2014 [18]	Three SIMS comparison randomized controlled trials

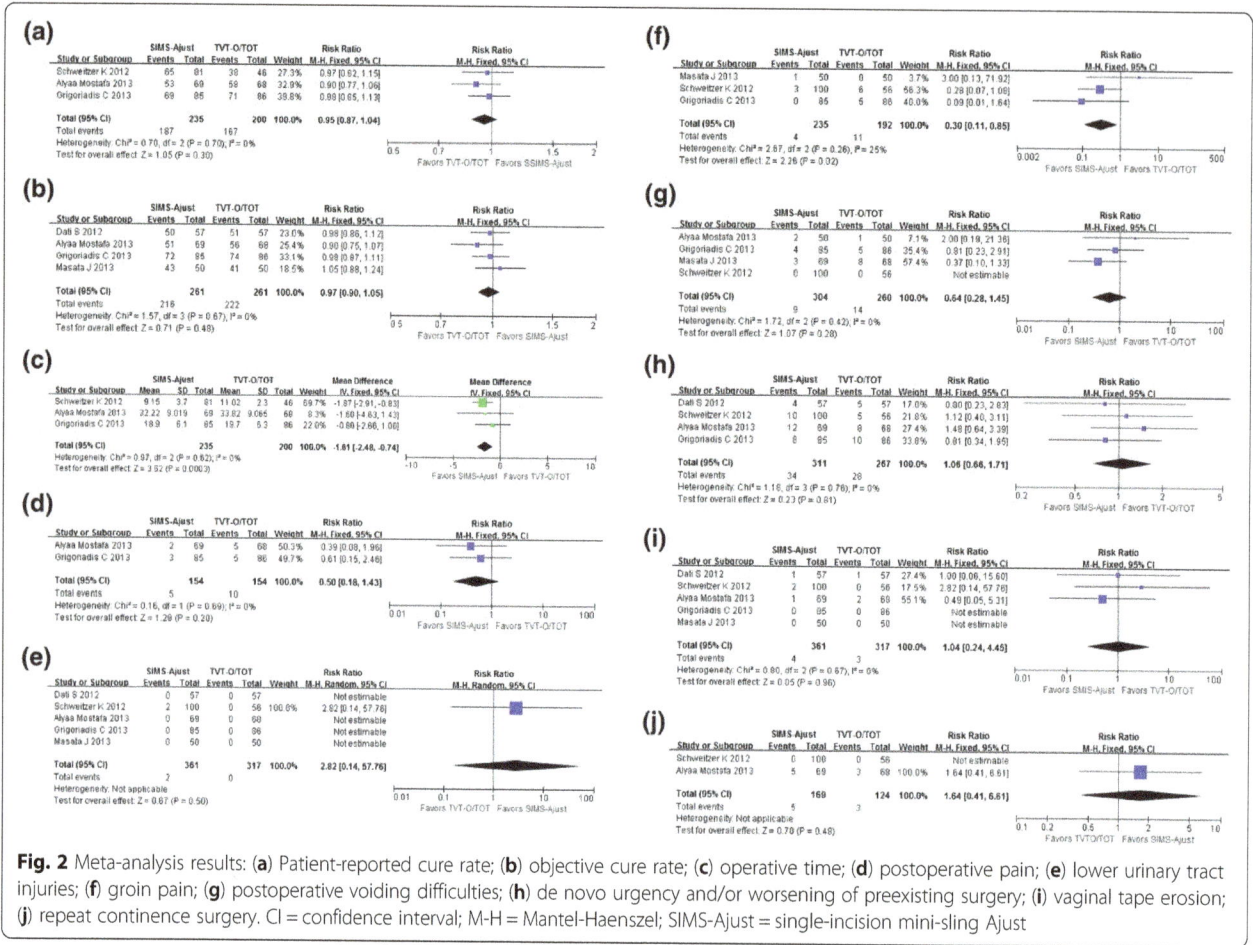

Fig. 2 Meta-analysis results: (**a**) Patient-reported cure rate; (**b**) objective cure rate; (**c**) operative time; (**d**) postoperative pain; (**e**) lower urinary tract injuries; (**f**) groin pain; (**g**) postoperative voiding difficulties; (**h**) de novo urgency and/or worsening of preexisting surgery; (**i**) vaginal tape erosion; (**j**) repeat continence surgery. CI = confidence interval; M-H = Mantel-Haenszel; SIMS-Ajust = single-incision mini-sling Ajust

then used for the statistical analysis, and the results show no significant difference in the patient-reported cure rate in the treatment of female stress urinary incontinence between SIMS-Ajust and TVT-O/TOT [RR = 0.97, 95 % CI (0.90 to 1.05), P > 0.05] (see Fig. 2b).

Surgical Information

A total of three studies were used for the statistical analysis of operation time, with 235 cases in the SIMS-Ajust group and 200 cases in the TVT-O/TOT group. Heterogeneity test $I^2 = 0$ %, $P > 0.1$; therefore, the included reports can be considered homogeneous, and the analysis results show that SIMS-Ajust has a shorter operation time than TVT-O/TOT in the treatment of female stress urinary incontinence [WMD = −1.61 min, 95 % CI (−2.48 to −0.88), P < 0.05] (see Fig. 2c). A total of two studies were used for the statistical analysis of postoperative pain: 154 cases are in the SIMS-Ajust group with five cases having postoperative pain, and 154 cases are in the TVT-O/TOT group with 10 cases having postoperative pain. Heterogeneity test $I^2 = 0$ %, $P > 0.1$, and therefore, the included reports can be considered homogeneous, and a fixed model is used for the

statistical analysis. The results show that there is no significant difference in the incidence rate of postoperative pain between SIMS-Ajust and TVT-O/TOT [RR = 0.50, 95 % CI (0.18 to 1.43), P > 0.05] (see Fig. 2d).

Complications

The statistics on five postoperative complications show that the incidence rate of postoperative groin pain by SIMS-Ajust is significantly less than for TVT-O/TOT [RR = 0.30, 95 % CI (0.11 to 0.85), <0.05]. The statistics on lower urinary tract injuries, postoperative voiding difficulties, de novo urgency and/or worsening of preexisting surgery, and vaginal tape erosion show no significant difference between the two operations [RR = 0.50, 95 % CI (0.18 to 1.43), P > 0.05; RR = 2.82, 95 % CI (0.14 to 57.76), P > 0.05; RR = 0.64, 95 % CI (0.28 to 1.45), P > 0.05; RR = 1.06, 95 % CI (0.66 to 1.71), P > 0.05; RR = 1.04, 95 % CI (0.24 to 4.45), P > 0.05] (see Fig. 2e-i).

Repeat of continence surgery

In total, three studies performed statistical analysis on repeated continence surgery. In the 169-case SIMS-Ajust group, five cases had repeated continence surgery; in the

124-case SMUS group, three cases required repeated continence surgery. Heterogeneity test $I^2 = 0$ %, $P > 0.1$, so the included reports can be considered homogeneous. A fixed model is used for statistical analysis, and the results showed no significant difference in the incidence rate of repeated continence surgery between these two groups [$RR = 1.64$, 95 % CI (0.41 to 6.61), $P > 0.05$] (Fig. 2j).

Publication bias

A total of five (<10) RCTs were included in this study, so funnel plot analysis was not performed to detect publication bias.

Discussion

A tension-free midurethral sling is a grade A recommendation according to the guide for stress urinary incontinence treatment [19]. Midurethral slings can be divided into three generations [20]: In 1995, Ulmsten and Petros [21] established retropubic tension-free vaginal tape (TVT) as the first generation of sling operations to treat urinary incontinence, and it was soon widely accepted and considered the standard operation for the treatment of female stress urinary incontinence (SUI). Although this operation has effective results, bladder perforation and other complications [22] prompted people to continue to search for other sling methods. The second generation of sling operations for the treatment of urinary incontinence is the transobturator TVT-O and TOT operation, and meta-analysis [23] showed no significant difference in efficacy between retropubic vaginal tape operation and transobturator operation. Although this operation avoids bladder perforation, postoperative thigh pain or groin pain becomes a common complication, and its incidence rate is between 1.6 % and 8.2 % [24,25]. Various vaginal single-incision midurethral sling operations are the third generation of urinary incontinence operations [20]. Compared with traditional operations, single-incision vaginal sling operations 1) have a shorter sling, with less foreign material being inserted into human body, thereby reducing the adverse reactions to foreign material; 2) have less injury to the patient, thereby reducing possible perforation infections; 3) avoid having bladder, obturator nerves, and blood vessels in the puncture path, which is therefore safer than the traditional retropubic midurethral sling (RP-TVT) and TVT-O/TOT.

The Ajust sling is one of the single-incision vaginal slings that appeared on the market in 2009 [5]. Its puncture method is to use a specially designed anchor to fix the sling on the obturator membrane without letting both ends penetrate through the skin. After implantation, the tightness of the sling is adjusted through the device. In comparison, a TVT-O/TOT sling penetrates through the inner side of the thigh. Therefore, anatomically, it seems that SIMS-Ajust might have a lower cure rate or increased cases of repeat continence surgery due to its weaker anchor force. However, in reality, SIMS-Ajust has turned this factor entirely into an advantage. Our meta-analysis of the two tapes showed that SIMS-Ajust had enough anchor force in practice and with low groin pain. After comparing the five studies included in this meta-analysis, we found no significant difference in the patient-reported cure rate and objective cure rate between SIMS-Ajust and TVT-O/TOT. In addition, there is no significant difference in the comparison of the incidence rate of repeat continence surgery between SIMS-Ajust and TVT-O/TOT. The follow-up periods of both the reports included in this study are longer than 12 months. It is reasonable to say that the mid-term efficacy of SIMS-Ajust is reliable. This result indicates that although the SIMS-Ajust puncture path is short, its anchor has enough force to fix the sling in the midurethral position and cure stress urinary incontinence. In a 90-sample study by Mohamed Abdel-Fattah et al. [6], there were two cases of less effective slings that failed when removed, which corroborates the reliability of the anchor force from the side. The effectiveness of SIMS-Ajust is similar to the effectiveness of traditional TVT-O/TOT.

Similar to other single incision slings, the Ajust puncture does not require an incision on the inner side of the thigh or suprapubic, which reduces the risks of blood vessel, nerve, and visceral injuries. There are no cases of blood vessel or nerve injuries and other serious complications in the studies included in this meta-analysis. SIMS-Ajust has a low postoperative groin pain incidence rate. In the RCT study of Grigoriadis C. [7], SIMS-Ajust has no cases of postoperative groin pain, while TVT-O/TOT has five cases of postoperative groin pain, which disappeared 15 days after the operation. Therefore, in terms of the appearance of groin pain, the advantage of SIMS-Ajust is obvious. The included studies show that SIMS-Ajust has a shorter operation time than SMUS by 1–3 min, indicating that its operation is simpler and more convenient, this shorter may have no contribution to improvement of the safety of the operation. In the comparison of other complications, postoperative pain, lower urinary tract injuries, postoperative voiding difficulties, de novo urgency and/or worsening of preexisting surgery, and vaginal tape erosion are similar for both operation methods. Therefore, we can say that SIMS-Ajust is a safe operation for treating female stress urinary incontinence. Meanwhile, Dwayne Boyers et al. [8] performed statistical analysis on the health services and patient quality adjusted life-years (QALYs) of the same group of people in Alyaa Mostafa's study to assess the health costs, and the results showed that because SIMS-Ajust is performed under local anesthesia, the cost is reduced according to one-year follow-up cost-effectiveness.

There are limitations of this study: (1) the number of included RCT studies is small (5), and none of them are double-blind studies; (2) observation indicators and assessment methods are different, resulting in the loss of some study data; (3) the 95 % confidence interval of some observation indicators is too wide, which requires more studies; and (4) possible gray literature may exist and lead to publication bias.

Conclusions

In summary, SIMS-Ajust surgical treatment for female stress urinary incontinence is safe and effective. SIMS-Ajust surgery, compared with TVT-O/TOT surgery, has the same high patient-reported and objective cure rates and low perioperative complications incidence rate. In addition, it has a short operation time and a low incidence rate of groin pain. However, as some of the studies included in this meta-analysis have a short follow up time, and meta-analysis requires continuous updates, the long-term efficacy needs further observation.

Consent

Written informed consent was obtained from the patient's guardian/parent/next of kin for the publication of this report and any accompanying images.

Abbreviations
SIMS-Ajust: Adjustable single-incision mini-sling; TVT-O/TOT: Transobturator tension-free vaginal tape; RCTs: Randomized controlled trials; SUI: Stress urinary incontinence; SMUS: Standard midurethral slings.

Competing interests
Financial disclosures: Peng Zhang certifies that all conflicts of interest, including specific financial interests and relationships and affiliations relevant to the subject matter or materials discussed in the manuscript (eg, employment/affiliation, grants or funding, consultancies, honoraria, stock ownership or options, expert testimony, royalties, or patents filed, received, or pending), are the following: None.

Authors' contributions
Author contributions: PZ had full access to all the data in the study and takes responsibility for the integrity of the data and theaccuracy of the data analysis. Study concept and design: PZ, BF. Acquisition of data: BF, HH. Analysis and interpretation of data: PZ, BF, HH, YX, BW. Drafting of the manuscript: PZ, BF. Critical revision of the manuscript for important intellectual content: 9 PZ, BF. Statistical analysis: BF, YX. Obtaining funding: None. Administrative, technical, or material support: PZ, XZ. Supervision: PZ. Other (specify): None. All authors read and approved the final manuscript.

Authors' information
Peng Zhang and Bohan Fan are first author.

Acknowledgement
The authors would like to thank all authors who kindly provided their data and made this review possible: Drs. Alyaa Mostafa, Schweitzer, Dati, Grigoriadis, Masata.

Funding/Support and role of the sponsor
None.

Author details
[1]Urology department, Beijing Chaoyang hospital, Capital Medical University, 8 Gongren Tiyuchang NanluChaoyang District, Beijing 100020, China.
[2]Urology department, Beijing Chaoyang hospital Capital Medical University, 8 Gongren Tiyuchang NanluChaoyang District, Beijing 100020, China.
[3]Urology department, Beijing Chaoyang hospital Capital Medical University, 8 Gongren Tiyuchang Nanlu,Chaoyang District, Beijing 100020, China.

References
1. Fultz NH, Herzog AR. Prevalence of urinary incontinence in middle aged and older women: a survey based methodological experiment. J Aging Health. 2000;12:459–69.
2. Novielli K, Simpson Z, Hua G, Diamond JJ, Sultana C, Paynter N. Urinary incontinence in primary care: a comparison of older African-american and Caucasian women. Int Urol Nephrol 2003;35(3):423–8.
3. Osborn DJ, Strain M, Gomelsky A, Rothschild J, Dmochowski R. Obesity and female stress urinary incontinence. Urology 2013;82(4):759–63.
4. Thüroff JW, Abrams P, Andersson KE, Artibani W, Chapple CR, Drake MJ, et al. EAU Guidelines on Urinary Incontinence. Actas Urol Esp. 2011;35(7):373–88.
5. Kennelly MJ, Myers EM. Retropubic and Transobturator Slings: Still Useful or Should All Patients Be Treated with Mini-slings? Curr Urol Rep. 2011;12:316–22.
6. Abdel-Fattah M, Agur W, Abdel-All M, Guerrero K, Allam M, Mackintosh A, et al. Prospective multi-centre study of adjustable single-incision mini-sling (Ajust ®) in the management of stress urinary incontinence in women: 1-year follow-up study. BJUI 2011;109:880–6.
7. Grigoriadis C, Bakas P, Derpapas A, Creatsa M, Liapis A. Tension-free vaginal tape obturator versus Ajust adjustable single incision sling procedure in women with urodynamic stress urinary incontinence. Eur J Obstet Gynecol Reprod Biol. 2013;170(2):563–6.
8. Boyers D, Kilonzo M, Mostafa A, Abdel-Fattah M. Comparison of an adjustable anchored single-incision mini-sling, Ajust®, with a standard mid-urethral sling, TVT-OTM: a health economic evaluation. BJU Int, 2013;112:1169–77.
9. Mostafa A, Lim CP, Hopper L, Madhuvrata P, Abdel-Fattah M. Single-Incision Mini-Slings Versus Standard Midurethral Slings in Surgical Management of Female Stress Urinary Incontinence: An Updated Systematic Review and Meta-analysis of Effectiveness and Complications. Eur Urol. 2014;65(2):402–27.
10. Mostafa A, Agur W, Abdel-All M, Guerrero K, Lim C, Allam M, et al. Multicenter prospective randomized study of single-incision mini-sling vs tension-free vaginal tape-obturator inmanagement of female stress urinary incontinence: a minimum of 1-year follow-up[J]. Urology. 2013;82(3):552–9.
11. Jadad AR, Rennie D. The randomized controlled trial gets a middleaged checkup. JAMA 1998;279:319–20.
12. Higgins JPT, Green S, editors. Cochrane Handbook for Systematic Reviews of Interventions, v.5.1.0. http://www.cochrane.org/. Accessed October 14, 2012.
13. Dati S, Rombola P, Cappello S, Piccione E. Single-incision minisling (AJUST) vs obturator tension-free vaginal shortened tape (TVTABBREVO) in surgical management of female stress urinary incontinence. Int J Gynecol Obstet 2012;119:S670.
14. Schweitzer KJ, Cromheecke GJ, A. L. Milani, H. W. Van Eijndhoven, D. Gietelink 4, E. Hallenleben, et al. A randomized controlled trial omparing the TVT-O® with the Ajust® as primary surgical treatment of female stress urinary incontinence[J]. Int Urogynecol J. 2012;23(2):S77–78.
15. J. Masata, K. Svabik, P. Hubka, R. Elhaddad, A. Martan. Comparison of the safety and peri-operative complications of transobturator introduced tension-free vaginal tape (TVT-O) and single-incision tape with adjustable length and anchoring mechanism (Ajust) in a randomized trial: short term results[J]. Int Urogynecol J. 2013;24(1):S114–5.
16. Mostafa A, Agur W, Abdel-All M, Guerrero K, Lim C, Allam M, et al. A multicentre prospective randomised study of single-incision mini-sling (Ajust®) versus tension-free vaginal tape-obturator (TVT-O™) in the management of female stress urinary incontinence: pain profile and short-term outcomes. Eur J Obstet Gynecol Reprod Biol. 2012 ,165(1):115–21.
17. Alois M, Jan K, Jaromir M, Kamil S, Michael H A,Lukas H, et al. Prospective Randomized Study of MiniArc and Ajust Single Incision Sling Procedures. LUTS, 2013;6(3):172–4.
18. Palomba S, Falbo A, Oppedisano R, Torella M, Materazzo C, Maiorana A, et al. A randomized controlled trial comparing three single-incision minislings for stress urinary incontinence. Int Urogynecol J. 2014;25(10):1333–41.

19. Lucas MG, Bosch RJ, Burkhard FC, Cruz F, Madden TB, Nambiar AK, et al. EAU guidelines on surgical treatment of urinary incontinence. Actas Urol Esp. 2013;37(8):459–72.

20. Maslow K, Gupta C, Klippenstein P, Girouard L. Randomized clinical trial comparing TVT Secur system and trans vaginal obturator tape for the surgical management of stress urinary incontinence. Int Urogynecol J 2014;25:909–14.

21. Ulmsten U, Petros P. Intravaginal slingplasty (IVS):an ambulatory surgical procedure for treatment of female urinary incontinence. Scand J Urol Nephrol, 1995;29:75–82.

22. Deng DY, Rutman M, Raz S, Rodriguez LV. Presentation and management of major complications of midurethral slings: Are complications under-reported? Neurourol Urodyn 2007;26:46–52.

23. Novara G, ArtibaniVW, Barber MD, Chapple CR, Costantini E, Ficarra V, et al. Updated Systematic Review and Meta-Analysis of the Comparative Data on Colposuspensions, Pubovaginal Slings, and Midurethral Tapes in the Surgical Treatment of Female Stress Urinary Incontinence. Eur Urol, 2010; 58(2):218–38.

24. Bianchi-Ferraro AM, Jarmy-Dibella ZI, de Aquino Castro R, Bortolini MA, Sartori MG, Girão MJ. Randomized controlled trial comparing TVT-O and TVT-S for the treatment of stress urinary incontinence: 2-year results. Int Urogynecol J, 2014;25(10):1343–8.

25. Tincello DG, Botha T, Grier D, Jones P, Subramanian D, Urquhart C, et al. The TVT Worldwide Observational Registry for Long-Term Data: safety and efficacy of suburethral sling insertion approaches for stress urinary incontinence in women. J Urol, 2011;186(6):2310–5.

[−2]proPSA versus ultrasensitive PSA fluctuations over time in the first year from radical prostatectomy, in an high-risk prostate cancer population

S. De Luca[1], R. Passera[2]* ⓘ, A. Sottile[3], C. Fiori[1], R. M. Scarpa[1] and F. Porpiglia[1]

Abstract

Background: [−2]proPSA and its derivatives have an higher diagnostic accuracy than PSA in predicting prostate cancer (PCa). In alternative to PSA, ultrasensitive PSA (uPSA) and [−2]proPSA could be potentially useful in recurrent disease detection. This research focused on [−2]proPSA and uPSA fluctuations over time and their possible clinical and pathological determinants, in the first year after RP.

Methods: A cohort of 106 consecutive patients, undergoing RP for high-risk prostate cancer (pT3/pT4 and/or positive margins), was enrolled. No patient received either preoperative/postoperative androgen deprivation therapy or immediate adjuvant RT, this latter for patient choice. [−2]proPSA and uPSA were measured at 1, 3, 6, 9, 12 months after RP; their trends over time were estimated by the mixed-effects linear model. The uPSA relapse was defined either as 3 rising uPSA values after nadir or 2 consecutive uPSA >0.2 ng/ml after RP.

Results: The biochemical recurrence (BCR) rate at 1 year after RP was either 38.6 % (in case of 3 rising uPSA values) or 34.9 % (in case of PSA >0.2 ng/ml after nadir), respectively. The main risk factors for uPSA fluctuations over time were PSA at diagnosis >8 ng/ml ($p = 0.014$), pT ($p = 0.038$) and pN staging ($p = 0.001$). In turn, PSA at diagnosis >8 ng/ml ($p = 0.012$) and pN ($p < 0.001$) were the main determinants for [−2]proPSA trend over time. In a 39 patients subgroup, uPSA decreased from month 1 to 3, while [−2]proPSA increased in 90 % of them; subsequently, both uPSA and [−2]proPSA increased in almost all cases. The [−2]proPSA trend over time was independent from BCR status either in the whole cohort as well in the 39 men subgroup.

Conclusions: Both uPSA and [−2]proPSA had independent significant fluctuations over time. PSA at diagnosis >8 ng/ml and pathological staging significantly modified both these trends over time. Since BCR was not confirmed as determinant of [−2]proPSA fluctuations, its use as marker of early biochemical relapse may not be actually recommended, in an high-risk prostate cancer patients population.

Keywords: Prostate cancer, (−2)pro-prostate-specific antigen, Prostate-specific antigen, Biochemical recurrence

Background

After a successful radical prostatectomy (RP), a serum detectable Prostate Specific Antigen (PSA) may be considered a marker of residual prostate tissue, presumably anticipating either locoregional or systemic disease [1].

However, approximately 20 % of patients experience biochemical recurrence (BCR) after RP [2–4]; around 30 % of them will ultimately develop a clinical progression [5, 6].

Several trials proved that adjuvant radiation therapy (RT) after RP decreases BCR risk and provides survival benefit, in high-risk disease patients. An early and reliable BCR detection is therefore crucial, since postoperative RT is more effective when given to subjects having low PSA levels [7].

* Correspondence: passera.roberto@gmail.com
[2]Division of Nuclear Medicine, San Giovanni Battista Hospital and University of Torino, Corso AM Dogliotti 14, 10126 Torino, Italy
Full list of author information is available at the end of the article

New PSA ultrasensitive methods detect levels <0.1 ng/ml, and some assays even minimal ones (1 pg/ml) [8, 9]. A classical definition for ultrasensitive PSA (uPSA) relapse is 3 rising uPSA values after nadir [10]; recurrence seldom occurs in patients with uPSA <0.04 ng/ml, 3 years after RP [11].

In recent years, many efforts were made to improve the biomarkers diagnostic accuracy for prostate cancer (PCa); at the same time, an alternative to PSA as BCR marker is still unavailable. Some studies showed that [–2]proPSA and its derivatives improve PSA accuracy in predicting PCa at prostate biopsy (Bx), being associated to PCa aggressiveness either at Bx or at final pathology after RP [12, 13]. Moreover, [–2]proPSA could be potentially useful in recurrent disease detection, a virtually unexplored field.

To our knowledge, no study investigated the [–2]proPSA trend over time post-RP. We enrolled at RP a sequential cohort of high-risk PCa patients (extra prostate disease and/or positive margins), eligible for adjuvant RT but not being given for patient choice.

The primary endpoint of this research was to longitudinally investigate either [–2]proPSA and uPSA time trends as well their clinical and pathological determinants, in the first year after RP, at a single high-volume institution. The secondary endpoint was to elucidate a [–2]proPSA possible role in early BCR detection.

Methods

A cohort of 106 consecutive patients, undergoing robot assisted radical prostatectomy (RARP) for a pathological high-risk PCa (pT3/pT4 and/or positive margins), was enrolled at San Luigi Gonzaga Hospital - Orbassano (Italy) from September 2013 to October 2014. Among them, 83 patients (81.3 %) underwent robot-assisted extended pelvic lymph nodes dissection prior to RARP (external iliac artery/vein, obturator fossa, obturator nerve, internal iliac artery/presacral lymph nodes) [14]. Lymphadenectomy was planned according to Briganti nomogram [15]. Pathological staging was performed according to the TNM Classification of Malignant Tumors seventh edition [16]; histological grading was assessed according to the Gleason grading system [17]. No patient received either preoperative/postoperative androgen deprivation therapy or immediate adjuvant RT, this latter for patient choice.

The follow-up was scheduled at 1/3/6/9/12 months after RARP; it included a complete physical and digital rectal examination (DRE), as like [–2]proPSA and uPSA measurements. The uPSA relapse was defined either as 3 rising uPSA values after nadir [10] or two consecutive uPSA >0.2 ng/ml rising after RP [18].

Due to the observational nature of this research and according to Italian regulation, no formal IRB/IEC approval was needed [19].

uPSA and [–2]proPSA serum concentrations measurement

Serum samples were analysed by the Access 2 Immunoassay System on a UniCell DxI800 instrument (Beckman Coulter, USA). The calibration procedure was performed by a 7-point recombinant [–2]proPSA curve (0–5000 pg/ml). The blank and quantitation limits (according to the Clinical Laboratory Standards Institute document EP17-A) were 0.5 and 3.23 pg/ml, respectively. uPSA results were obtained by a single determination, while that from [–2]proPSA by a duplicate one; the analyses were repeated in case of coefficient of variation >20 %. All analyses were performed in the same laboratory (Candiolo Cancer Institute).

Statistical methods

The primary outcomes were the uPSA and [–2]proPSA trends over time after RARP and their potential modifications by independent covariates. uPSA and [–2]proPSA were longitudinally measured at five time-points (1/3/6/9/12 months after RP), and these repeated measures were used as dependent variables in univariate and multivariate mixed-effects linear models [20]. Due to the not-Gaussian distribution of uPSA and [–2]proPSA, all models were estimated using their log-transformed values [ln(uPSA) and ln [–2]proPSA]. At first, the univariate analyses were performed for the following covariates: age (>65 vs. ≤65 years), Body Mass Index [BMI, (>26 vs. ≤26)], DRE (positive vs. negative), PSA at diagnosis (>8 vs. ≤8 ng/ml), number of positive Bx samples (>5 vs. ≤5), GS at Bx (8–9 vs. ≤7), number of lesions at Magnetic Resonance Imaging [MRI (≥2 vs. 1)], prostate volume (>40 vs. ≤40 ml), tumor percentage (>10 % vs. ≤10 %), GS at surgery (8–9 vs. ≤7), capsule/vesicles/neural/vascular/marginal involvement (any vs. none), pT (pT3b vs. pT3a vs. pT2), pN (pN+ vs. pN0) and BCR (any vs. none). Two different definitions of BCR were used: either uPSA value >0.2 ng/ml or 3 rising uPSA values after nadir. The multivariate mixed-effects linear models for uPSA and [–2]proPSA trends over time were estimated by the restricted maximum likelihood method, using a first-order autoregressive covariance matrix: both ln(uPSA) and ln([–2]proPSA) variances at each time-point were considered comparable and constant, while the correlations between subsequent measures similar. Patient characteristics were analyzed by the Fisher's exact test for categorical variables, while for continuous ones by the Mann–Whitney and Kruskal-Wallis tests (for independent measures) or by the Wilcoxon and Friedman ones (for repeated measures). All results for continuous variables were expressed as the median (range). All reported p-values were obtained by the two-sided exact method, at the conventional 5 % significance level. Data were analysed as of September 2015 by R 3.2.1 (R Foundation for Statistical Computing, Vienna-A, http://www.R-project.org).

Table 1 Main patient characteristics

Age at diagnosis, years	65 (48–77)
PSA at diagnosis, ng/ml	7.8 (4.0–81.0)
BMI at diagnosis, kg/m^2	26.3 (17.4–34.6)
Prostate volume, ml	41.2 (22.4–103.9)
Tumor percentage, %	10.2(2.3–52.9)
Cancer familiarity,	
neg	6 (5.7 %)
pos	100 (94.3 %)
DRE,	
neg	71 (67.6 %)
pos	34 (32.4 %)
GS at biopsy,	
6	31(29.5 %)
7(3 + 4)	29(27.6 %)
7(4 + 3)	21(20.0 %)
8	16(15.2 %)
9	8(7.6 %)
Lesions at MRI,	
1	31 (53.4 %)
2+	27 (46.6 %)
GS at surgery,	
6	4(3.8 %)
7(3 + 4)	37(37.4 %)
7(4 + 3)	37(37.4 %)
8	15(15.2 %)
9	6(6.1 %)
Margins,	
neg	53 (50.0 %)
pos	53 (50.0 %)
Capsule involvement,	
neg	25 (23.6 %)
pos	81 (76.4 %)
Neural involvement,	
neg	8 (7.5 %)
pos	98 (92.5 %)
Vascular involvement,	
neg	65 (68.4 %)
pos	30 (31.6 %)
pT2	9 (8.5 %)
pT3a	83 (78.3 %)
pT3b	14 (13.2 %)
pN0	69 (79.3 %)
pN+	18 (20.7 %)

Table 1 Main patient characteristics *(Continued)*

uPSA, ng/ml 1/3/6/9/12 months	0.010 (0–1.15)/0.018 (0–0.67)/ 0.051 (0.01–0.52)/0.100 (0.01–0.56)/ 0.154 (0–0.89)
[–2]proPSA, pg/ml 1/3/6/9/12 months	0.22 (0–2.14)/0.57 (0–2.84)/0.89 (0–3.97)/ 1.25 (0.03–3.72)/1.38 (0–4.86)

For continuous variables, all the results are expressed as median (range)

Results

The main patient characteristics (106 patients) are reported in Table 1. The 1-year after surgery BCR rate was 34.9 % using uPSA value > 0.2 ng/ml, while 38.6 % using 3 rising uPSA values after nadir; at the same time, no subject had an imaging-confirmed metastatic disease.

The uPSA values sequentially increased in 43.4/69.8/83.1/89.0 % patients, at 3/6/9/12 months after RARP, respectively. The uPSA trend over time was confirmed by the Friedman test ($p < 0.001$); using the Wilcoxon one, all the differences between two adjacent time-points were extremely significant ($p < 0.001$), except that between 1 vs. 3 months ($p = 0.833$).

The mixed-effects linear model was used to confirm the uPSA time trend (within-subject factor) and to estimate its potential risk factors (between-subject factors) (Table 2, Fig. 1a). This approach confirmed that uPSA fluctuations over time were statistically significant ($p < 0.001$). In the multivariate mixed-effects linear model, the main determinants for uPSA fluctuations were PSA at diagnosis >8 ng/ml ($p = 0.014$), pT ($p = 0.038$) and pN ($p = 0.001$).

The [–2]proPSA values sequentially increased in 86.8/93.4/90.4/91.5 % patients, at 3/6/9/12 months after surgery, respectively. The difference among the median [–2]proPSA repeated measures was highly significant at the Friedman test ($p < 0.001$); all the differences between adjacent time-points were extremely significant ($p < 0.001$), when investigated by the Wilcoxon test.

Using the mixed-effects linear model as for uPSA, [–2]proPSA fluctuations over time were statistically significant ($p < 0.001$) (Table 2, Fig. 1b). Their main predictors were PSA at diagnosis >8 ng/ml ($p = 0.012$) and pN ($p < 0.001$); the interaction between them was marginal ($p = 0.099$).

In 39 patients, uPSA decreased from month 1 to 3, conversely [–2]proPSA increased in 90 % of them; in the further follow-up, both uPSA and [–2]proPSA increased in almost all cases.

Of note, [–2]proPSA trend over time was independent from BCR status ($p = 0.096$ and 0.194 according to BCR definitions, respectively; Fig. 2a, b) in the whole cohort as well in the 39 men subgroup (its BCR rate was 33.3 %). When BCR was calculated as uPSA >0.2 ng/ml, the 1-year [–2]proPSA was around double for BCR patients

Table 2 Mixed linear models for uPSA and [–2]proPSA repeated measures

uPSA	Univariate model	Multivariate model	[–2]proPSA	Univariate model	Multivariate model
Covariate	p	p	Covariate	p	p
Time trend	**<0.001**	**<0.001**	Time trend	**<0.001**	**<0.001**
Age >65 years	0.095	0.455	Age >65 years	0.472	
BMI >26	0.059	0.507	BMI >26	0.315	
PSA at diagnosis >8 ng/ml	**0.015**	**0.014**	PSA at diagnosis >8 ng/ml	**0.032**	**0.012**
Positive DRE	0.168		Positive DRE	0.241	
Biopsy samples >5	0.365		Biopsy samples >5	0.483	
GS at biopsy >7	0.419		GS at biopsy >7	0.349	
MRI lesions >1	0.178		MRI lesions >1	0.607	
Prostate volume >40 ml	0.214		Prostate volume >40 ml	0.472	
Tumor percentage >10 %	0.522		Tumor percentage >10 %	0.658	
Positive margins	**0.018**	0.214	Positive margins	0.822	
GS at surgery >7	0.209		GS at surgery >7	0.102	
Capsule involvement	**0.039**		Capsule involvement	0.077	
Neural involvement	0.216		Neural involvement	0.603	
Vascular involvement	0.110		Vascular involvement	0.083	0.952
pT	**<0.001**	**0.038**	pT	**0.008**	0.879
pN	**<0.001**	**0.001**	pN	**0.008**	**<0.001**
			BCR (uPSA +0,2 ng/ml)	0.096	
			BCR (3 rising uPSA values)	0.194	
pT*pN (interaction)	-	0.639	PSA at diagnosis*pN (interaction)	-	0.099

p-values

compared to no-BCR ones (its observed marginal means were 0.31–0.54–0.87–1.17–1.33 pg/ml for BCR subjects and 0.41–0.77–1.31–1.64–2.17 pg/ml for no-BCR ones). When BCR was calculated as 3 rising uPSA values after nadir, [–2]proPSA increased over time with a superimposable pattern (0.31–0.60–0.93–1.35–1.50 pg/ml for BCR subjects and 0.37–0.61–1.09–1.32–1.65 pg/ml for no-BCR ones).

Discussion
Recently, while many efforts have been made to improve the biomarkers diagnostic accuracy for PCa, an alternative to PSA as BCR marker is still lacking.

A persistently elevated or rising PSA after RP identifies an heterogeneous patient population, having highly variable prognosis and controversial management. Several trials showed that adjuvant RT after RP decreases BCR risk and provides survival benefit for high-risk patients [21–23]. Conversely, surgical treatment would not have failed in up to 50 % of patients receiving adjuvant RT: thus, they would have been unnecessarily exposed to radiations. To minimize overtreatment, RT should be reserved only for confirmed recurrences; however, an early salvage RT has not been proven to be equivalent to adjuvant RT yet.

uPSA is an interesting tool, whose variations could foresee a BCR [11]; this finding rarely occurs in patients with very low uPSA nadir after RP [24]. However, the uPSA role after RP is not fully defined yet. Recently, Seikkula investigated uPSA after RP and the possible correlation of uPSA doubling time (uPSA-DT) with traditional PSA doubling time (PSA-DT); uPSA >0.03 ng/ml emerged as good relapse predictor, while the above correlation between was marginal [25].

Therefore, new biomarkers for risk stratification after RP are required. Several studies demonstrated that the [–2]proPSA truncated form is detectable in tumor extracts and its serum values are markedly associated with PCa [26–30]. Sokoll demonstrated that [–2]proPSA may improve PCa detection: its raising is associated with an aggressive disease [31]. Le showed that this biomarker was able to discriminate PCa from benign disease, in males with PSA 2.5–10 ng/ml and negative DRE [27]. Recently, Guazzoni confirmed that [–2]proPSA and its derivatives are associated with PCa volume and aggressiveness [13].

Nevertheless, well considering that [–2]proPSA and its derivatives have an higher diagnostic performance than PSA, the potential usefulness of this PSA isoform in the detection of recurrent disease post radical treatment is still quite unexplored.

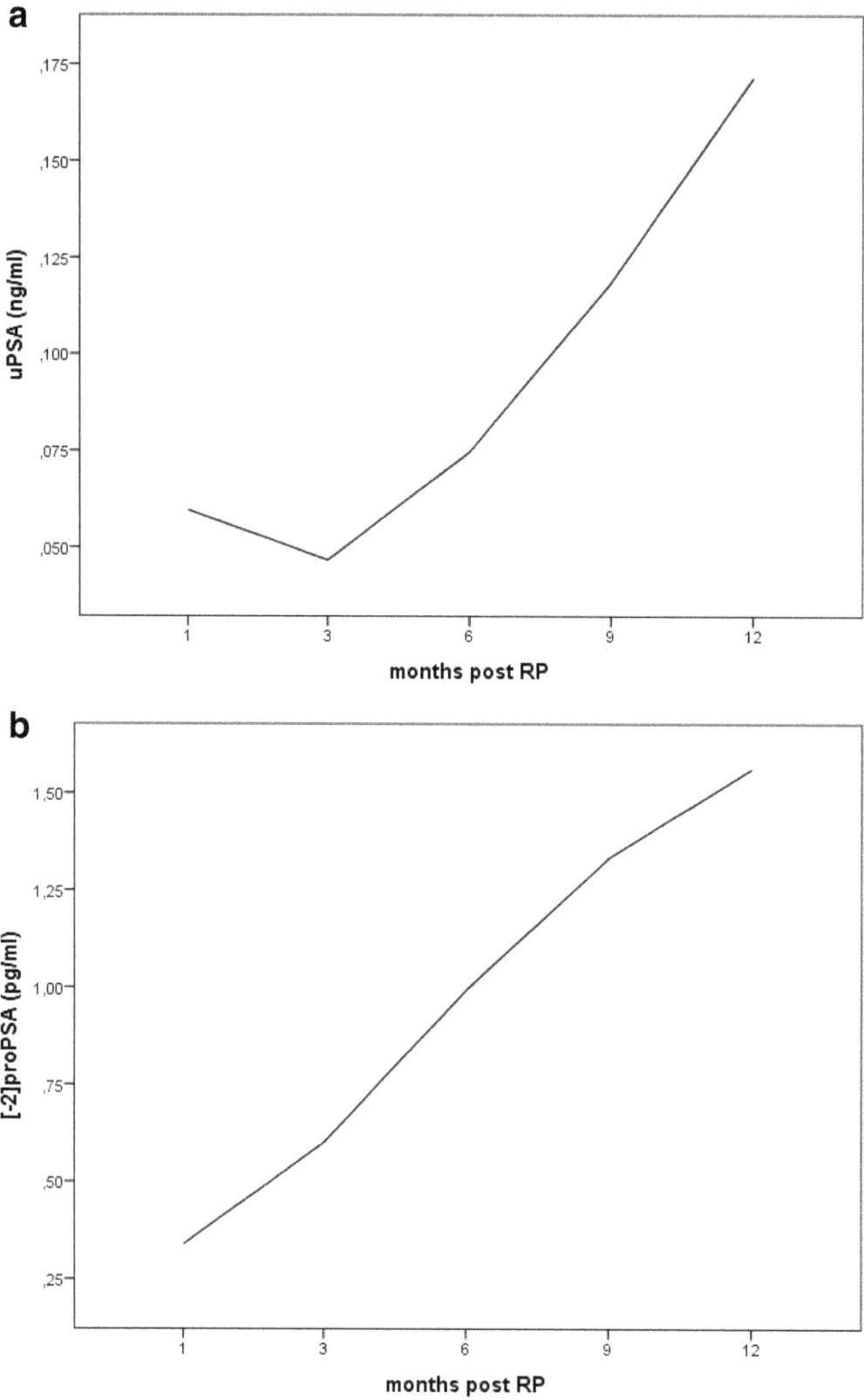

Fig. 1 a, b uPSA and [−2]proPSA mean observed values at 1–3–6–9–12 months after radical prostatectomy

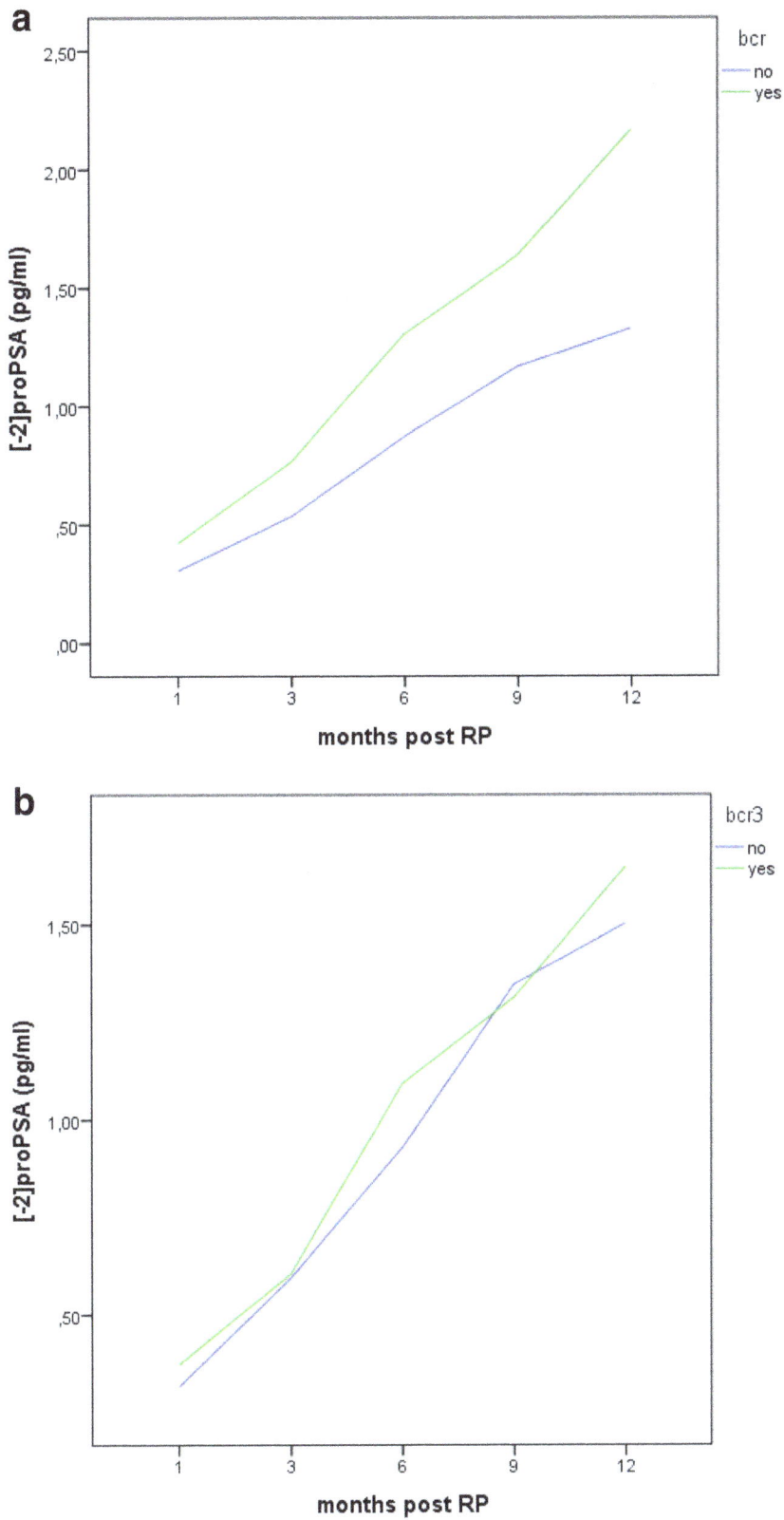

Fig. 2 a, **b** [−2]proPSA mean observed values at 1–3–6–9–12 months after radical prostatectomy by both BCR definitions (bcr = uPSA value increasing 0.2 ng/ml; bcr3 = 3 rising uPSA values after nadir)

Sottile investigated the role of [−2]proPSA in the identification of patients with metastatic progression after RP [32]. In this study, 76 patients with BCR were retrospectively studied; the imaging performed at BCR time confirmed metastatic disease in 31 out of them. Serum samples were collected at the time of imaging-confirmed metastatic progression. Median PSA, free PSA (fPSA), %fPSA, [−2]proPSA and PHI were compared between metastatic and non-metastatic patients; [−2]proPSA was a statistically significant predictor of imaging-proven metastatic PCa. However, [−2]proPSA was assessed only at BCR time, so no information may be derived on its potential role, in predicting subsequent clinical progression, when measured at BCR time [32].

The current trial is the first investigating [−2]proPSA fluctuations over time post-RP, and their possible determinants in an high-risk PCa patients cohort.

The [−2]proPSA time trend in the first 3 months showed a different pattern, compared to uPSA one. While uPSA had quite stable levels in two thirds of cases (slowly increasing only in the next period), [−2]proPSA showed a constant linear increase.

The main risk factors for uPSA fluctuations were PSA at diagnosis, pT and pN staging, being PSA at diagnosis and pN the only ones for [−2]proPSA variations.

A secondary endpoint was to investigate [−2]proPSA potential role as BCR early biomarker, in comparison to uPSA: in our series, the [−2]proPSA trend over time was independent from BCR status.

Our study has some points of strengths. The main one is that our results may suggest a stop in further researches for [−2]proPSA in the post RP arena. Second, it was designed as observational study in a homogeneous cohort of men with high-risk PCa, candidates for RP. Finally, we adopted a standardized centralised pathological evaluation; all blood samples were managed in the same laboratory according to Semjonow guidelines: no archived serum were used [33].

Conclusions

[−2]proPSA and uPSA showed significant fluctuations over time after RP, with an independent pattern. PSA at diagnosis and pathological staging significantly modified both these trends. Since BCR was not confirmed as a modifier of [−2]proPSA time trend, its use as marker of an early biochemical relapse may not be actually recommended, among high-risk prostate cancer patients.

Ethics approval and consent to participate

Due to the observational nature of this research and according to Italian regulation, the San Luigi Gonzaga Hospital (Orbassano-Italy) IRB/IEC was notified about this research proposal, while no formal ethics approval was needed [19].

Abbreviations

[−2]proPSA: [−2]pro-prostate specific antigen; BCR: biochemical recurrence; BMI: Body Mass Index; Bx: biopsy; DRE: digital rectal examination; DT: doubling time; GS: Gleason score; LNI: lymph nodes invasion; MRI: magnetic resonance imaging; PCa: prostate cancer; PSA: prostate specific antigen; RARP: robot assisted radical prostatectomy; RP: radical prostatectomy; RT: radiotherapy; uPSA: ultrasensitive prostate specific antigen.

Competing interests
The authors declare that they have no competing interests.

Authors' contributions
SDL and RP designed the study; SDL and CF collected the clinical data; RP performed the statistical analyses; AS performed the laboratory analyses; RMS and FP supervised the research team. All authors read and approved the final manuscript.

Acknowledgements
None.

Funding
The authors did not receive any financial support

Author details
[1]Division of Urology, San Luigi Gonzaga Hospital and University of Torino, Orbassano, Italy. [2]Division of Nuclear Medicine, San Giovanni Battista Hospital and University of Torino, Corso AM Dogliotti 14, 10126 Torino, Italy. [3]Division of Laboratory Medicine, Candiolo Cancer Institute, Candiolo, Italy.

References
1. Minardi D, Galosi AB, Dell'Atti L, et al. Detectable serum PSA after radical prostatectomy. Clinical and pathological relevance of perianastomotic biopsies. Anticancer Res. 2004;24:1179–85.
2. Polascik TJ, Oesterling JE, Partin AW. Prostate specific antigen: a decade of discovery - what we have learned and where we are going. J Urol. 1999; 162:293–306.
3. Moul JW. Prostate specific antigen only progression of prostate cancer. J Urol. 2000;163:1632–42.
4. Freedland SJ, Humphreys EB, Mangold LA, et al. Risk of prostate cancer-specific mortality following biochemical recurrence after radical prostatectomy. J Am Med Assoc. 2005;294:433–9.
5. Ward JF, Blute ML, Slezak J, et al. The long-term clinical impact of biochemical recurrence of prostate cancer 5 or more years after radical prostatectomy. J Urol. 2003;170:1872–6.
6. Pound CR, Partin AW, Eisenberger MA, et al. Natural history of progression after PSA elevation following radical prostatectomy. J Am Med Assoc. 1999; 281:1591–7.
7. Eggener SE, Scardino PT, Walsh PC, et al. Predicting 15-year prostate cancer specific mortality after radical prostatectomy. J Urol. 2011;185:869–75.
8. Hudson MA, Bahnson RR, Catalona WJ. Clinical use of prostate specific antigen in patients with prostate cancer. J Urol. 1989;142:1011–7.
9. Ferguson RA, Yu H, Kalyvas M, et al. Ultrasensitive detection of prostate-specific antigen by a time-resolved immunofluorometric assay and the immulite immunochemiluminescent third-generation assay: potential applications in prostate and breast cancers. Clin Chem. 1996;42:675–84.
10. Fumitaka S, Tanaka S, Matsuyama Y, et al. Efficiency of ultra-sensitive prostate-specific antigen assay in diagnosing biochemical failure after radical prostatectomy. Jpn J Clin Oncol. 2007;37:446–51.
11. Malik RD, Goldberg JD, Hochman T, et al. Three-year postoperative ultrasensitive prostate-specific antigen following open radical retro-pubic prostatectomy is a predictor for delayed biochemical recurrence. Eur Urol. 2011;60:548–53.
12. Lazzeri M, Haese A, de la Taille A, et al. Serum isoform [−2]proPSA derivatives significantly improve prediction of prostate cancer at initial biopsy in a total PSA range of 2–10 ng/ml: a multicentric European study. Eur Urol. 2013;63(6):986–94.

13. Guazzoni G, Lazzeri M, Nava L, et al. Preoperative prostate-specific antigen isoform p2PSA and its derivatives, %p2PSA and prostate health index, predict pathologic outcomes in patients undergoing radical prostatectomy for prostate cancer. Eur Urol. 2012;61(3):455–66.

14. Porpiglia F, Bertolo R, Manfredi M, et al. Total anatomical reconstruction during robot-assisted radical prostatectomy: implications on early recovery of urinary continence. European Urology. 2015. doi: 10.1016/j.eururo.2015.08. 005. [Epub ahead of print]

15. Briganti A, Larcher A, Abdollah F, et al. Updated nomogram predicting lymph node invasion in patients with prostate cancer undergoing extended pelvic lymph node dissection: the essential importance of percentage of positive cores. Eur Urol. 2012;61(3):480–7.

16. Sobin LH, Gospodarowicz MK, Wittekind C. Prostate. In: Sobin LH, Gospodarowicz MK, Wittekind C, editors. UICC TNM classification of malignant tumors. 7th ed. New York: Wiley; 2009. p. 243–8.

17. Epstein JI, Allsbrook Jr WC, Amin MB, et al. ISUP Grading Committee. The 2005 international society of urological pathology (ISUP) consensus conference on Gleason grading of prostatic carcinoma. Am J Surg Pathol. 2005;29:1228–42.

18. Guidelines of prostate cancer. European Association of Urology 2015 (http://uroweb.org/wp-content/uploads/09-Prostate-Cancer_LR.pdf)

19. Agenzia Italiana del Farmaco-AIFA, Guidelines for observational studies, March 20 2008 (http://www.agenziafarmaco.gov.it/it/content/linee-guida-studi-osservazionali)

20. Singer JD, Willett JB. Applied longitudinal data analysis: modeling change and event occurrence. New York: Oxford University Press; 2003.

21. Stephenson AJ, Shariat SF, Zelefsky MJ, et al. Salvage radiotherapy for recurrent prostate cancer after radical prostatectomy. JAMA. 2004;291(11):1325–32.

22. Stephenson AJ, Scardino PT, Kattan MW, et al. Predicting the outcome of salvage radiation therapy for recurrent prostate cancer after radical prostatectomy. J Clin Oncol. 2007;25(15):2035–41.

23. King CR. The timing of salvage radiotherapy after radical prostatectomy: a systematic review. Int J Radiat Oncol Biol Phys. 2012;84(1):104–11.

24. Kang JJ, Reiter RE, Steinberg ML, et al. Ultrasensitive Prostate Specific Antigen after Prostatectomy Reliably Identifies Patients Requiring Postoperative Radiotherapy. J Urol. 2014. [Epub ahead of print]

25. Seikkula H, Syvänen KT, Kurki S, et al. Role of ultrasensitive prostate-specific antigen in the follow-up of prostate cancer after radical prostatectomy. Urol Oncol. 2014. [Epub ahead of print]

26. Stephan C, Kahrs AM, Cammann H, et al. A [−2]proPSA-based artificial neural network significantly improves differentiation between prostate cancer and benign prostatic diseases. Prostate. 2009;69:198–207.

27. Le BV, Griffin CR, Loeb S, et al. [−2]Proenzyme prostate specific antigen is more accurate than total and free prostate specific antigen in differentiating prostate cancer from benign disease in a prospective prostate cancer screening study. J Urol. 2010;183:1355–9.

28. Jansen FH, VanSchaik RHN, Kurstjens J, et al. Prostate-specific antigen (PSA) isoform p2PSA in combination with total PSA and free PSA improves the diagnostic accuracy in prostate cancer detection. Eur Urol. 2010;57:921–7.

29. Guazzoni G, Nava L, Lazzeri M, et al. Prostate-specific antigen (PSA) isoform p2PSA significantly improves the prediction of prostate cancer at initial extended prostate biopsies in patients with total PSA between 2.0 and 10 ng/ml: results of a prospective study in a clinical setting. Eur Urol. 2011;60:214–22.

30. Catalona WJ, Partin AW, Sanda MG, et al. A multicenter study of [−2]pro-prostate specific antigen combined with prostate specific antigen and free prostate specific antigen for prostate cancer detection in the 2.0 to 10.0 ng/ml prostate specific antigen range. J Urol. 2011;185:1650–5.

31. Sokoll LJ, Sanda MG, Feng Z, et al. A prospective, multicenter, National Cancer Institute Early Detection Research Network study of [−2]proPSA: improving prostate cancer detection and correlating with cancer aggressiveness. Cancer Epidemiol Biomarkers Prev. 2010;19:1193–200.

32. Sottile A, Ortega C, Berruti A, et al. A pilot study evaluating serum pro-prostate-specific antigen in patients with rising PSA following radical prostatectomy. Oncol Lett. 2012;3(4):819–24.

33. Semjonow A, Köpke T, Eltze E, et al. Pre-analytical in-vitro stability of [−2]proPSA in blood and serum. Clin Biochem. 2010;47:926–8.

Pure retroperitoneal natural orifice translumenal endoscopic surgery (NOTES) transvaginal nephrectomy using standard laparoscopic instruments

Dechao Wei, Yili Han, Mingchuan Li, Yongxing Wang, Yatong Chen, Yong Luo and Yongguang Jiang[*]

Abstract

Background: Among the different organs used for NOTES (natural orifice translumenal endoscopic surgery) technique, the transvaginal approach may be the optimal choice because of a simple and secure closure of colpotomy site. Pure and hybrid NOTES transvaginal operations were routinely performed via transperitoneal access. In this study, we investigate the safety and feasibility of pure retroperitoneal natural orifice translumenal endoscopic surgery (NOTES) transvaginal nephrectomy using conventional laparoscopic techniques in a porcine model.

Methods: Six female pigs, weighing an average of 30 kg, were used in this study. Under general anesthesia, pure retroperitoneal NOTES transvaginal nephrectomy was conducted using standard laparoscopic instruments. Posterolateral colpotomy was performed, and the incision was enlarged laterally using blunt dissection and pneumatic dilation. A single-port device was inserted to construct the operative channel. The retroperitoneal space was created using sharp and blunt dissection under endoscopic guidance up to the level of the kidney. Dissection and removal of the kidney were performed according to standard surgical procedure, and the colpotomy site was closed using interrupted sutures. The survival and complications were observed 1 week postoperatively.

Results: Our results showed that two cases failed because of peritoneal rupture. One case was successful, but required the assistance of an extra 5 mm laparoscopic trocar inserted in the flank. Three cases of pure retroperitoneal NOTES transvaginal nephrectomy were completed, and survived 1 week after the operation. In these three cases, no intra- or postoperative complications were observed.

Conclusions: All findings confirmed the safety and feasibility of the retroperitoneal pure retroperitoneal NOTES transvaginal nephrectomy using standard laparoscopic instruments, which suggested the possibility of clinical application in human beings in the future.

Keywords: models, Animal, Natural orifice translumenal endoscopic surgery/method, Retroperitoneal space, Transvaginal surgery, Nephrectomy

* Correspondence: jyg-azyy@sohu.com
Department of Urology, Beijing Anzhen Hospital, Capital Medical University,
Beijing 100029, People's Republic of China

Background

The introduction of minimally invasive surgery has promoted the development of new surgical techniques, including the natural orifice transluminal endoscopic surgery (NOTES). The NOTES technique allows the use of hollow organs (i.e. stomach, bladder, rectum, or vagina) to access the peritoneal cavity during abdominal surgery [1, 2]. There are some theoretical advantages of this technique over open and conventional laparoscopic surgery, including avoidance of incision-related complications (wound infections, adhesions, and hernias), less postoperative pain, improved aesthetics, and a diminished immunologic impact [3, 4]. As the NOTES progress, there is a potential to make a paradigm shift in urological surgery.

Among the different organs used for NOTES technique, the transvaginal approach may be the optimal choice for female patients because of the simple and secure closure of colpotomy site. Animal studies have showed the feasibility and safety of this access route of NOTES procedures [5, 6]. Kaouk et al. also reported the use of NOTES transvaginal nephrectomy in human beings for the first time [7].

In urology, the traditional laparoscopic surgery can be performed in a minimally invasive manner using the retroperitoneal access route. Operations including lymphadenectomy for testicular cancer, nephrectomy, and adrenalectomy have been successfully conducted with this method. The benefits of this approach include less pain, less analgesic requirement, shorter convalescence, and shorter hospital stay [8].

Pure and hybrid NOTES transvaginal operations were routinely performed via the transperitoneal route. However, theoretically, the transvaginal approach to the retroperitoneal space may further reduce the invasiveness of surgery. Zorron et al. first completed excision of cyst of the kidney using flexible transvaginal retroperitoneoscopy with the assistance of two laparoscopic 5-mm trocars inserted in the left flank in human beings [9]. Moreover, robotic retroperitoneal NOTES transvaginal nephrectomy was completed in a cadaver model [10]. All of which suggested the feasibility of the retroperitoneal route in NOTES technique. In this study, we aimed to combine the transvaginal and retroperitoneal access routes to carry out pure NOTES nephrectomy in a porcine model using standard laparoscopic instruments and investigate the feasibility of this novel technique.

Methods

Animals

Six female pigs (Chinese experimental minipig, average weight 30 kg) were used in this study. All the pigs were got from Beijing Beiqijia Meile Farm (Beijing, China, license number: SCXK 2013-0005). All experimental procedures were complied with the Guidelines of Animal Care of Capital Medical University, and were approved by the Ethics Committee of Capital Medical University, China.

Procedures

The animals were anesthetized by general endotracheal anesthesia, and then were secured to the operating table in a modified flank position. The animals were positioned in lateral decubitus position with abducted lower limbs. A lateral decubitus position could reduce the negative effects of the intestinal tract to make it easier to create a larger retroperitoneal working space, and the abducted lower limbs could provide space for the surgeon to operate in the vagina. The bladder was decompressed by a 12-Fr Foley catheter.

First, the anterior and posterior vaginal walls were incised longitudinally, and fixed to the skin with reverse sutures. Afterwards, posterolateral colpotomy was performed according to the right or left kidney. With a finger, we stretched the incision to divide the tissue. In this step, the important anatomic landmarks were the deep inguinal ring and the psoas muscle. When the finger touched upon the deep inguinal ring, blunt dissection was performed digitally to create a retroperitoneal space while maintaining contact with the psoas muscle in the posterolateral direction. Pneumatic dilation (150 mL) was used to further enlarge this cavity, and a self-designed multi-channel Triport (with our modifications) was implanted and fixed on the skin to construct the operative channel. The Triport embraced one 10-mm and two 5-mm standard channels (Fig. 1).

The retroperitoneal cavity was insufflated with CO_2 gas to get 15 mmHg pressures. A 5-mm hard laparoscope was subsequently inserted into retroperitoneum. With the guidance of endoscopy, the dissection of the retroperitoneal space was performed up to the plane of the kidney with two extra-long instruments. During this step, we could easily identify abdominal aorta, the iliac

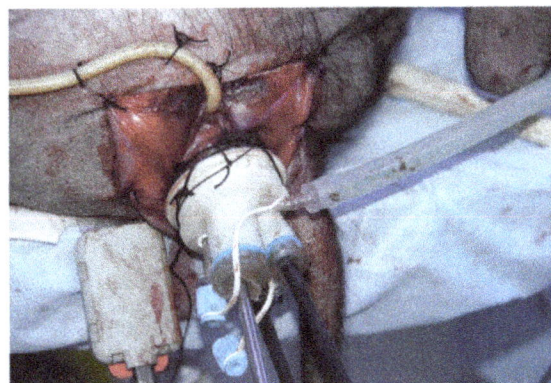

Fig. 1 Construction of the operative channel

vessels, iliac lymph nodes, ureter, kidney, and adrenal gland (Fig. 2).

The kidney was initially dissected using sharp and blunt techniques. Dissection was performed along the posterior aspect of the kidney, close to the psoas muscle in a medial-to-lateral direction towards the upper pole. The appropriate division of medial attachments to the kidney allowed clear visualization of the renal hilum. Finally, the superior and lateral attachments of the kidney were freed. The ureter was transected after firmly controlled with titanium clips or Hem-O-Lok clips. The renal artery and vein were also treated in the same way. In the porcine model, renal vessels could be transected directly with an ultrasonic scalpel (Fig. 3). The kidney was extracted through the existing vaginal incision in a laparoscopic retrieval bag. The incision was closed with interrupted sutures (Fig. 4). Survival and postoperative complications were observed one week after the operation.

Results

Among six cases, two failed because of peritoneal rupture. One case was successful but required the assistance of an extra 5 mm laparoscopic trocar inserted in the flank (Fig. 5). Pure retroperitoneal NOTES transvaginal nephrectomy using standard laparoscopic instruments was completed successfully in three cases, without conversion to multiport laparoscopy or open surgery (right nephrectomy [n = 1], left nephrectomy [n = 2]) (Table 1). The mean size of the removed kidneys was 10.4 cm × 5.1 cm × 3.0 cm, and the mean weight was 117 g (range, 109–125 g). After the operation, no death and postoperative complications were observed in the porcine.

Because of improved experience and identification of the anatomic landmarks, the operation time was dramatically reduced from 240 to 180 min. No intraoperative complications, bleeding, or injury to any retroperitoneal organs occurred. Estimated blood loss was 100 mL in each case.

Discussion

In urology, retroperitoneal laparoscopy has become the preferred option for some surgeons because of its many advantages when compared to transperitoneal access. This approach avoids intestinal disturbance and injury, allowing for quick patient recovery and short hospital stays; postoperative adhesions are minimized for the above-mentioned reasons; retroperitoneal laparoscopy avoids the negative effects of previous abdominal surgery, and the risk of wound complications are also reduced [11–13]. In addition, retroperitoneal anatomy is simpler than that of the abdominal cavity, and operative time is less than that required for the transperitoneal access [11–14]. Based on these advantages, retroperitoneal laparoscopy is widely applied in urological procedures.

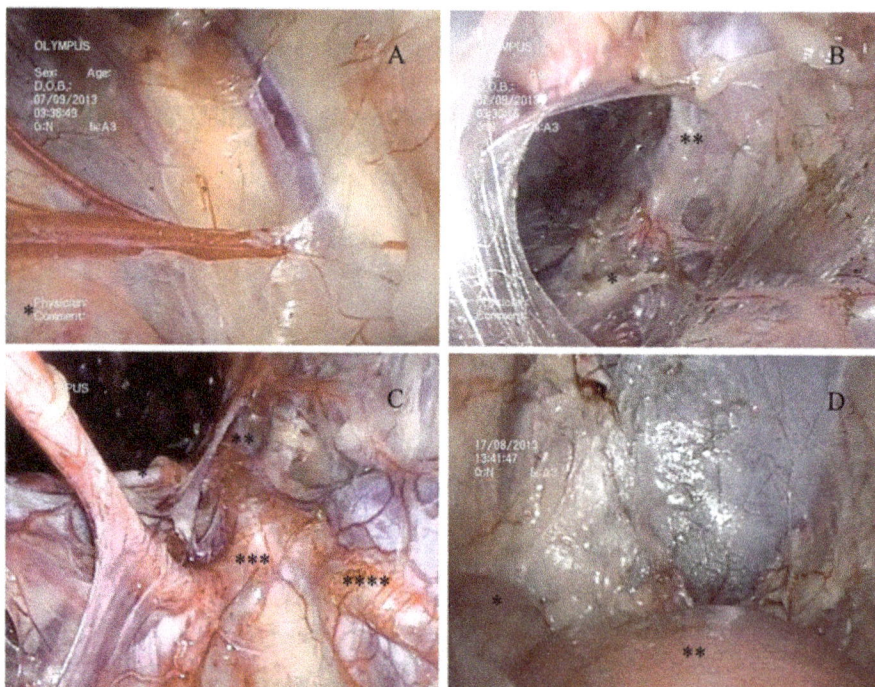

Fig. 2 Construction of the retroperitoneal space. a The left side. * Rectum. b The left enlarged retroperitoneal space. * Medial iliac lymph nodes. ** Left external iliac vessels. c The right side. * Right external iliac artery. ** Aorta. *** Right internal iliac artery. **** Left internal iliac artery. d The left side. * Adrenal. ** Renal

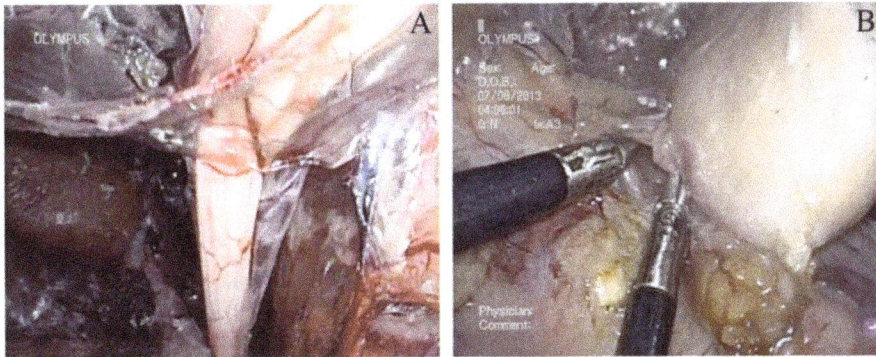

Fig. 3 The nephrectomy procedure. **a** The treatment of the right renal vein. **b** The treatment of the left renal vein

In recent years, minimally invasive surgery techniques are being developed due to similar diagnostic and therapeutic effect to open surgery with less operative trauma, reduced morbidity, shorter hospital stays, minimal scarring and lower cost. Using this new technique, surgeons can employ the natural orifices such as the vagina to enter the abdominal cavity to conduct operations. This technique completely eliminates the need for abdominal incisions, and decreases the wound complications. These potential benefits of NOTES are receiving increased attention [15].

In this study, we combine the transvaginal and retroperitoneal access routes to carry out pure NOTES nephrectomy in a porcine model using standard laparoscopic instruments and investigate the feasibility of this novel technique. The aim of the study was to explore a novel laparoscopic technique and determine its feasibility and safety.

Three cases were completely successful and survived after the procedures without any operative complications such as serious bleeding. One case was successful but required assistance of an extra laparoscopic port in the flank. The first two cases failed because of peritoneal rupture. It is well known that the peritoneal membrane is very thin, peritoneal rupture commonly occurred during the step of initial dissection. It was frustrating that we failed

to repair the peritoneal membrane in the two cases due to narrow space and unclear visualization. Consequently, the CO2 gas would leak into the peritoneal cavity when we tried to enlarge and maintain retroperitoneal space for operation. Finally, we have no choice but to abort the first two cases. Fortunately, with increased experience, we prevented this issue successfully. We summarized that the deep inguinal ring and psoas muscle are important landmarks when dissecting the peritoneum. Finger dissection ought to touch the deep inguinal ring first, and maintains contacting with the psoas muscle to dissect. Subsequent peritoneal dissection was simple with the guidance of video endoscope.

Another key of the procedures was the placement of the access port. To facilitated the implantation of operative instruments and prevented gas leakage, we modified the conventional soft Triport to a hard Triport, Improvement of all these measures ensured the smooth implementation of the operation. Furthermore, the length of instruments also had an effect on the operation. In this study, we used extra-long instruments (45 cm). If this technique was applied to humans, longer laparoscopic instruments would be required.

Based on successful peritoneal dissection, placement of the access port, and clear anatomic landmarks, freeing and removal of the kidney was not difficult. In this

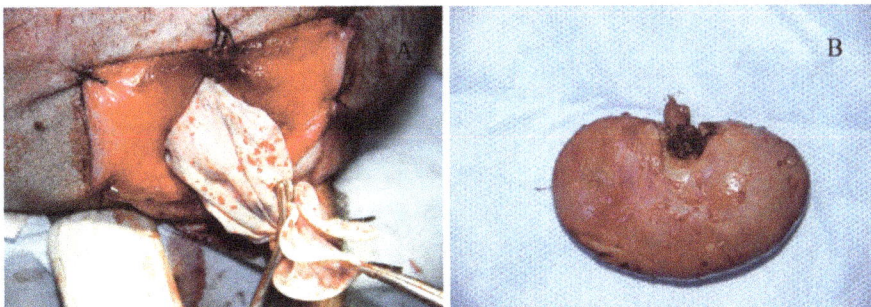

Fig. 4 Transvaginal removal of the resected kidney, **a** Transvaginal removal of specimen. **b** Left kidney

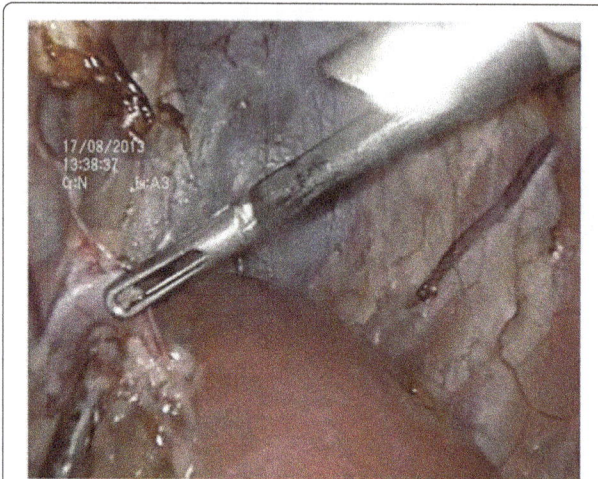

Fig. 5 Assisted nephrectomy with an additional laparoscopic trocar in the flank

study, we found that right side of nephrectomy was easier than the left because of the rectal interference. The whole procedure was performed without any intraoperative complications such as serious bleeding or injuries to organs. No postoperative complications were observed.

Even though our research has confirmed the safety and feasibility of transvaginal laparoscopic nephrectomy through retroperitoneal access preliminarily, we are yet unable to define the explicit intraoperative and postoperative complications, given that it is the first report of pure retroperitoneal NOTES transvaginal nephrectomy using standard laparoscopic instruments. The major complications of transperitoneal NOTES transvaginal access include the risk of pelvic infection, bowel perforation, transient brachial plexus injury, and dyspareunia vaginal cuff hematoma [16, 17]. We speculate that these two accesses have similar complications.

There are still some limitations in this new technique. First, this procedure can be used only in women. However, women's view on this new technique is still inconsistent [18, 19]. Second, it is essential to design new instruments to perform the operation successfully. Although we are able to perform the operation smoothly

in the porcine model, it would require considerable improvement of laparoscopic instruments before this new technique moving on to human trials.

Pure and hybrid transperitoneal NOTES transvaginal nephrectomy in human has been reported in recent years [20–23]. Bazzi et al. successfully performed transvaginal hybrid NOTES partial nephrectomy in the porcine model by the SPIDER Surgical System [24]. The signification of retroperitoneal space through transvaginal access has also been identified in the literature [25]. Allemann et al. have performed transvaginal nephrectomy, adrenalectomy, and lymphadenectomy through retroperitoneal access in a porcine model and human cadaver in the recent years [26]. In their procedure, they completed the operation with one flexible endoscope and one laparoscopic instrument, but failed to retrieve the renal specimen due to the discrepancy between the size of the kidney and the width of the vaginal incision. Zorron et al. performed hybrid NOTES transvaginal retroperitoneoscopy to treat left renal cyst in one human case for the first time using a flexible two-channel colonoscope and two conventional laparoscopic instruments [9]. Robotic retroperitoneal NOTES transvaginal nephrectomy was also explored in a cadaver model [10]. Differing from these researchers, we performed the operation with the conventional laparoscopic technique and instruments (one 5 mm hard endoscope and two laparoscopic instruments), and removed the kidney through the transvaginal access. To our knowledge, we present the first report of pure NOTES transvaginal nephrectomy with conventional laparoscopic technique through a retroperitoneal access.

Conclusions

Our data suggest the safety and feasibility of pure retroperitoneal NOTES transvaginal nephrectomy in a porcine model using conventional laparoscopic instruments for the first time. The potential applications of this surgical procedure include nephrectomy, adrenalectomy, and lymphadenectomy in urology, as well as surgery of the retroperitoneal organs in other field.

Table 1 Summary of the cases

Sequence	Nephrectomy side	EBL (ml)	Operative time (min)	Result	Complication
1	L	–	–	Aborted	peritoneal rupture
2	R	–	–	Aborted	peritoneal rupture
3	L	100	240	Completed with additional laparoscopic port	None
4	R	100	200	Completed	None
5	L	100	195	Completed	None
6	R	100	180	Completed	None

L left; R right, EBL estimated blood lose

This new technique should be further explored before be moved on human trials.

Abbreviations
NOTES, orifice translumenal endoscopic surgery.

Acknowledgements
This study was supported by the Beijing Science and Technology plan (Grant number z121107001012153).

Authors' contributions
DW participated in the study design, coordination, and data analysis, performed statistical analysis of the data, prepared figures and description of figures, and helped to draft the manuscript. YH participated in the study design, and data interpretation, and critically revised the manuscript for important intellectual content. YW and ML provided a statistical description of the manuscript. YC participated in collection of data. YL participated in collection of data. YJ conceptualized and planned the study, provided the clinical data, participated in the study design, coordination, and data interpretation, and wrote and revised the manuscript. All authors read and approved the final manuscript. This new technique should be further explored before moving on to human trials.

Competing interests
The authors declare that they have no competing interests.

References
1. Gettman MT, Box G, Averch T, et al. Consensus statement on natural orifice transluminal endoscopic surgery and single-incision laparoscopic surgery: heralding a new era in urology? Eur Urol. 2008;53(6):1117–20.
2. Box G, Averch T, Cadeddu J, et al. Nomenclature of natural orifice translumenal endoscopic surgery (NOTES) and laparoendoscopic single-site surgery (LESS) procedures in urology. J Endourol. 2008;22(11):2575–81.
3. McGee MF, Rosen MJ, Marks J, et al. A primer on natural orifice transluminal endoscopic surgery: building a new paradigm. Surg Innov. 2006;13(2):86–93.
4. Halim I, Tavakkolizadeh A. NOTES: the next surgical revolution? Int J Surg. 2008;6(4):273–6.
5. Clayman RV, Box GN, Abraham JB, et al. Rapid communication: transvaginal single-port NOTES nephrectomy: initial laboratory experience. J Endourol. 2007;21(6):640–4.
6. Ryou M, Fong DG, Pai RD, Tavakkolizadeh A, Rattner DW, Thompson CC. Dual-port distal pancreatectomy using a prototype endoscope and endoscopic stapler: a natural orifice transluminal endoscopic surgery (NOTES) survival study in a porcine model. Endoscopy. 2007;39(10):881–7.
7. Kaouk JH, White WM, Goel RK, et al. NOTES transvaginal nephrectomy: first human experience. Urology. 2009;74(1):5–8.
8. Garg M, Singh V, Sinha RJ, Sharma P. Prospective randomized comparison of transperitoneal vs retroperitoneal laparoscopic simple nephrectomy. Urology. 2014;84(2):335–9.
9. Zorron R, Goncalves L, Leal D, Kanaan E, Cabral I, Saraiva P. Transvaginal hybrid natural orifice transluminal endoscopic surgery retroperitoneoscopy– the first human case report. J Endourol. 2010;24(2):233–7.
10. Laydner H, Autorino R, Isac W, et al. Robotic retroperitoneal transvaginal natural orifice translumenal endoscopic surgery (NOTES) nephrectomy: feasibility study in a cadaver model. Urology. 2013;81(6):1232–7.
11. Xu W, Li H, Ji Z, et al. Comparison of retroperitoneoscopic versus transperitoneoscopic resection of retroperitoneal paraganglioma: a control study of 74 cases at a single institution. Medicine. 2015;94(7), e538.
12. Li QY, Li F. Laparoscopic adrenalectomy in pheochromocytoma: retroperitoneal approach versus transperitoneal approach. J Endourol. 2010;24(9):1441–5.
13. Viterbo R, Greenberg RE, Al-Saleem T, Uzzo RG. Prior abdominal surgery and radiation do not complicate the retroperitoneoscopic approach to the kidney or adrenal gland. J Urol. 2005;174(2):446–50.
14. Ren T, Liu Y, Zhao X, et al. Transperitoneal approach versus retroperitoneal approach: a meta-analysis of laparoscopic partial nephrectomy for renal cell carcinoma. PLoS One. 2014;9(3), e91978.
15. Flora ED, Wilson TG, Martin IJ, O'Rourke NA, Maddern GJ. A review of natural orifice translumenal endoscopic surgery (NOTES) for intra-abdominal surgery: experimental models, techniques, and applicability to the clinical setting. Ann Surg. 2008;247(4):583–602.
16. Wood SG, Panait L, Duffy AJ, et al. Complications of transvaginal natural orifice transluminal endoscopic surgery: a series of 102 patients. Ann Surg. 2014;259(4):744–9.
17. Bazzi WM, Raheem OA, Cohen SA, et al. Natural orifice transluminal endoscopic surgery in urology: review of the world literature. Urology Annals. 2012;4(1):1.
18. Fei YF, Fei L, Salazar M, et al. Transvaginal surgery: do women want it? J Laparoendosc Adv Surg Tech A. 2014;24(10):676–83.
19. Strickland AD, Norwood MGA, Behnia-Willison F, et al. Transvaginal natural orifice translumenal endoscopic surgery (NOTES): a survey of women's views on a new technique. Surg Endosc. 2010;24(10):2424–31.
20. Branco AW, Branco Filho AJ, Kondo W, et al. Hybrid transvaginal nephrectomy. Eur Urol. 2008;53(6):1290–4.
21. Sotelo R, de Andrade R, Fernandez G, et al. NOTES hybrid transvaginal radical nephrectomy for tumor: stepwise progression toward a first successful clinical case. Eur Urol. 2010;57(1):138–44.
22. Kaouk JH, Haber GP, Goel RK, et al. Pure natural orifice translumenal endoscopic surgery (NOTES) transvaginal nephrectomy. Eur Urol. 2010;57(4):723–6.
23. Xue Y, Zou X, Zhang G, et al. Transvaginal natural orifice transluminal endoscopic nephrectomy in a series of 63 cases: stepwise transition from hybrid to pure NOTES. Eur Urol. 2015;68(2):302–310.
24. Bazzi WM, Stroup SP, Cohen SA, et al. Comparison of transrectal and transvaginal hybrid natural orifice transluminal endoscopic surgery partial nephrectomy in the porcine model. Urology. 2013;82(1):84–9.
25. Zacharopoulou C, Nassif J, Allemann P, et al. Exploration of the retroperitoneum using the transvaginal natural orifice transluminal endoscopic surgery technique. J Minim Invasive Gynecol. 2009;16(2):198–203.
26. Allemann P, Perretta S, Marescaux J. Surgical access to the adrenal gland: the quest for a "no visible scar" approach. Surg Oncol. 2009;18(2):131–7.

4

Characteristics and repair outcome of patients with Vesicovaginal fistula managed in Jimma University teaching Hospital, Ethiopia

Demisew Anemu Sori[*], Ahadu Workineh Azale and Desta Hiko Gemeda

Abstract

Background: In Ethiopia, about 9000 fistula cases are estimated to occur every year with an incidence of 2.2/1000 women. This study was aimed to determine obstetric fistula characteristics and surgical repair outcomes among patients with fistula surgical repair.

Methods: A Hospital based cross sectional study design was conducted on all patients with Obstetric vesicovaginal Fistula, who were admitted to Gynecology ward, and had surgical repair from January 2011 to December 2014. Data was collected from patients' chart, operation logbook and discharge logbook which were filled up from the entry of the patient to the hospital till her discharge. At discharge, a dye test was done to determine the outcome of repair.

Results: One hundred sixty eight patients with obstetric vesicovaginal fistula were repaired during the study period. The age of the women ranged from 12 to 45 years with mean of 25 ($\pm$6) years and 10.1 % were younger than 18 years. Eighty percent of patients were laboring for two or more days, 46.4 % delivered abdominally (cesarean section 24.4 %, hysterectomy for uterine rupture 22 %), and 85.7 % ended up in stillbirth. Most patients (56 %) had mid-vaginal vesicovaginal fistula. Route of repair was vaginal among 95.8 % of patients, and spinal anesthesia was applied among 70.8 % of patients. Out of 93.4 % patients who had successful closure of their fistula, 84.5 % of patients had their fistula healed and continent, 8.9 % of them developed urinary incontinence while 6.5 % of fistula repair had failed at the time of discharge.

Conclusions: Most fistula patients in this study are older than 18 years, referred from health centers either for cephalopelvic disproportion or obstructed labor after prolonged labor at home. In this study, Spinal anesthesia as well as vaginal route was widely employed and high success rates were achieved with surgical repair. Therefore, increasing access to comprehensive emergency obstetric and new born care is essential to minimize the delay contributing to perinatal mortality and obstetric fistula. In addition use of spinal anesthesia and vaginal route of repair is essential for the high success of repair outcome and low postoperative morbidities.

Keywords: Vesicovaginal fistula, Obstetric fistula, Surgical repair

* Correspondence: demisame5@gmail.com
Jimma University College of Public Health and Medical Sciences, Jimma, Ethiopia

Background

Obstetric fistula is a significant cause of maternal morbidity (maternal near-miss) sustained mostly by teenage women due to prolonged obstructed labor, in the majority labor obstructed for three or more days and delivery ended up in stillbirth in 78–93 % [1–5]. Globally, the exact prevalence of obstetric fistula is not known, however, in 2006, the WHO estimated that more than 2 million young women throughout the world live with untreated fistula and between 50,000 and 100,000 new women are affected each year [6]. In Ethiopia, where the maternal mortality ratio is high (676 per 100,000 live births), the overall prevalence of obstetric fistula among women of reproductive age (15–49 years) was estimated at 2.2–7.3 per 1000 women [4], with a total of 142,387 fistula cases and 9000 new cases occurring a year [7–9].

Though Classifications of obstetric vesicovaginal fistula (VVF) vary, based on anatomic classification, midvaginal vesical fistula is the commonest. In low income countries where access to maternity care is restricted, fistulae are associated with a prolonged or obstructed labor, most commonly occurring when a baby's head becomes lodged in the mother's pelvis cutting off blood flow to the surrounding tissues. Prolonged obstruction can cause the tissues to necrotize leading to fistula formation [10–15]. Though most obstetric fistulas are from the natural course of obstructed labor, iatrogenic fistula at the time of obstetric surgery is also rising [16, 17].

Obstetric fistula is a devastating maternal morbidity which leaves a woman with uncontrollable leaking of urine and/or feces or both from her vagina. Untreated obstetric fistula leads to debilitating physical, health and social problems including divorce, isolation and stigma by their husband and families, and economic dependency [18, 19]. Although surgical repair is the main stay of treatment of obstetric fistula with closure rate of 85 to 95 % and severe stress incontinence rate of 15–20 %, the repair outcome will be affected by different factors like; type of fistula, experience of the surgeon, route of repair, postoperative care and type of anesthesia [8, 13, 14, 16, 18–22].

In Ethiopia there are few health facilities including Jimma University teaching Hospital (JUTH) performing obstetric fistula repair with limited capacity and few expertise. The Hospital has been performing surgical repair since the past four years and it is crucial to determine the clinical characteristics and surgical outcomes of obstetric fistula repair.

In this study we sought to establish the clinical characteristics and outcomes in patients undergoing fistula repair at our facility.

Methods

A Hospital based cross sectional study design was conducted on all patients with Obstetric vesicovaginal Fistula using a retrospective review of charts, who were admitted to Gynecology ward, Fistula treatment center and had surgical repair from January 2011 to December 2014 and who meet the inclusion criteria. English version pretested data collection format was used to collect Data on Socio-demographic, obstetric variables and physical examination findings by trained gynecology and obstetrics residents and fistula surgeons from a patient chart, operation logbook and discharge logbook which were filled up from the entry of the patient to the hospital till her surgery, postoperative period until discharge. All patients with obstetric fistula (Additional file 1) stayed in the ward for 14 days (for patients with vesical fistula without urethral involvement) to 21 days (for patients with vesical fistula with urethral involvement) with an indwelling urinary catheter after surgery and were followed up daily till discharge. At discharge, a dye test was done to determine the outcome of repair as almost all women will not comply to the three months follow up if there is no problem. In this study the outcome variables were Successful repair, Successful repair with incontinence and failure or unsuccessful closure. Successful repair was considered when a woman is continent and dry following fistula surgery after 14–21 days before discharge. Successful repair with incontinence was considered when a woman is wet of urine on stress but had a negative dye test. Failure or unsuccessful closure was considered when a woman is wet of urine and had a positive dye test after 14–21 days of continuous bladder drainage following fistula repair.

The Collected data was entered in to Epidata version 3.1, cleaned and analyzed using SPSS version 20 and interpretation, discussion and recommendations were made based on the findings.

An official letter was obtained from the Institutional Review Board of Jimma University to conduct this research and get permission from the Hospital. After permission was obtained, data was collected from patients' chart, operation logbook, and from discharge logbook which was filled up during the study period. The outcome of this study has been communicated to the Department of Obstetrics and Gynecology and to the Hospital.

Results

Among the total 200 vesicovaginal fistula patients repaired from January 2011 to December 2014 in Jimma University Teaching Hospital, 32 were excluded as their data was incomplete; and data of the remaining 168 were analyzed.

The age of the patients ranged from 12 to 45 years with mean of 25 (±6) years and 17 (10.1 %) were younger than 18 years. Sixty six (39.3 %) were primipara, 102 (60.7 %) were multiparous of which 40 (23.8 %) were grand multipara. One hundred thirty three (79.2 %) patients were laboring for two or more days while 24 (14.3 %) were laboring for more than three days during the causative pregnancy. One hundred twenty one (72 %) of patients delivered in the health facility, and 144 (85.7 %) of deliveries ended up in still birth. Regarding the mode of delivery, 67 (39.9 %) of patients delivered vaginally which may be spontaneous or after prolonged labor at home, 78 (46.4 %) had abdominal delivery out of which 41 (24.4 %) and 37 (22 %) were managed by cesarean section and hysterectomy respectively. Three patients had uterine repair after uterine rupture.

Based on anatomic classification, 94 (56 %) had mid-vaginal vesicovaginal fistula followed by circumferential vesicovaginal fistula (where bladder neck is totally detached from the urethra in these cases) 38 (22.6 %), juxta cervical 25 (14.9 %), juxta urethral 4 patients. For the majority, repairs were approached vaginally, among 161 (95.8 %), and under spinal anesthesia, among 119 (70.8 %). Fourteen (8.3 %) patients had failed previous fistula repair (Table 1).

According to the Goh classification, most patients had simple fistula and were in the class Ibi among 30.7 % of patients followed by Iai among 17.3 % of patients, however 4.8 % of patients had IVbiii (Fig. 1).

Seventy eight (46.4 %) patients had operative abdominal delivery of which uterine rupture was the commonest indication among 40 (51.3 %) patients followed by obstructed labor among 35 (44.9 %) patients and fetopelvic disproportion among 3 patients. Fifteen out of 40 (37.5 %) patients presented with uterine rupture had bladder rupture and 4 (2.4 %) had iatrogenic bladder injury during cesarean section. Seven patients had neurologic injury at the time of admission and of which 6 patients had foot drop.

Regarding the postoperative complications, 16 (9.5 %) patients had urinary tract infection (cystitis and pyelonephritis) for which they were treated and get cured. Bladder was catheterized for 21 days for circumferential vesicovaginal fistulae, among 38 (22.8 %), and juxtaurethral fistulae, among 4 patients and for 14 days for mid-vaginal fistula, among 94 (56 %) patients. Out of 157 (93.4 %) patients who had successful closure of their fistula, 142 (84.5 %) had healed and continent, 15 (8.9 %) had developed urinary incontinence after their fistula was closed and healed while 11 (6.5 %) had failed fistula repair (Table 2).

Discussion

This study showed that most women with vesicovaginal fistula were older than 18 years. This finding is different from the previous studies where majority were teenage and predisposed to contracted pelvis and as a result obstructed labor which is the commonest cause of obstetric fistula in sub Saharan Africa [2, 3, 23]. Though

Table 1 Socio-demographic characteristics and obstetric variables of vesicovaginal fistula patients Repaired between 2011 and 2014

Variable		Number ($n = 168$)	Percent
Age in years	<18 years	17	10.1
	≥18 years	151	89.9
Parity	I	66	39.3
	II-IV	62	36.9
	≥V	40	23.8
Duration of labor	1 day	35	20.8
	2–3 days	109	64.9
	>3 days	24	14.3
Place of delivery	Health facility	121	72.0
	Home	47	28.0
Mode of delivery	Vaginal delivery	67	39.9
	Instrumental	23	13.7
	Cesarean Section	41	24.4
	Hysterectomy	37	22.0
Special consideration (Goh classification)	Previous repair	14	8.3
	Circumferential	38	22.6
	Ureteric fistula	2	1.2
	No special consideration	114	67.9
Surgery approach	abdominal	7	4.2
	Vaginal	161	95.8
Type of anesthesia	General Anesthesia	49	29.2
	Spinal Anesthesia	119	70.8
Duration of bladder catheter	10 days	2	1.2
	14 days	124	73.8
	21 days	42	25.0
Type of obstetric fistula (anatomic classification)	Mid-vaginal VVF	94	56.0
	Circumfrential VVF	38	22.6
	Juxta cervical VVF	25	14.9
	Ureteric fistula	2	1.2
	Juxta urethral VVF	4	2.4
	Other	5	2.9
Fetal outcome	Alive	24	14.3
	Still birth	144	85.7

the great proportion of patients gave birth for two or more times, more than a third gave birth for the first time. This might be explained by the fact that both primigravidity and multiparity were identified risk factors for obstetric fistula [20]. In this study, majority of patients had prolonged labor (80 %) which lasted for two or more days, delivered in the health facility (72 %), and about 86 % of deliveries were ended up in still births.

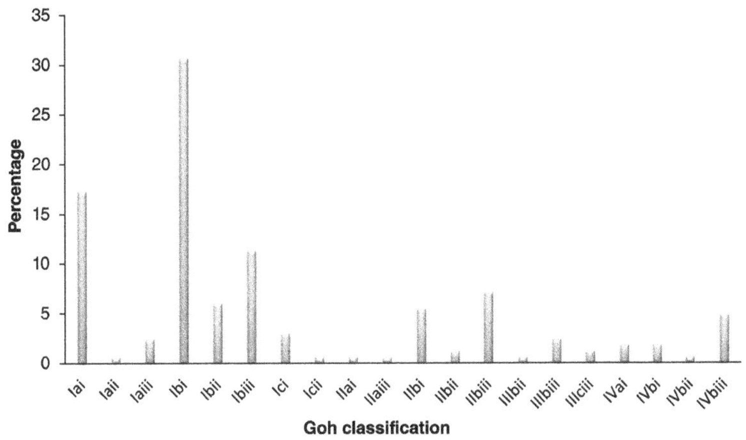

Fig. 1 Goh classification of Vesicovaginal fistula patients repaired between 2011 and 2014

These findings are similar with studies from sub-Saharan Africa [3, 4] except for the high rate of still birth in this study, which can be explained by the low health facility delivery rate of Ethiopia (10 %) [4], and in the current study, majority of patients were referred after prolonged labor either for uterine rupture or obstructed labor or feto-pelvic disproportion. These complications could have been averted by availing comprehensive emergency obstetric and new born care in each district [10, 24]. However, the still birth rate in the current study is lower than the previous study done in Ethiopia and Nigeria

Table 2 Obstetric variables and repair outcomes of vesicovaginal fistula patients repaired between 2011 and 2014

Variable		Number (N = 168)	Percentage
Bladder rupture	Yes	15	8.9
	No	153	91.1
Iatrogenic vesical fistula	Yes	4	2.4
	No	164	97.6
Postoperative complications	Anemia	3	15.8
	Pyelonephritis	4	21.1
	Cystitis	12	63.1
Indications for abdominal delivery	Fetopelvic disproportion	3	3.8
	Obstructed labor	35	44.9
	Uterine rupture	40	51.3
Neurologic injury	Foot drop	6	85.7
	Joint contracture	1	14.3
Fistula repair outcomes	Fistula healed and continent	142	84.5
	Fistula healed but incontinent	15	8.9
	Fistula not healed/failed	11	6.6

where the still birth rate is reported to be 93 % and 91.7 % respectively [3, 5].

From among forty six percent of abdominal deliveries, uterine rupture accounted for 23.8 %. This rate is very high when compared to other studies in Africa [20] and explained by the fact that most mothers had stayed laboring at home for long time and decided to seek health care late after complications has already developed [10, 11]. Fifty six percent of patients had mid-vaginal vesicovaginal fistula followed by circumferential vesicovaginal fistula and eight percent of patients had previous one fistula repair. These findings are similar with other studies done in Africa where 47 % of fistula was midvaginal [12, 14]. However, patients having previous failed repair are lower in this study compared to a study in Nigeria [16]. This may be explained by the fistula patients' characteristics in the current study whereby most patients had simple fistula by Goh of Ibi (30.7 %) followed by Iai (17.3 %), though 4.8 % had IVbiii.

One aspect of surgical repair in particular, the route of repair undertaken, is critical as the abdominal (versus vaginal) approach may be associated with longer term hospitalization, Urinary tract infection (UTI) and increased blood loss [13, 21]. Type of anesthesia used is also an important factor which affects postoperative morbidities. In the current study, nearly 96 % had their repair transvaginally, 71 % under spinal anesthesia, when compared with most studies in other African countries [16]. Transvaginal route and spinal anesthesia is most widely used in the current study. This difference might be related to the background and experience of the fistula surgeon whereby some can perform almost all repairs vaginally including juxta cervical fistulas while others may prefer abdominal approach. However it is similar with a multistage study done in developing countries [14] where the vaginal approach accounts for 95.52 %. These might have contributed to the low postoperative morbidity (9.5 %) in the present study.

Nearly 38 % (15/40) of patients presented with uterine rupture had bladder rupture and only 4 patients had iatrogenic vesical fistula during cesarean section. In general, surgical skill of operating surgeon at the time of cesarean section is critical to avoid iatrogenic bladder fistula. The iatrogenic vesical fistula in this study is by far lower than the reports in most studies in Africa [16, 17]. Presence of neurologic injury mostly shows the severity of obstructed labor complex and may affect the repair outcome as well. In our study, the neurologic injury rate is 4 % which is very low when compared with a previous study done in East Africa [2, 17]. The difference can be explained by the fact that most patients in our study had simple fistula Goh Ibi followed by Iai which tells the degree of injury to the birth canal.

The overall fistula closure rate varies from center to center which may be affected by fistula characteristics and the experience of the surgeon. In the present study the overall closure rate was 93.4 % and 8.9 % of the patients developed urinary incontinence though their fistula was healed at discharge. This finding is comparable with studies in Africa [3, 17, 22] though there are reports of low fistula closure rate in another study [2, 20, 12].

In this study, some socio-demographic and Obstetric characteristics of fistula patients were missed because it was not filled up at the time of admission. In addition long term outcome was not assed because almost all patients would not come back for subsequent visits.

Conclusions

Most fistula patients in this study are older than 18 years, referred from health centers either for cephalopelvic disproportion or obstructed labor after prolonged labor at home. In this study, Spinal anesthesia as well as vaginal route was widely employed and high success rates were achieved with surgical repair of vesicovaginal fistula. Therefore, increasing access to comprehensive emergency obstetric and new born care (CEmONC) at all levels of health system is essential. In addition use of spinal anesthesia and vaginal route of repair is essential for the high success of repair outcome and low postoperative morbidities.

Abbreviations
CEmONC, comprehensive emergency obstetric and new born care; JUTH, Jimma University teaching Hospital; UTI, Urinary tract infection; VVF, vesicovaginal fistula

Acknowledgements
We would like to acknowledge the residents involved in data collection, United Nation Population Fund (UNFPA) for funding the write up.

Authors' contributions
DA: is the principal investigator and contributed to the development of the Concept, collected data, analyzed data and wrote the draft and final article. AW: contributed to development of concept, data collection, data analysis and reviewed the draft and final article. DH: contributed to development of concept, and data analysis and reviewed the draft and final article. All authors read and approved the final manuscript.

Competing interests
We declare that there are no financial and non-financial competing interests.

Ethics approval and consent to participate
An official letter was obtained from the Institutional Review Board of Jimma University to conduct this research and get permission from the Hospital. After permission was obtained, data was collected from patients' chart, operation logbook, and from discharge logbook which was filled up during the study period. The outcome of this study has been communicated to the Department of Obstetrics and Gynecology and to the Hospital. Consent to participate was not required.

References
1. Wall LL. Obstetric vesico vaginal fistula as an international public-health problem. Lancet. 2006;368(9542):1201–9.
2. Holme A, Breen M, MacArthur C. Obstetric fistulae: a study of women managed at the Monze Mission Hospital, Zambia. BJOG. 2007;114:1010–7.
3. Muleta M. Obstetric fistulae: a retrospective study of 1210 cases at the Addis Ababa Fistula Hospital. J Obstet Gynaecol. 1997;17(1):68–70.
4. Central Statistical Agency [Ethiopia] and ICF International. Ethiopia Demographic and Health Survey 2011. Addis Ababa, Ethiopia and Calverton, Maryland, USA: Central Statistical Agency and ICF International; 2012.
5. Wall LL, Karshima JA, Kirschner C, Arrowsmith SD. The obstetric vesicovaginal fistula: Characteristics of 899 patients from Jos, Nigeria. Am J Obstet Gynecol. 2004;190:1011–9.
6. WHO. Obstetric fistula: guiding principles for clinical management and programme development. Geneva: World Health Organization; 2006.
7. Muleta M, Fantahun M, Tafesse B, Hamlin EC, Kennedy RC. Obstetric fistula in rural Ethiopia. East Afr Med J. 2007;84(11):525–33.
8. Hancock B, Browning A. Practical obstetric fistula surgery. Royal society of medicine press Ltd 1Wimpole street, London W1G0AE,UK: Royal Society of Medicine Press Ltd; 2009.
9. Biadgilign et al. A population based survey in Ethiopia using questionnaire as proxy to estimate obstetric fistula prevalence: results from demographic and health survey. Reprod Health. 2013; 10:14.
10. Roka et al. Factors associated with obstetric fistulae occurrence among patients attending selected hospitals in Kenya, 2010: a case control study. BMC Pregnancy Childbirth. 2013; 13:56.
11. Danso KA, Martey JO, Wall LL, Elkins TE. The epidemiology of genitourinary fistulae in Kumasi, Ghana, 1977-1992. Int Urogynecol J Pelvic Floor Dysfunct. 1996;7(3):117–20.
12. Olusegun AK, Akinfolarin AC, Olabisi LM. A Review of Clinical Pattern and Outcome of Vesicovaginal Fistula. J Natl Med Assoc. 2009;101:593–5.
13. Kapoor R, Ansari MS, Singh P, Gupta P, Khurana N, Mandhani A, et al. Management of vesicovaginal fistula: an experience of 52 cases with a rationalized algorithm for choosing the transvaginal or transabdominal approach. Indian J Urol. 2007;23:372–6.
14. Frajzyngier V, Ruminjo J, Asiimwe F, Barry T, Bello A, Danladi D, et al. Factors influencing choice of surgical route of repair of genitourinary fistula, and the influence of route of repair on surgical outcomes: findings from a prospective cohort study. BJOG. 2012;119:1344–53.
15. Goh JT. A new classification for female genital tract fistula. Aust N Z J Obstet Gynecol. 2004;44(6):502–4.
16. McFadden E, Taleski SJ, Bocking A, Spitzer RF, Mabeya H. Retrospective Review of Predisposing Factors and Surgical Outcomes in Obstetric Fistula Patients at a Single Teaching Hospital in Western Kenya. J Obstet Gynaecol Can. 2011;33(1):30–5.
17. Raassen TJIP, Ngongo CJ, Mahendeka MM. Iatrogenic genitourinary fistula: an 18-year retrospective review of 805 injuries. Int Urogynecol J. 2014;25:1699–706.

Characteristics and repair outcome of patients with Vesicovaginal fistula managed in Jimma University...

27

18. Mselle et al. waiting for attention and care: birthing accounts of women in rural Tanzania who developed obstetric fistula as an outcome of labor. BMC Pregnancy Childbirth. 2011, 11:75.

19. WHO Department of Making Pregnancy Safer. Obstetric Fistula: Guiding principles for clinical management and programme development. Geneva: WHO Library cataloguing-in-publication data; 2006. p.11-30.

20. Hawkins L, Spitzer RF, Christoffersen-Deb A, Leah J, Mabeya H. Characteristics and surgical successes of patients presenting for repair of Obstetric fistula in Western Kenya. Int J Gynecol Obstet. 2013;120:178–82.

21. Morhason-Bello IO, Ojengbede OA, Adedokun BO, Okunlola MA, Oladokun A. Uncomplicated midvaginal vesico-vaginal fistula repair in Ibadan: a comparison of the abdominal and vaginal routes. Ann Ibadan Postgrad Med. 2008;6:39–43.

22. Waaldijk K. The immediate management of fresh obstetric fistulas. Am J Obstet Gynecol. 2004;191(3):795–9.

23. Zheng AX, Anderson FWJ. Obstetric fistula in low-income countries. Int J Gynecol Obstet. 2009;104:85–9.

24. Wall LL, Arrowsmith SD, Briggs ND, Browning A, Lassey A. The obstetric vesicovaginal fistula in the developing world. Obstet Gynecol Surv. 2005; 60(7 Suppl 1):S3–51.

5

Surgical treatment of Peyronie's disease with autologous tunica vaginalis of testis

Bianjiang Liu[1], Quan Li[2], Gong Cheng[1], Ninghong Song[1*], Min Gu[1] and Zengjun Wang[1]

Abstract

Background: To investigate the feasibility and safety of surgical treatment for Peyronie's disease (PD) by excising and repairing plaque using autologous tunica vaginalis of testis.

Methods: From March 2007 to December 2012, total 19 patients with PD underwent surgical treatment at our center. All patients had significant phallocampsis during erection. All patients complained of decreased sexual function. During the operation, the fibrotic plaque was excised and neurovascular bundle (NVB) was spared. A size-matching autologous tunica vaginalis of testis was harvested as the graft and patched to the defect. All patients received follow up every 3 months in the first year and 6 months in the following years. Data on sexual function before and after the operation was collected and compared.

Results: All operations were completed successfully without serious complications. The mean operative time was 74 min. The mean size of excised plaque was 3.0 cm^2. Postoperative pathological studies revealed the fibroplastic hyperplasia of excised tissue. All patients had satisfactory correction of penile appearance. The erectile penile length between pre- and post-operation didn't show significant difference. Postoperative intercourse satisfaction and overall satisfaction measured by IIEF-5 were significant improved.

Conclusions: Our surgical treatment is feasible and safe for patients with PD. It can effectively improve the penile cosmetic appearance and patients' intercourse/overall satisfaction on sexual life.

Keywords: Peyronie's disease, Tunica vaginalis, Autologous, Sexual function

Background

Peyronie's disease (PD) is a progressive fibrotic tissue disorder of the penile tunica albuginea. PD can lead to the formation of fibrous plaques, penile deformity, painful erection, loss of penile flexibility, and finally sexual dysfunction [1]. It is generally recognized that PD contains two inflammatory phase: acute and chronic phase. Medical therapy is used for the acute phase or those unfit for surgery [2]. Surgical treatment is the gold standard for PD due to the most reliable and sustained correction of phallocampsis. There are many surgical options for PD such as Nesbit procedure, Yachia procedure, Plication procedures, and grafting procedures. Grafting procedures are the focus of recent studies for effectively preserving penile length. Three types of graft have been reported: autologous graft, xenograft and synthetic graft [3]. Considering the higher rate of infection, regional inflammation reaction and allergic reaction, synthetic graft is not the main stream [4]. A variety of autologous grafts have been used including vein wall, rectus sheath, and buccal mucosa. The testicular tunica vaginalis was first reported as autologous graft in 1980. However, the technique has not been widely applied [5]. In present study, we reported our experience of surgical repair on 19 patients with PD using autologous tunica vaginalis of testis. The aim of the study was to investigate the feasibility and safety of our surgical treatment for PD.

Methods

Approval for the study was granted by the ethics committee of Nanjing Medical University (China) and informed written consent was received from patients, including acquiring essential medical images for publication.

* Correspondence: nh_song@163.com
[1]Department of Urology, The First Affiliated Hospital of Nanjing Medical University, Nanjing 210029, China
Full list of author information is available at the end of the article

Patients

From March 2007 to December 2012, total 19 patients with PD were recruited to our center. The mean age of patients was 40 (32-61) years. All patients had phallocampsis during erection. Preoperative measurement by goniometer revealed that the mean penile curvature was 36° (25–50°). All patients complained of decreased sexual function. Physical examinations revealed 11 plaques at the dorsal penis, 3 plaques at the lateral penis, and 5 plaques at the ventral penis. Surgical indications included in the stable history at least for 12 months, significant phallocampsis, and decreased erectile function related to PD after ineffective medical treatment.

Procedures

All operations were performed by the same experienced urologists at our center. After induction of general anesthesia, the patients were placed in the supine position. A tourniquet was secured at the base of penis (Fig. 1a). A circumferential skin incision was made along the coronary sulcus to deglove penile shaft to the base

of penis (Fig. 1b and c). The deep dorsal vein was isolated and clipped at both arms of the curvature. The ligated segmental vein was transected and removed. Then meticulous dissection was performed to preserve the neurovascular bundle (NVB) and to fully expose the foci on the tunica albuginea. A transverse incision was made to cut off the proximal fibrous plaque. Two longitudinal incisions were made along its bilateral sides. From the proximal end, the plague was excised deeply into the whole albugineous wall till the distal end. When the plaque was removed, the curvature could be corrected with no significant dorsal tension. The size of the defect was measured. A 2–3 cm longitudinal incision was made at the anterior wall of the scrotum. The parietal wall of tunica vaginalis was exposed for entry of the tunica cavity. To obtain a sufficient size of the graft, a rectangle tunica flap was harvested along the epididymal side (Fig. 1d). The flap was trimmed for suitable length and width to cover the defect. Then the flap and normal tunica albuginea were sutured together with 5-0 absorbable sutures (Fig. 1e and f). Artificial erection with saline

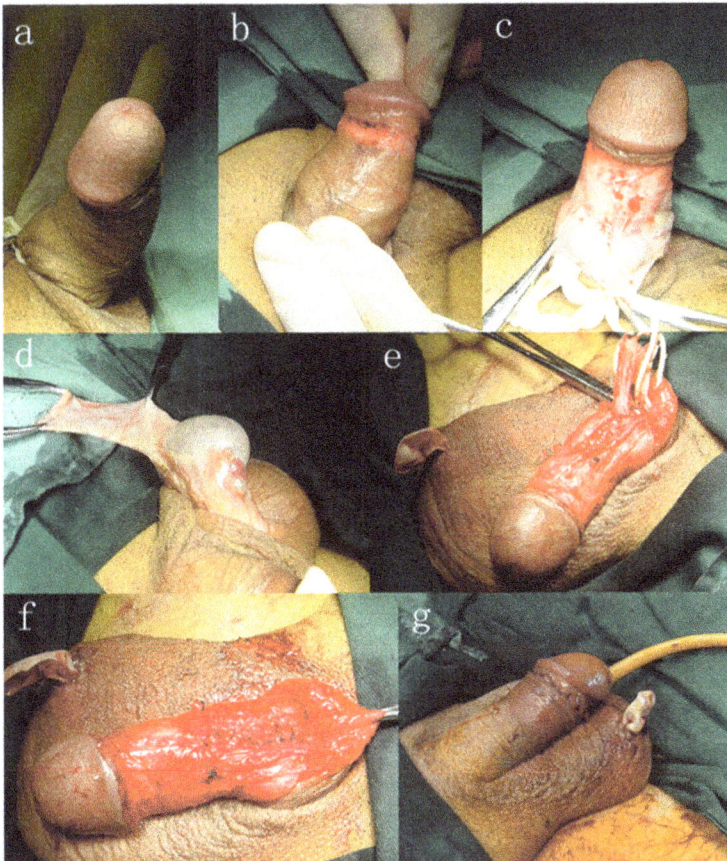

Fig. 1 The main surgical steps of repairing PD using autologous tunica vaginalis of testis. **a** Dorsal curvature of penis. **b** Circumcision proximal to the glans coronal. **c** Degloving of penile skin to the base of the penis. **d** Harvesting tunica vaginalis of testius. **e** Suturing the flap to the albugineous defect. **f** Completion of defect repairing. **g** suturing the penile and testicular incisions and indwelling routinely the drainage tube and Foley catheter

injection was performed to confirm the satisfactory correction of phallocampsis. Lastly, the incisions were sutured with indwelling routinely the drainage tube and Foley catheter (Fig. 1g). During suturing penile incision, the relative position of penile shaft and degloved prepuce were determined carefully to avoid penile rotation. After operation, oral antibacterial was used. The drainage tube and catheter were removed within 24 h.

Outcomes analysis

During the follow up, all patients received interview and physical examination every 3 months in the first year and 6 months in the following years. The International Index of Erectile Function (IIEF-5) questionnaire was made at 6 months postoperatively. Data on sexual function before and after operation was collected and compared. Data were expressed as mean ± SD. Paired T-test was performed for the comparison of pre- and post-opersation. Statistical analysis was made using SPSS 17.0 (SPSS Inc., Chicago, IL, U.S.). A p value < 0.05 was considered statistically significant.

Results

Demographic and preoperative clinical characteristics of 19 patients were presented in Table 1. All operations were completed successfully without serious complications. The mean operative time was 74 (55–100) min. The mean size of excised plaque was 3.0 (1.7–4.5) cm^2. Postoperative pathological studies revealed the fibroplastic hyperplasia of excised tissue. All patients had satisfactory correction of phallocampsis. The erectile penile length between pre- and post-operation didn't show significant difference (11.23 ± 2.32 cm vs 11.34 ± 2.20 cm; $p = 0.21$). During 12-43 months follow up, all patients had no abnormal penile appearance and recurrent fibrous plaque.

To explore the surgical influence on sexual function, we quantified and compared different aspects of sexual function using IIEF-5 questionnaire between pre- and post-operation (Table 2). Although the postoperative

Table 1 Demographic and preoperative clinical characteristics of 19 patients

Variable	Mean (range)
Age (year)	40 (32–61)
BMI	24.3 (21.1–26.7)
History of disease (year)	2.8 (1–5)
Affected location	
Dorsal	11
Lateral	3
Ventral	5
Curvature	36° (25–50°)

Table 2 IIEF-5 scores of sexual function before and after operation

	Pre-operation	Post-operation	p value
Erectile function	18.6 ± 3.1	18.7 ± 2.2	0.88
Orgasmic function	7.5 ± 1.0	7.6 ± 1.0	0.64
Sexual desire	8.0 ± 0.9	8.5 ± 1.1	0.13
Intercourse satisfaction	7.7 ± 1.1	9.0 ± 2.0	0.02*
Overall satisfaction	6.5 ± 1.1	7.2 ± 0.9	0.007*

Data were shown as Mean ± SD
*p value < 0.05

scores of erectile function, orgasmic function, and sexual desire improved, there had no significant differences compared with the preoperative status ($p = 0.88$, 0.64, and 0.13, respectively). However, the postoperative scores of intercourse satisfaction and overall satisfaction improved significantly than pre-operation ($p = 0.02$ and 0.007, respectively).

Discussion

Surgical treatment for PD is necessary if the patients had significant phallocampsis, decreased sexual function related to PD, or ineffective medical treatment. Three surgical methods can be used for PD: penile tunica albuginea placation, grafting procedures, and penile prosthesis implantation [6–8]. Tunica albuginea placation is a relatively simple surgical procedure. However, it may lead to postoperative penile shortening. Penile prosthesis implantation is technically complicated and expensive. Grafting procedures are now the focus of surgical treatment for PD. The material selection is currently controversial. Autologous graft, xenograft and synthetic graft can be used [4, 9, 10]. The ideal graft material should be readily available, pliable, inexpensive, resistant to infection and able to preserve erectile function. Autologous graft are most common used due to their easy incorporation into host tissue and few incidence of local inflammatory reaction [11, 12].

In current study, we chose autologous tunica vaginalis of testis for repairing PD. The first is that tunica vaginalis is relatively superficial and convenient to harvest. It has good blood supply and histocompatibility after transplanting. Compared with synthetic graft, the autologous graft is more economical and has lower risk of graft removal due to postoperative infection [13, 14]. Second, tunica vaginalis has uniform thickness and good pliability and elasticity to guarantee the penile erection. In present study, we observed that the tunica vaginalis had a good viability and satisfactory function exertion. Furthermore, tunica vaginalis incision is more safe and simple than other autologous graft such as vein wall, rectus sheath, and buccal mucosa. No significant surface scars, pains, and regional complications occurred after operation. During the follow up, all patients had no recurrence of fibrotic plaque or curvature at the graft site. No recurrent phallocampsis during the erection was observed. The correction of penile deformity during erection promoted the sexual quality and correspondent sexual satisfaction. Only one patients thought that the surgery bring slight shortening of penile length despite the curvature had been corrected. Our data showed the short- and mid-term effectiveness of autologous graft. Most significant benefits for patients receiving surgery were the improvement on penile appearance and sexual satisfaction.

ED is a well-recognized co-morbidity of PD. PD, due to penile deformity, may make intercourse less enjoyable, more awkward, and even impossible [15]. Although improving the sexual function, the surgery could also lead to de novo ED [6]. The possible causes of postoperative ED include in the progression or recurrence of the disease, injury of NVB and psychological influence. In our study, 79 % of patients had their erectile function moderately affected. After operation, the sexual function was improved generally. Although there were no significant differences between preoperative and postoperative scores of erectile function, orgasmic function, and sexual desire, postoperative intercourse satisfaction and overall satisfaction were improved obviously. The results should be attributed to the correction of penile deformity and enhancement of patients' self-confidence. There is no single parameter or combination of medical comorbidities to adequately predict the development of ED after PD. Strictly complying with surgical rules, careful preoperative counseling, and post-operative physiological caring are essential to decrease de novo ED. There was no postoperative ED in our study. The result confirmed the safety of our method in treating PD.

One limitation of our study includes its retrospective design. We can't compare with the clinical outcomes between tunica vaginalis and autologous grafts or xenografts. In addition, although the short- and mid-term outcomes of our surgical treatment are good, the long-term outcomes, especially the influence on the sexual function, remain to be seen.

Conclusions

Our surgical treatment is feasible and safe for patients with PD. It can effectively improve the penile cosmetic appearance and patients' intercourse/overall satisfaction on sexual life.

Abbreviations
IIEF-5: International Index of Erectile Function; NVB: neurovascular bundle; PD: Peyronie's disease.

Competing interests

Authors' contributions
All authors participated in the study conception, design and coordination. LB and LQ performed the surgery and wrote the paper. CG, GM and WZ performed the data analysis. SN designed the study. All authors read and approved the final manuscript.

Acknowledgements
This work is supported by a grant from National Natural Science Foundation of China (81200467) and by A Project Funded by the Priority Academic Program Development of Jiangsu Higher Education Institutions (JX10231802).

Author details
[1]Department of Urology, The First Affiliated Hospital of Nanjing Medical University, Nanjing 210029, China. [2]Department of Urology, Suzhou Municipal Hospital, Suzhou 215000, China.

References
1. Ralph D, Gonzalez-Cadavid N, Mirone V, Perovic S, Sohn M, Usta M, et al. The management of Peyronie's disease: evidence-based 2010 guidelines. J Sex Med. 2010;7:2359–74.
2. Gur S, Limin M, Hellstrom WJ. Current status of the surgical management of Peyronie's disease: medical, minimally invasive and surgical treatment options. Expert Opin Pharmacother. 2011;12:931–44.
3. Smith JF, Walsh TJ, Lue TF. Peyronie's disease: a critical appraisal of current diagnosis and treatment. Int J Impot Res. 2008;20:445–59.
4. Kadioglu A, Sanli O, Akman T, Ersay A, Guven S, Mammadov F. Graft materials in Peyronie's disease surgery: a comprehensive review. J Sex Med. 2007;4:581–95.
5. Das S. Peyronie's disease: Excision and autografting with tunica vaginalis. J Urol. 1980;124:818–9.
6. Hatzimouratidis K, Eardley I, Giuliano F, Hatzichristou D, Moncada I, Salonia A, et al. European Association of Urology: EAU guideline on penile curvature. Eur Urol. 2012;62:543–52.
7. Kadioglu A, Sanli O, Akman T, Cakan M, Erol B, Mamadov F. Surgical treatment of Peyronie's disease:a single center experience with 145 patients. Eur Urol. 2008;53:432–9.
8. Chaudhary M, Sheikh N, Asterling S, Ahmad I, Greene D. Peyronie's disease with erectile dysfunction: penile modeling over inflatable penile prostheses. Urology. 2005;65:760–4.
9. Kelemen Z. Reconstructive surgery of penile deformities and tissue deficiencies. Orv Hetil. 2009;150:1023–9.
10. Richardson B, Pinsky MR, Hellstrom WJ. Incision and grafting for severe Peyronie's disease (CME). J Sex Med. 2009;6:2084–7.
11. Lentz AC, Carson CC. Peyronie's surgery: graft choices and outcomes. Curr Urol Rep. 2009;10:460–7.
12. Djinovic R. Penile corporoplasty in Peyronie's disease: which technique, which graft? Curr Opin Urol. 2011;21:470–7.
13. Kumar R, Nehra A. Surgical and minimally invasive treatments for Peyronie's disease. Curr Opin Urol. 2009;19:589–94.
14. Dublin N, Stewart LH. Oral complications after buccal mucosal graft harvest for urethroplasty. BJU Int. 2004;94:867–9.
15. Dibenedetti DB, Nguyen D, Zografos L, Ziemiecki R, Zhou X. A Population-Based Study of Peyronie's Disease: Prevalence and Treatment Patterns in the United States. Adv Urol. 2011;2011:282503.

6

10-Year experience regarding the reliability and morbidity of radio guided lymph node biopsy in penile cancer patients and the associated radiation exposure of medical staff in this procedure

Ulf Lützen[1][*][†] [ID], Carsten Maik Naumann[2][†], Jens Dischinger[3], Marlies Marx[1], René Baumann[4], Yi Zhao[1], Michael Jüptner[1], Daniar Osmonov[2], Katrin Bothe[2], Klaus-Peter Jünemann[2] and Maaz Zuhayra[1]

Abstract

Background: The guidelines of the European Association of Urologists (EAU), of the German Society of Nuclear Medicine (DGN), and the European Society for Medical Oncology (ESMO) recommend sentinel lymph node biopsy (SLNB) for lymph node staging in penile cancer with non-palpable inguinal lymph nodes as one diagnostic method. Despite this, the method is neither widely nor regularly applied in Germany – the same applies to many other countries, which may be due to insecurity in dealing with open radioactive tracers. This study aims to assess the reliability and morbidity of this method, as well as the associated radioactive burden for clinical staff.

Methods: Between 2006 and 2016, 34 patients with an invasive penile carcinoma and inconspicuous inguinal lymph node status underwent SLNB in 57 groins after application of a radiotracer (Tc-99 m nanocolloid). We collected the results prospectively. The reliability of the method was assessed by determining the false-negative rate. In addition, we evaluated complication rates and determined the radioactive burden for the clinical staff both pre- and intraoperatively.

Results: SLNB was performed in 34 patients with penile cancer with non-palpable inguinal lymph nodes in 57 groins. In two patients inguinal lymph node metastases were detected by means of SLNB. In one patient recurrent inguinal lymph node disease was found after negative SLNB in both groins. Thus, the false negative rate was 3.13 % per patient (1/32 patients) and 3.51 % per groin (2/57 groins). The morbidity rate was 2.94 % per patient (1/34 patients) and 1.75 % per groin (1/57 groins). Radiation exposure for the clinical staff during this procedure was low at a maximum of ca. four μSV per intervention.

Conclusions: SLNB is a reliable method with low morbidity that is associated with a low radiation burden for clinical staff. Due to the enhanced methodological and logistic demands, this intervention should be performed in specialized centres and in an interdisciplinary approach.

Keywords: Penile carcinoma, Sentinel lymph nodes, Lymph node staging, Tc 99 m-nanocolloid, Radiation exposure, Sentinel lymph node biopsy, SPECT/CT

* Correspondence: uluetzen@nuc-med.uni-kiel.de
[†]Equal contributors
[1]Department of Nuclear medicine, Molecular Imaging Diagnostics and Therapy, University Hospital Schleswig Holstein, Campus Kiel, Kiel, Germany
Full list of author information is available at the end of the article

Background

Application of Tc-99 m-labelled nanocolloid for pre- and intraoperative imaging of the sentinel lymph nodes (SLN) is a fully established standard method in malignant melanoma and breast cancer, both in Germany and internationally, and it is rooted firmly in the national and international guidelines of expert societies [1, 2].

For penile cancer, the European Association of Urologists (EAU), the German German Society of Nuclear Medicine (DGN), and the European Society for Medical Oncology (ESMO) also recommend sentinel lymph node biopsy (SLNB) in invasive primary tumours with a moderate degree of differentiation and non-palpable inguinal lymph nodes [3–5]. The former EAU categorization of the penile carcinoma as high-risk, intermediate-risk and low-risk is no longer in use [6].

In some few countries like the United Kingdom and the Netherlands, SLNB using open radioactive nuclides is an established and widely used procedure for penile cancer. In other countries like Germany, this procedure is neither regularly nor widely used. Despite the fact that urologists frequently deal with ionizing radiation from other sources, there is a lack of familiarity with the technique and the high methodological demands of SLN-procedures, therefor this could be one reason. A further cause could lie in former publications stating unreliability of the method of up to 15 % [7].

The aim of this prospective study is to establish both the reliability and the morbidity associated with SLNB after radio-labelling of sentinel lymph nodes with Tc-99 m nanocolloid. In addition, we aim to determine and assess the radiation burden for clinical staff resulting from the application of this method, and to compare it to similar procedures in other tumour entities.

Methods

Being a university-based cancer center, we treat all types of penile cancer, as well as other tumour entities in an interdisciplinary team. Out of all patients who suffer from an invasive penile carcinoma and were assigned to our center by regional and national physicians, only those with non-palpable inguinal lymph nodes – this being the only pre-selection criterion – were included in this study in the period 2006 to 2016. During this period, 34 patients with an inconspicuous inguinal lymph node status in 57 groins were included in this study. 23 patients showed non-palpable inguinal lymph nodes bilaterally, 11 patients only unilaterally. The latter patients presented palpable inguinal lymph nodes in the contra lateral groin in the physical examination. All groins without palpable inguinal lymph nodes underwent SLNB with Tc-99-labelled nanocolloid, regardless of the palpation status in the contra lateral groin. The

applied tracer was a pure gamma emitter with a half-life of six hours and energy of 141 keV.

All patients included in this study underwent initial preoperative physical screening, including palpation and additional ultrasound examination of the inguinal region. Preoperative cross-section images via magnetic resonance imaging (MRI) and computer tomography (CT) of the pelvic region, including the inguinal region, were not mandatory.

The median age of the patients was 63.5 (34–84) years. The details of the malignant disease, the tumour characteristics as well as the SLN diagnostic results and the results of the follow-up are presented in Table 1.

Nuclear medical imaging of SLN was done following a-two-day protocol [8]. On the preoperative day, the patients received an intradermal peritumoural injection of the radio tracer under local anesthesia (Fig. 1). We applied an overall activity of 150 MBq, Tc-99 m-labelled nanocolloid. We performed lymphatic drainage scintigraphies in several projections (at least four): at the earliest on the injection day at least one hour p. i., – or, in the case of lacking or retarded lymphatic drainage, on the morning before the surgical intervention. For indirect body contouring, the emission measurements for generation of planar images were performed additionally by means of a Co-57 planar source (Fig. 2). Image acquisition was done with a twin head gamma camera (Siemens, ECAM and Symbia T).

In addition we performed single-photon-emission computed tomography/computed tomography (SPECT/CT) of the lower abdomen, the pelvic abdomen and the inguinal region with a twin head SPECT/CT-hybrid camera (Siemens, Symbia T and Symbia Intevo). CT-data were acquired in a so-called low-dose technique. The scans of the functional imaging were fused with the co-registered CT-scans (Fig. 3). In this context, morphological imaging enabled attenuation correction of the emission data on the one hand, as well as easier

Table 1 Tumourstaging/-grading of patients with SLNB- and follow-up results

Tumourstaging/-grading	Patients (n)	Positive SLN	False-negative SLN
T1G1	2	0	1
T1G2	13	0	0
T1G3	4	1	0
T2G1	0	0	0
T2G2	9	1	0
T2G3	0	0	0
T3G1	2	0	0
T3G2	2	0	0
T3G3	2	0	0

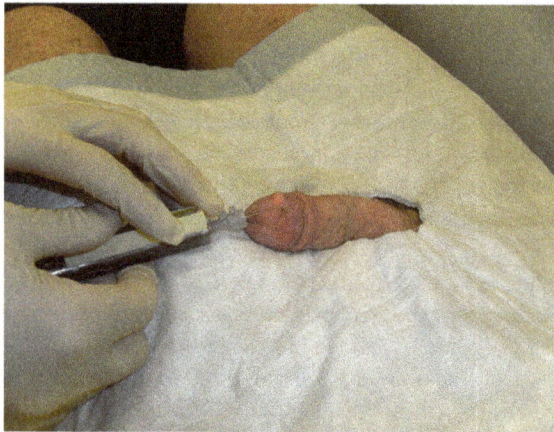

Fig. 1 Pre-operative peritumoural intracutaneous injection of the radioactive tracer (Tc 99 m-labelled nanocolloid)

anatomical allocation of the radio-marked lymph nodes, thus facilitating better surgical planning, on the other.

Subsequent to the imaging process, we identified and marked the SLN by means of a Co-57 pen as well as a felt-tip pen on the skin surface. In addition we performed a perilesional intradermal injection of patent blue immediately before the surgical intervention. Intraoperatively, the SLN were identified both visually, via the blue hue accrued in the lymph nodes, as well as by measuring the radioactivity by means of a gamma probe. In the case of preoperative non-visualization of radioactive labeled lymph nodes in scintigraphy the day before surgery, an intraoperative exploration, augmented by the gamma probe, was done the following day. All detectable radioactive-labeled, blue stained as well as clinically suspicious lymph nodes that were not detected by preoperative physical examination (e.g. due to obesity) were removed as recommended [8].

Each enrolled patient of this study received a prophylactic antibiotic therapy as a single shot application of cephalosporin prior to surgery. Incisions of approximately four

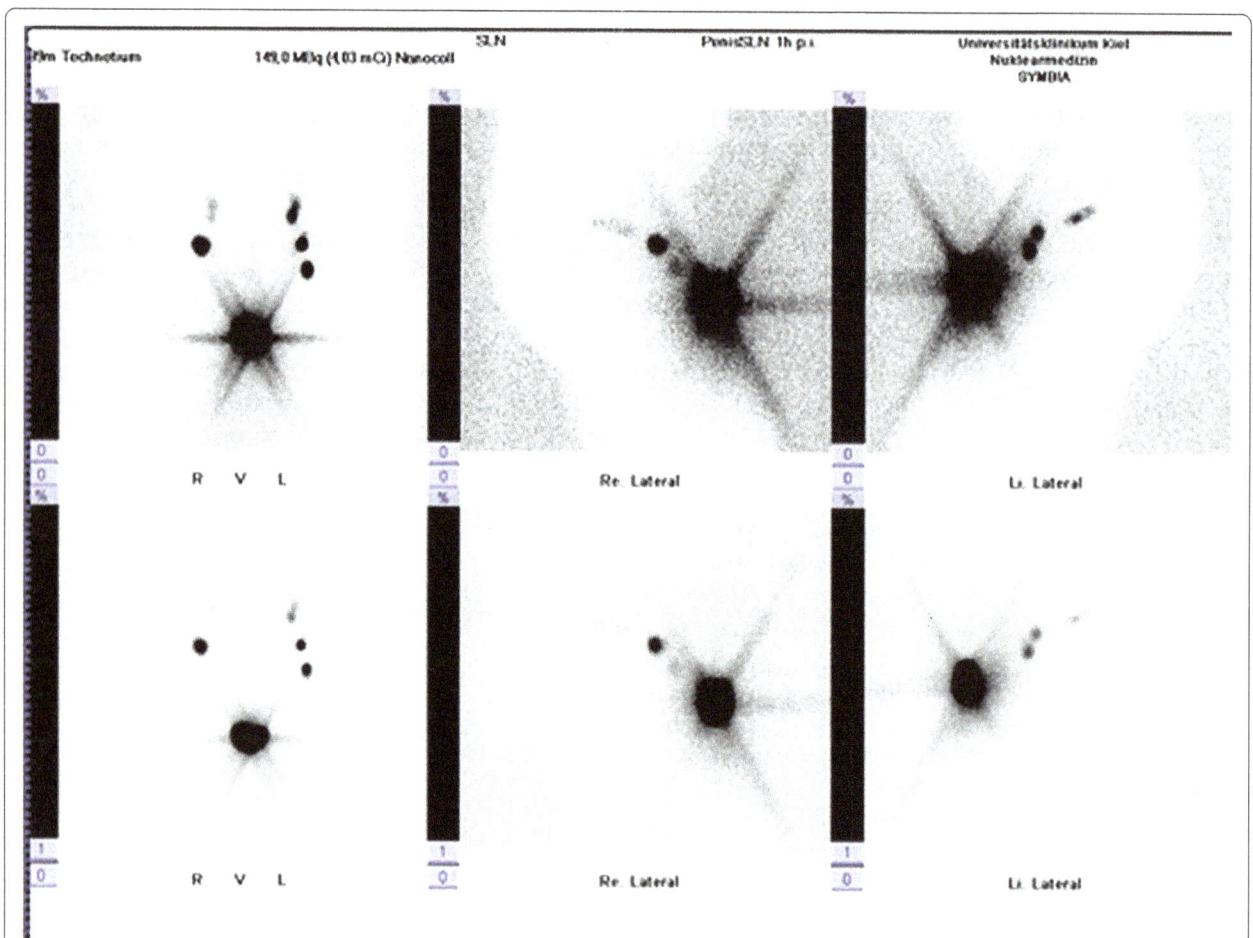

Fig. 2 Pre-operative scans of Sentinel-lymph nodes by means of planar scintigraphy in several projections and indirect body contouring via a Co 57-planar source: Evidence of so-called "hot spots" in the inguinal region bilaterally (3 SLN left, 2 SLN right) as well as in the region of the tumour

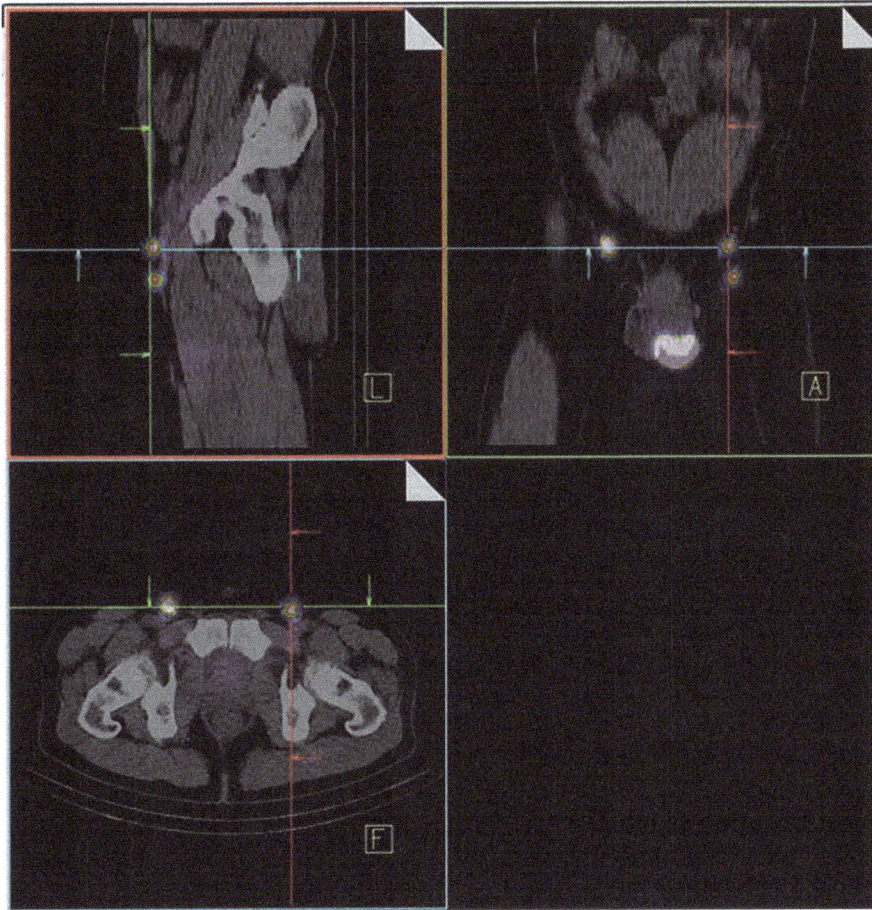

Fig. 3 Pre-operative scans of sentinel lymph nodes by means of SPECT/CT: Evidence of so-called "hot spots" in the inguinal region bilaterally (2 SLN left, 1 SLN right) as well as in the region of the tumour

cm were made for extirpation of the lymph nodes, following the relaxed skin tension lines. All patients were provided with drains at the end of surgery. The drains were left until the flow-rate was equal or smaller than 20 ml per 24 h. The mean respectively median operation time was 130.3 min respectively 120 min. On average, 3.2 lymph nodes (median 2/range 1–11) per patient were resected. Neither compression bondages nor stockings were applied. The mean, respectively median length of the postoperative hospitalization was 5.6, respectively 5.0 days. Histopathological examination of the entire SLNs was done in 100 micrometer (μm) sections under additional hematoxylin-eosin staining. In case there was evidence of positive SLNs with malignant tumour cells, we performed a radical lymphadenectomy (LAE) in a two-stage surgical intervention in the affected inguinal region and if necessary a systemic cytotoxic therapy. In our cohort, inguinal LAE was necessary in two cases. In one case, chronic lymphedema of the lower extremity resulted. In the other case, there were no unexpected events in terms of morbidity.

Three different urologists performed the SLNB-procedures. Preoperatively, also three different nuclear medicine physicians performed the applications of the radioactive tracer. Morbidity and disease-free survival (DFS) after SLNB was evaluated during clinical outpatient follow-up examinations.

As a reference standard, a negative groin was defined as a histologically negative SLN status and uneventful follow-up without nodal recurrence. A positive groin was defined as a histologically positive SLN status or lymph node recurrence during the follow-up period. Based on this definition, we compared SLNB to the reference standard of follow-up examinations. Follow-up was done in the same way in all histologically negative SLN-patients i.e. by physical examination, including inguinal node palpation of the groins in three-monthly intervals for the first two years, every four months in year three and in six-monthly intervals in the fourth and fifth year after diagnosis.

For assessment of the radiation exposure of the involved medical staff in this procedure, we performed both pre- and intraoperative measurements. To this end, we applied a dose rate meter (Berthold, LB123 and Berthold, TOL F) to measure the dose rate (DR) and the time needed for each procedural step. Using these two measured parameters we calculated the effective dose and the hand dose of the involved staff. As a control we used an additional digital personal dosimeter (Polimaster, PM1621MA) for determination of the effective dose of the surgeon. During the measurements, the digital personal dosimeter was placed in the breast pocket of the surgeons' shirt. Prior to radiation measurements during the SLN-procedures, the background radiation in all rooms was determined and subtracted. In view of the fact that the lower detection limit of the thermoluminescence ring dosimeter (TLD) of fingers is >100 µSv, we abstained from using TLD finger rings during pre- and intraoperative measurements. TLD is only of limited use due to the low applied activity and the required pre- and intraoperative times during the procedure, and it is inferior to measurement via sensitive dose rate meters. The assessment comprises the following: preoperatively, the identification of dose values for the staff from nuclear medicine, and intraoperatively, that for anesthetists, surgical staff and the surgeon, taking into account the required time span, the distance to the radiation source, and the intensity of applied activity.

Prior to the procedure, all patients were duly informed about the details of the measures and gave their written informed consent for this guideline-conform procedure. In addition, the study was approved by the Ethics Committee of Kiel University (AK D 426/07).

Results
Reliability and morbidity
In two patients, metastatic disease in the SLN was proven by means of SLNB with subsequent histological examination (Table 1). There were no false-positive results. In one patient, bilateral recurrence of inguinal lymph node metastases was diagnosed four months after histologically negative SLNB. After clinical suspicion of the inguinal lymph node recurrence a bilateral inguinal LAE was conducted. The mean resp. median disease-free survival of patients with a negative SLN result was 52.26 resp. 51 (4–109) months. One patient died from the consequences of a stroke ca. five months after the intervention. A further patient died from the consequences of a renal cell carcinoma ca. twelve months after treatment of penile carcinoma. All other patients were examined as part of the regular follow-up.

The current data, which covers a period of ten years, shows a false-negative rate of 3.13 % in relation to the number of patients (1/32 patients) and 3.51 % in relation to number of investigated groins (2/57 groins). Assessment of morbidity after SLNB alone showed one case of

a prolonged inguinal lymphorrhea, which disappeared spontaneously by leaving the intraoperatively placed drain. SLNB-associated morbidity was thus calculated as 2.94 % per patient (1/34 patients) and 1.75 % per groin (1/57 groins).

The patient who had a false-negative SLNB result during follow-up had a rather unusual clinical course and deserves special attention. In this patient, SLNB was performed during a secondary resection, i. e. after resection of the primary tumour ex domo with an unclear resection status. Despite a unilaterally unsuccessful visualization of a radio-labelled SLN, we performed follow-up investigations on the basis of the T1 stadium diagnosed ex domo and the G1 differentiation as well as a R0 resection according to the guidelines. Unfortunately in this case tumour specimens were not available for our pathologists for re-evaluation.

During a sonographic follow-up examination four months after surgery, we found a bilateral lymph node recurrence, which was successfully resolved by surgical intervention as mentioned above. The patient has been disease-free during further follow-up.

Based on cross-counting (Table 2) and chi-square test we calculated for SLNB a sensitivity of 66.67 % and a specificity of 100.00 %, with a 95 % confidence interval (CI) of 9.5 to 99.2 % (sensitivity) respectively of 88.8 to 100.0 % (specificity).

Radiation exposure of involved staff
Table 3 shows the pre- and intraoperatively measured mean DR of the applied radioactivity at various distances to the radiation source.

In consideration of the measured exposure time of 45 min with a mean distance of 30 cm to the patient prior to resection of the primary tumour, and a exposure time of 120 min after resection of the primary tumour, we calculated a mean effective dose for the surgeon of ca. four µSv per patient (2.2 µSv/h × 0.75 h + 1.1 µSv/h × 2 h), based on the measured mean dose rate values presented in Table 2. The mean effective dose for the surgeon as controlled by the digital dosimeter is ca. 4.06 µSv for the entire surgical intervention. The values thus concur closely with the estimated values.

Table 2 Cross-table of the results of SLNB and follow-up and of SLNB alone

		Results of SLNB and follow-up (n)		
		Histo. positive	Histo. negative	Sum
Results of SLNB alone (n)	histo. positive	true positive 2	false positive 0	all positive 2
	histo. negative	false negative 1	true negative 31	all negative 32
	sum	all true findings 3	all false findings 31	all findings 34

Table 3 Pre- and intraoperative mean dose rates during SLN procedure (2-day protocol) with a 150 MBq Tc-99 m nanocolloid at various distances to the radiation source/patient

Distance	Mean dose rate (μSv/h)
Preoperatively	
Directly on the injection needle (0 cm)	200
Hands of nuclear medicine physician (10 cm)	100
Position of nuclear medicine physician (30 cm)	10
Position assisting staff (50 cm)	2
Intraoperatively (prior to resection of the tumour)	
Hands of surgeon (10 cm)	20
Surgeon (30 cm)	2.2
Surgical staff/physician (50 cm)	0.5
Anesthetist (200 cm)	0.13
Intraoperatively (after resection of the tumour)	
Directly on the sample (0 cm)	15
Hands of surgeon (10 cm)	1.5
Surgeon (30 cm)	1.1
Surgical staff/physician (50 cm)	0.3

The mean hand dose of the surgeon is calculated to be ca. 18 μSv per patient (20 μSv/h × 0.75 h + 1.5 μSv/h × 2 h).

The surgical staff can keep a distance of at least 50 cm to the patient resp. the surgical area during the entire procedure. In the worst case, this can result in a mean effective dose of 0.98 μSv per patient (0.5 μSv/h × 0.75 h + 0.3 μSv/h × 2 h) for these persons. The hand dose is negligible here.

Table 4 shows a summary of the mean pre- and intraoperative radiation exposure for the clinical staff as has been measured or estimated above for penile carcinoma SLNB, in comparison with the mean dose values that apply in malignant melanoma or breast cancer SLNB procedures.

Discussion
Reliability and morbidity
The indication for an LAE in penile carcinomas has been under controversial discussion for many years, especially with respect to clinically and sonographically inconspicuous inguinal lymph nodes [9]. The degree of metastatic spread and the respective appropriate therapeutic management have a significant impact on patient survival. Classic inguinal LAE is associated with a substantial morbidity rate of up to 87.5 % according to the literature (e. g. wound healing problems, generation of seroma or lymphorrhea, etc.) [9, 10].

Only 20 to 25 % of patients with clinically negative inguinal lymph node status harbour occult metastases. By reverse logic, this means that ca. 75 to 80 % of patients with clinically inconspicuous inguinal lymph nodes undergo the increased of morbidity risk going through this surgical intervention in vain. A tentative watchful waiting approach, however, involves a high risk of tumour-related mortality. Results from the literature show that resection of metachronous, clinically evident metastases during follow-up procedures significantly diminishes the long-term survival chances of these patients, compared to immediate resection of occult metastases, from 84 to 35 % [9, 11]. Thus we did not choose the tentative approach in the patients included in this study.

Alternative, non-invasive functional and morphological imaging procedures such as positron-emission tomography/computed tomography (PET/CT) or MRI and CT alone do not have sufficient sensitivity in patients with clinically inconspicuous inguinal lymph node status

Table 4 Pre- and intraoperative mean radiation exposure of the clinical staff by SLNB in different tumour entities

	Tumour entity					
	Penile carcinoma		Malignant melanoma		Breast cancer	
applied activity [MBq] Tc-99 m-labelled nanocolloid	150 2-day protocol		45 1-day protocol		150 2-day protocol	
	mean Effective Dose E [μSv]	mean Organ-dose of the hands H_hands [μSv]	mean Effective Dose E [μSv]	mean Organ-dose of the hands H_hands [μSv]	mean Effective Dose E [μSv]	mean Organ-dose of the hands H_hands [μSv]
clinical staff						
nuclear medicine physician	105	20	2	10	0.6	10
nuclear medicine technologist	0.5	10	0.5	10	0.2	10
surgeon	4.0	100	0.5	7	0.6	5
anesthetist	1.0	-	0.7	-	0.4	-
surgical staff	1.0	-	0.5	-	0.4	-

[12–15]; they are not seen as useful and have thus not been used as obligatory imaging tools in this study.

EAU guidelines recommend performance of SLNB in penile carcinomas with a tumour stadium ≥ T1G2 and non-palpable inguinal lymph nodes (cN0) [6]. If SLN-labelling with radioactive tracers is not available, the guidelines alternatively recommend a fine needle aspiration biopsy (FNAB) of the inguinal lymph nodes with subsequent cytopathological examination.

Regarding FNAB, however, the low sensitivity of only 39 % in penile cancer has to be taken into consideration [16]. A further alternative is to base the treatment strategy on individual risk factors [6]. A decision in favor or against inguinal SLNB based on risk factors like tumour stage and/or tumour differentiation for metastatic risk assessment involves substantial uncertainties. All patients with proven or clinically evident invasive penile cancer without palpable inguinal lymph nodes underwent SLNB. In case of uncertainty concerning the invasiveness of the tumor, we performed preoperative radioactive lymph node labeling including scintigraphy. SLNB was only performed if rapid frozen section during surgery showed at least a T1-carcinoma. However, the reliability of histopathological tumour grading based solely on rapid frozen section is unclear and has not been described in literature yet. Even paraffin-embedded specimens show a high degree of inter-observer variability among pathologists with respect to tumour staging and tissue differentiation [17, 18]. Taking these facts into account, we accepted a possible over diagnosis/-treatment in a very low number of patients with T1G1-tumours by SLNB. As mentioned before, the remarkable thing was that the only relapse due to a false-negative SLNB-procedure was proven in a patient with a T1G1-disease, who had undergone primary surgery ex domo. For this reason, we performed SLNB in each invasive carcinoma of this entity.

The results from our study show that SLNB after radio-labelling with Tc 99 m-nanocolloid is a reliable method for lymph node-diagnostics.

The false-negative rate of 3.13 % in relation to the number of patients (1/32 patients) and 3.51 % in relation to number of investigated groins (2/57 groins) is comparable to that of the results of the Dutch workgroup around Leitje et al. [8], but significantly better than the results of the Swedish workgroup around Kirrander et al. [7], whose false-negative rate was 15 % in a study published in 2012. In the aforementioned Dutch study the false-negative rate was seven percent [8]. In the study by Leitje et al. the results are based on the number of the examined inguinal regions and have not been calculated per patient as in our study. The Dutch study observes that the metastases rate of ten percent is comparatively low, which implies the question whether the

high logistic and methodic demands of SLNB with radio-active nuclides can be justified.

Compared to other studies e.g. Lam et al. [19] or Kroon et al. [20] who report rates of 28 respectively 22 % of histologically positive lymph nodes under employment of SLNB, our rate of metastatic disease is lower. The reason might be that the patients enrolled in the study of Lam et al. had a significantly higher risk of metastatic disease, as can be seen in the lower number of T1-tumours (42 %) compared to our study (56 %). More importantly, the study of Lam et al. included a higher rate of G3-tumours (53 %). In our study the G3-tumour rate is only 18 %. Moreover, the study by Kroon et al. included only patients with T2- and T3-tumours, while T1-tumours were not taken into account, in contrast to our study. These facts and the criteria leading to the low number of primarily positive lymph nodes using the SLNB-procedure might be responsible for our statistical results of sensitivity, specificity, and the 95 % CI. Although our study includes a large patient cohort compared to other German studies, the number is rather small by international standards [8]. It is well possible that higher rates of metastases are found in larger patient cohorts in the future.

The following consideration shows the clinical implication of radio-labelled SLNB: in the current study, we were able to prove a negative nodal status by SLNB with sufficiently long follow-up periods in 31 patients.

Based on the now obsolete risk classification stated in the 2004 EAU-guidelines [21], 19 high-risk patients would have undergone obligatory LAE and further 13 intermediate-risk patients would have been candidates for a facultative classic inguinal LAE without any further diagnostic gain. In this context it has to be mentioned that the patient who had a bilateral inguinal lymph node recurrence after negative SLNB was a low-risk patient (T1G1/Table 1) and was diagnosed and underwent R0 resection ex domo where SLNB was not indicated. Unfortunately, tumor specimens were not available for re-evaluation by our pathologist.

Based only on the SLNB result, we were able to spare these patients the severe morbidity associated with classic inguinal LAE while guarding diagnostic safety. As a consequence we were able to reduce morbidity in our patient cohort to 2.94 % per patient (1/34 patients) and 1.75 % per groin (1/57 groins) by using SLNB.

In view of the results of our study, especially the case of the patient who underwent ex domo surgery of the primary tumour, the question arises whether SLNB after application of radioactive lymphogenic tracers can also be safely applied as a secondary intervention, i.e. after resection of the primary tumour.

Graafland et al. [22] performed a metachronous SLNB in 40 patients after earlier resection of the primary tumour. The reported results of a two-stage procedure are comparable to those of primary SLNB.

Our results cannot be used to confirm the findings by Graafland et al. as we encountered lymph node recurrence after a false-negative SLN-procedure four months after secondary SLNB during follow-up. In the currently described patient collective after primary SLNB the false-negative rate is zero percent.

Risks and benefits of SLNB and classic inguinal LAE

As mentioned the morbidity of a classic inguinal LAE is as high as 87.5 % [9, 10]. Due to the fact that lymph node metastases can only be proven in ca. 20 to 25 % of patients with clinically non-palpable inguinal lymph nodes [3], this treatment later reveals itself to have been unnecessary in 75 to 80 % of these patients.

As already stated, the Dutch workgroup around Horenblas, like some other workgroups, reported false negative rates of approximately 15 % during the early implementation phase of the SLNB-procedure [7, 23]. Data from an analysis by Neto et al. require a critical view [24]. These comprise studies examining the results of SLNB including patients with palpable inguinal lymph nodes. SLNB is not recommended by the expert society guidelines in patients with palpable inguinal lymph nodes due to its high unreliability [3]. In our study, we could show excellent reliability of SLNB, with a false negative rate of only 3.51 % (2/57) per groin respectively 3.13 % (1/32) per patient. Like us, Lam and coworkers report a false negative rate of 5 % (in relation to the groins) respectively 6 % (in relation to the patients) in a cohort of 264 patients. The faulty procedures occurred mainly during the implementation of the method [19]. Concerning the false negative rates of classic inguinal LAE for staging, no data in the literature are available yet.

One of the limitations of SLNB might be that tumour cells can lead to obstruction or occlusion of the lymphatic drainage pathways and can either cause a complete blockage or a rerouting of the radio tracer [23, 25]. This aspect can lead to restraints of SLNB. The risk of a relevant modification of lymphatic and thus tracer drainage depends on the metastatic load in the lymphatic pathways and in the lymph nodes. The risk of lymph node metastases in patients with palpable lymph nodes is about 50 % and therefore much higher than in those with an inconspicuous inguinal lymph node status during palpation of the groins (20 to 25 %). For this reason, expert society guidelines do not recommend SLNB in patients with palpable inguinal lymph nodes, as has been mentioned before [3].

The validity of clinical groin palpation within the physical examination is influenced by the physical constitution of the patient on one hand, and by the experience of the examiner on the other. In our study, one patient

developed a bilateral lymph node recurrence four months after histologically negative SLNB. The assessment of the inguinal lymph node status was impeded by corpulence. Obesity is capable of veiling otherwise palpable and potentially tumour-infested lymph nodes, thus wrongly leading to the conclusion that the patient is eligible for SLNB, which presents another limitation of this staging procedure. This risk of misjudgment could be minimized by preoperative sonography of the groins, as a supplement to clinical palpation.

As mentioned, a further possible source of errors in the application of this procedure is associated with the two-stage approach of SLNB after surgical removal of primary tumour. While Graafland et al. [22] report uniform results in 40 cases of a metachronously performed SLNB, we believe that surgery-related modifications of the tracer drainage, e.g. through scar formation or edema, might be a reason for the false-negative SLNB in one patient of this study.

Radiation exposure of the involved staff

German radiation protection laws prescribe that any indication for the application of ionizing radiation, also that of open radioactive nuclides, is mandatorily bound to a medical indication identified by a physician with the necessary expertise [26]. Thus the resulting benefit of this procedure for the patient outweighs the potential risk of ionizing radiation.

Based on the specifications of the German radiation protection commission (Strahlenschutzkommission, SSK), we have calculated an effective dose of 0.5 to 1.5 Millisievert (mSv) in patients undergoing the SLN procedure according to a so-called two-day protocol under application of the above-described tracer with an activity of 150 MBq [27]. Our dosimetric calculations fit to the data from the literature. Application of an additional low-dose CT in the pelvic region leads to an additional effective dose of 1–2 mSv [27]. We were able to confirm this by our calculations (CT Expo Version 2.4/2015/ G. Stamm, H. D. Nagel).

According to our measurements and calculations, the effective dose for the nuclear-medical staff of 0.5 µSv (nuclear medicine technologists) resp. 1.5 µSv (nuclear medicine physicians) is relatively low, which is owed to the fact that preoperative application of the tracer, despite its high radioactive load of 150 MBq, requires little time, and thus makes the exposure time much shorter than the intraoperative exposure. The effective dose values for the nuclear medical staff are comparable to those occurring during application of this kind of procedure in other tumour entities like breast cancer or malignant melanoma.

Compared to other procedures in nuclear medicine, sentinel lymph node diagnostics with radioactive tracers is associated with a relatively low radiation burden for the nuclear medical staff.

Physicians and technologists in nuclear medicine are allowed to be exposed to radiation by profession and are as such allocated to at least Category B with a maximum effective dosage of 6 mSv (6000 μSv)/a and a maximum hand dosage of 150 mSv (150000 μSv)/a. If the nuclear medicine physician was to only perform this kind of procedure, up to 4000 procedures per year would be eligible. If the nuclear medicine expert was allocated to category A of professional radiation exposure, maximum eligible effective dose would even be 20 mSv/a with a maximum hand dose of 500 mSv/a [26].

In this tumour entity, organ-preserving surgical resection of the primary tumour can be technically demanding and time-consuming. Thus the surgeon is the person with the highest effective dose exposure as shown by our pre- and intraoperative measurements (maximum of ca. four μSv per patient).

Compared to other tumour entities, the effective dose for the surgeon of penile carcinoma is higher (Table 3). This is due to the fact that more time is required in penile cancer surgery, – i.e. for the preparation of the primary tumour and subsequent functional reconstruction of the urethra -, compared to resection of malignant melanoma in unproblematic localizations or mastocarcinoma resection including the SLN; this considered, the radiation exposure time in penile cancer is longer.

Surgical staff including urologists is not classified as "radiation-exposed by profession" and is eligible for exposure up to a maximum effective dose of 1 mSv (1000 μSv)/a and a maximum hand dose of 50 mSv (50000 μSv)/a [26]. The effective dose for surgical staff measured by us amounts to ca. 1.0 μSv per patient (Table 3). Based on these results, this means that the surgical staff could perform ca. 1000 SLN interventions per year without exceeding the threshold value of German radiation protection regulations, while the surgeon could perform ca. 250 interventions per year [26, 28] In addition, it has to be taken into account that penile carcinomas both in Europe and in the U.S. are much more rare than for example breast cancer or malignant melanoma [29]. While the effective dose for the surgeon per patient is thus higher than in the other mentioned entities, the overall dose remains relatively low and far below the threshold of the radiation protection laws.

Our calculations and measurements as well as the data in the literature on staff radiation exposure [27] have shown that both the staff in nuclear medicine and the surgical staff can be expected to undergo only very limited radiation exposure, which is well within the legal boundaries. A tentative attitude towards SLNB with radioactive lymph node labelling cannot be justified on the basis of radiation protection aspects. Worries and fears on this score are unfounded. For more transparency, surgeons in Germany who perform SLNB with radioactive labelling have been obliged since 2011 to complete a 6 h–training in radiation protection [28]. Regardless of this, the procedure has high methodical demands and requires an experienced and interdisciplinary team consisting of a specialist in nuclear medicine, an urologist and a pathologist. This method could be facilitated through multidisciplinary centres or by collaborative clinical setups.

Conclusions

SLNB with SLN-labelling via Tc-99 m nanocolloids in penile cancer is a valuable diagnostic method associated with low morbidity rates. It offers a high degree of reliability, especially when performed during surgical resection of the primary tumour. The method has high methodological and logistical demands as it among other things requires an interdisciplinary team. In due consideration of radiation protection laws, the resulting radiation exposure for clinical staff during the SLN- procedure is low, and a tentative attitude towards this approach is not justified.

Acknowledgements
We thank Mrs. Almut Kalz for proofreading and editing the article, Mr. Bernhard Egeler for the technical support and Dr. Imme Haubitz for her advice and her expertise in statistical issues.

Funding
There is no funding in connection with this study.

Authors' contributions
MZ: Data analysis, Manuscript editing. CMN: Statistical analysis, Manuscript editing. JD: Acquisition of data. RB: Acquisition of data. MM: Acquisition of data. YZ: Statistical analysis. MJ: Statistical analysis. DO: contributed to conception. KB: contributed to conception. KPJ: Protocol development. UL: Protocol development, Manuscript writing. All authors read and approved the final manuscript.

Competing interests
All authors declare that they have no competing interests.

Author details
[1]Department of Nuclear medicine, Molecular Imaging Diagnostics and Therapy, University Hospital Schleswig Holstein, Campus Kiel, Kiel, Germany. [2]Department of Urology and Pediatric Urology, University Hospital Schleswig Holstein, Campus Kiel, Kiel, Germany. [3]Northern German Seminar for Radiation Protection gGmbH at the Christian-Albrechts-University Kiel, Kiel, Germany. [4]Department of Radio Oncology, University Hospital Schleswig Holstein, Campus Kiel, Kiel, Germany.

References

1. DGN-Handlungsempfehlung 031–033 - 031-033l_S1_Wächter_ Lymphknoten_Diagnostik_2014-10.pdf [Internet]. [cited 2015 Dec 28]. Available from: http://www.awmf.org/uploads/tx_szleitlinien/031-033l_S1_ W%C3%A4chter_Lymphknoten_Diagnostik_2014-10.pdf
2. S3 Leitlinie Melanom-Kurzfassung - 032-024k_S3_Melanom_Diagnostik_ Therapie_Nachsorge_2013-02.pdf [Internet]. [cited 2015 Dec 2 8]. Available from: http://www.awmf.org/uploads/tx_szleitlinien/032-024l_S3_Melanom_ Diagnostik_Therapie_Nachsorge_2013-verlaengert.pdf
3. Hakenberg OW, Compérat EM, Minhas S, Necchi A, Protzel C, Watkin N, et al. EAU guidelines on penile cancer: 2014 update. Eur Urol. 2015;67:142–50.
4. Vogt H, Schmidt M, Bares R, Brenner W, Grünwald F, Kopp J, et al. Procedure guideline for sentinel lymph node diagnosis. Nukl Nucl Med. 2010;49:167–72. quiz N19.
5. Poppel HV, Watkin NA, Osanto S, Moonen L, Horwich A, Kataja V, et al. Penile cancer: ESMO Clinical Practice Guidelines for diagnosis, treatment and follow-up. Ann Oncol. 2013;24:vi115–24.
6. Pizzocaro G, Algaba F, Horenblas S, Solsona E, Tana S, Van Der Poel H, et al. EAU penile cancer guidelines 2009. Eur Urol. 2010;57:1002–12.
7. Kirrander P, Andrén O, Windahl T. Dynamic sentinel node biopsy in penile cancer: initial experiences at a Swedish referral centre. BJU Int. 2013;111:E48–53.
8. Leijte JAP, Hughes B, Graafland NM, Kroon BK, Olmos RAV, Nieweg OE, et al. Two-center evaluation of dynamic sentinel node biopsy for squamous cell carcinoma of the penis. J. Clin. Oncol. Off. J. Am. Soc. Clin. Oncol. 2009;27:3325–9.
9. Kroon BK, Horenblas S, Lont AP, Tanis PJ, Gallee MPW, Nieweg OE. Patients with penile carcinoma benefit from immediate resection of clinically occult lymph node metastases. J Urol. 2005;173:816–9.
10. Bevan-Thomas R, Slaton JW, Pettaway CA. Contemporary morbidity from lymphadenectomy for penile squamous cell carcinoma: the M.D. Anderson Cancer Center Experience. J Urol. 2002;167:1638–42.
11. McDougal WS, Kirchner FK, Edwards RH, Killion LT. Treatment of carcinoma of the penis: the case for primary lymphadenectomy. J Urol. 1986;136:38–41.
12. Heyns CF, Fleshner N, Sangar V, Schlenker B, Yuvaraja TB, van Poppel H. Management of the lymph nodes in penile cancer. Urology. 2010;76:S43–57.
13. Kochhar R, Taylor B, Sangar V. Imaging in primary penile cancer: current status and future directions. Eur Radiol. 2010;20:36–47.
14. Hughes B, Leijte J, Shabbir M, Watkin N, Horenblas S. Non-invasive and minimally invasive staging of regional lymph nodes in penile cancer. World J Urol. 2009;27:197–203.
15. Mueller-Lisse UG, Scher B, Scherr MK, Seitz M. Functional imaging in penile cancer: PET/computed tomography, MRI, and sentinel lymph node biopsy. Curr Opin Urol. 2008;18:105–10.
16. Kroon BK, Horenblas S, Deurloo EE, Nieweg OE, Teertstra HJ. Ultrasonography-guided fine-needle aspiration cytology before sentinel node biopsy in patients with penile carcinoma. BJU Int. 2005;95:517–21.
17. Naumann CM, Alkatout I, Hamann MF, Al-Najar A, Hegele A, Korda JB, et al. Interobserver variation in grading and staging of squamous cell carcinoma of the penis in relation to the clinical outcome. BJU Int. 2009;103:1660–5.
18. Gunia S, Burger M, Hakenberg OW, May D, Koch S, Jain A, et al. Inherent grading characteristics of individual pathologists contribute to clinically and prognostically relevant interobserver discordance concerning Broders' grading of penile squamous cell carcinomas. Urol Int. 2013;90:207–13.
19. Lam W, Alnajjar HM, La-Touche S, Perry M, Sharma D, Corbishley C, et al. Dynamic sentinel lymph node biopsy in patients with invasive squamous cell carcinoma of the penis: a prospective study of the long-term outcome of 500 inguinal basins assessed at a single institution. Eur Urol. 2013;63:657–63.
20. Kroon BK, Horenblas S, Meinhardt W, van der Poel HG, Bex A, van Tinteren H, et al. Dynamic sentinel node biopsy in penile carcinoma: evaluation of 10 years experience. Eur Urol. 2005;47:601–6. discussion 606.
21. Solsona E, Algaba F, Horenblas S, Pizzocaro G, Windahl T. European Association of Urology. EAU Guidelines on Penile Cancer. Eur Urol. 2004;46:1–8.
22. Graafland NM, Valdés Olmos RA, Meinhardt W, Bex A, van der Poel HG, van Boven HH, et al. Nodal staging in penile carcinoma by dynamic sentinel node biopsy after previous therapeutic primary tumour resection. Eur Urol. 2010;58:748–51.
23. Kroon BK, Horenblas S, Estourgie SH, Lont AP, Valdés Olmos RA, Nieweg OE. How to avoid false-negative dynamic sentinel node procedures in penile carcinoma. J Urol. 2004;171:2191–4.
24. Neto AS, Tobias-Machado M, Ficarra V, Wroclawski ML, Amarante RDM, Pompeo ACL, et al. Dynamic sentinel node biopsy for inguinal lymph node staging in patients with penile cancer: a systematic review and cumulative analysis of the literature. Ann Surg Oncol. 2011;18:2026–34.
25. Leijte JAP, van der Ploeg IMC, Valdés Olmos RA, Nieweg OE, Horenblas S. Visualization of tumor blockage and rerouting of lymphatic drainage in penile cancer patients by use of SPECT/CT. J Nucl Med Off Publ Soc Nucl Med. 2009;50:364–7.
26. StrlSchV - Verordnung über den Schutz vor Schäden durch ionisierende Strahlen [Internet]. 2016. Available from: https://www.gesetze-im-internet. de/strlschv_2001/BJNR171410001.html
27. Die Strahlenschutzkommission - Beratungsergebnisse - Nuklearmedizinischer Nachweis des Wächter-Lymphknotens [Internet]. [cited 2015 Dec 28]. Available from: http://www.ssk.de/SharedDocs/Beratungsergebnisse/2001/ Nuklearmedizinischer_Nachweis.html
28. Strahlenschutz in der Medizin - Richtlinie zur Strahlenschutzverordnung (StrlSchV) vom 26. Mai 2011 (GMBl. 2011, Nr. 44–47, S. 867), zuletzt geändert durch RdSchr. des BMUB vom 11. Juli 2014 (GMBl. 2014, Nr. 49, S. 1020). Gemeinsames Ministerialblatt 2011; 2011. Available from: https://www.bfs. de/SharedDocs/Downloads/BfS/DE/rsh/3-bmub/3_17_0714.pdf?__ blob=publicationFile&v=1
29. Siegel RL, Miller KD, Jemal A. Cancer statistics, 2016. CA Cancer J Clin. 2016;66:7–30.

7

Biochemical recurrence-free survival and pathological outcomes after radical prostatectomy for high-risk prostate cancer

Jean-Baptiste Beauval[1*], Mathieu Roumiguié[1], Thomas Filleron[2], Thibaut Benoit[1], Alexandre de la Taille[3], Bernard Malavaud[1], Laurent Salomon[3], Michel Soulié[1] and Guillaume Ploussard[4]

Abstract

Background: We propose to improve the prognostic assessment after radical prostatectomy (RP) by dividing high-risk prostate cancer (hrPCa) (according to the d'Amico classification) into subgroups combining 1, 2 or 3 criteria of aggressiveness (cT2c-T3a, PSA >20 ng/ml, Gleason score (GS) > 7).

Methods: Data from 4795 hrPCa patients who underwent RP in two French university hospitals from 1991 to 2013 were analyzed. Subgroups were formed to determine whether an increasing number (1, 2 or 3) of criteria of tumor aggressiveness was associated with poorer oncological results and early biochemical recurrence (BCR) (PSA > 0. 2 ng/ml). These results were compared using Fisher's exact test and BCR was compared according to the Kaplan-Meier method.

Results: Eight hundred fifteen patients were treated by RP for hrPCa (8 %). Four hundred eleven patients (79.5 %) presented 1 RF (Risk Factor), 93 (18.0 %) 2 RF and 13 (2.5 %) 3 RF. Lymph node invasion and positive margin rates were 12.4 and 44.1 %, respectively. The prognostic sub-stratification based on these 3 factors was significantly predictive for adverse pathologic features and for oncologic outcomes. BCR free survival was respectively 56.4, 27.06 and 18.46 % for 1RF, 2RF and 3RF ($p < 0.0001$). However, no predominant negative criterion was found.

Conclusion: Oncologic results after RP are heterogenous within the hrPCa risk group. Sub-stratification based on three well-defined criteria leads to a better identification of the most aggressive cancers. On the other hand, RP provides both effective cancer control and satisfactory survival rates in patients with only one risk factor.

Keywords: High risk prostate cancer, Radical prostatectomy, BCR free-survival, Risk factors, Stratification

Background

Prostate cancer (PCa) is the most common form of malignant cancer in Europe and, the second leading of death attributable of cancer [1, 2]. Despite the widespread use of prostate specific antigen (PSA) individual screening, some patients are still diagnosed with locally advanced and/or high risk PCa. According to the D'Amico's classification, patient with PSA > 20 ng/mL and/or preoperative Gleason score of 8–10 and/or clinical stage ≥ T2c can be considered to be at high-risk of disease progression despite radical treatment with a curative intent [3].

In high-risk prostate cancer patients, the best course of treatment is often unclear, and the oncological outcomes appear heterogeneous among series and treatment options. Even though several treatment options, including RP, RT, and androgen deprivation therapy (ADT) alone or in combination, are available but the recurrence rate remains high regardless of the type of treatment [4]. Recently, long-term follow-up studies of high-risk PCa patients who underwent RP with or without adjuvant therapies have revealed good oncologic outcomes highlighting the potential underutilization of surgery in such cases [5, 6]. Retrospective population-based studies recently suggested that oncologic outcomes in terms of

* Correspondence: jbbeauval@gmail.com
[1]Department of Urology, Andrology and Renal Transplantation, CHU Rangueil, 1, av J Pouilhès, 31059 Toulouse, France
Full list of author information is available at the end of the article

disease-specific mortality were at least comparable in high risk PCa patients treated with RP as compared to those undergoing radiotherapy combined with androgen deprivation therapy [6–8]. Evidence also suggests that patients with high-risk PCa are those who benefit the most from RP [8–10].

Thus, large multicentric series have reported that a significant percentage (about 30 %) of PCa preoperatively defined as high risk, was organ-confined and favourable in RP specimens [11–13]. These findings highlight the interest of improving patients selection within the heteregeneous group of high risk PCa.

The aim of this study was to define subgroups combining 1, 2 or 3 criteria of aggressiveness (cT2c-T3a, PSA > 20 ng/ml, Gleason score (GS) > 7) among surgically treated hrPCa and to define their risk of progression.

Methods

Patient sample

After institutional review board approval (patient records/information were anonymized and de-identified prior to analysis, consent was not required for your study), we retrospectively examined data from 815 consecutive patients who underwent radical prostatectomy and bilateral extended pelvic nodes dissection (in 98.1 % cases) for clinical high-risk prostate cancer in D'Amico risk classification (PSA >20 ng/ml, clinical T2c or more stage, biopsy Gleason sum 8–10) between 1990 and 2013 in two French academic centers (overall cohort: 4795 RPs). Surgical procedures were performed by 7 different senior surgeons, who used standardized techniques (open, laparoscopic or robot-assisted RP) and applied the same anatomic template during pelvic lymph node dissection, as previously described [14]. We excluded 298 men because of incomplete information on preoperative PSA, Gleason score, clinical stage and pathologic T stage. Only patients with complete clinical and pathological data who did not receive neoadjuvant therapies were eligible. In the final analysis, the data on the 517 patients included the preoperative parameters such as age, prostatic specific antigen (PSA), clinical stage (CS) and biopsy Gleason score.

The clinical stage was assigned according to the 2002 TNM staging system, prostate biopsy cores were obtained with transrectal ultrasound guidance, using a >10-core biopsy protocol, and pretreatment PSA was measured before digital rectal examination. Genitourinary pathologists assessed the biopsy and pathologic gradings according to the Gleason gradings system before 2005 and the modified ISUP Gleason score after 2005. The pT stage was graded according to the 2002 AJCC staging system for PCa.

Biochemical recurrence (BCR) was defined as a PSA value 0.2 ng/ml after RP, confirmed by at least two consecutive measurements.

Statistical analysis

Data were summarized by frequency and percentage for categorical variables, and by median and range for continuous variables. Comparisons between groups were performed using the Mann–Whitney rank sum test for continuous variables and Chi square or Fisher's exact test for categorical variables.

Biochemical Recurrence Free Survival was calculated from the date of the surgery to the date of the diagnosis of the biochemical recurrence. BCR was estimated using Kaplan-Meier method and univariate analysis was performed using the log rank test. Logistic regression models were built to determine the independent predictive value of PSA, Gleason score and clinical stage at diagnosis.

All statistical tests were two sided, and differences were considered statistically significant when $p < 0.05$. Stata 13.0 software (StatCorp LP, College Statio, Texas) was used for all statistical analysis.

Results

Patients' descriptive characteristics are to be found on Table 1. 411 patients (79.5 %) presented 1 RF (Risk Factor), 93 (18.0 %) 2 RF and 13 (2.5 %) 3 RF. Median serum PSA level was 21.0 (1.7:158.0) ng/ml. According to the risk classification, median PSA was 15.7 (1.7-158.0) for 1RF, 30.0 (3.0-134.0) for 2RF, 31.7 (22.0-50.0) for 3RF, respectively ($p < 0.001$). The proportions of the clinical stage were different between the 3 groups: cT1c-cT2b: 91.2 % ($n = 375$), 35.5 % ($n = 33$) and 0 %; cT2c-cT3: 8.8 % ($n = 36$), 64.5 % ($n = 60$) and 100 % ($n = 13$)) respectively for 1RF, 2RF and 3RF ($p < 0.0001$). Furthermore, the proportions of Gleason sum >7 found into prostate biopsy was greater in population with less RF (43.6 % ($n = 179$), 62.4 % ($n = 58$) and 100 % ($n = 13$) respectively for 1RF, 2RF and 3RF ($p < 0.0001$). In overall population, the pT stage was pT2 in 29 % of patients, pT3a in 37.9 %, pT3b in 32.9 %, and pT4 in 0.2 %. Positive surgical margin was reported in 44.1 % of cases ($n = 228$) and increased within the risk sub-stratification: 40.6, 58.1, and 53.8 % for 1RF, 2RF and 3RF respectively ($p < 0.0007$)). Lymph node metastasis was noted in 12.4 % of patients: 9.2 % ($n = 37$), 22.6 % ($n = 21$) and 38.5 % ($n = 5$) for 1RF, 2RF and 3RF respectively ($p < 0.0001$). The number of nodes removed was exactly the same for the 3 groups of patients (median 10 LN (1–39). The majority of the patients had only one criterion of aggressiveness (79.5 %) (Additional file 1: Table S1).

Second-line treatments were adjuvant treatments before recurrence in only 29 cases as follows (5.6 %):

Table 1 Descriptive statistics of 523 patients with clinical high-risk prostate cancer treated with radical prostatectomy and pelvic node dissection

	Overall	1RF	2RF	3RF	p
No (%)	523	411 (79.5)	93 (18.0)	13 (2.5)	
Missing	3				
Age,yr					
Age,yr Median	64.0	64.0	64.0	59	0.02
Range	41.0:79.0	44.0:79.0	44.0:76.0	47.0:70.0	
PSA, ng/ml					
Median	21.0	15.7	30.0	31.7	<0.001
Range	1.7: 158.0	1.7:158.0	3.0:134.0	22.0:50.0	
Clinical stage					
cT1	266 (51.5)	246 (59.9)	20 (21.5)	0 (0)	<0.0001
cT2	193 (37.3)	150 (36.5)	39 (41.9)	4 (30.8)	
cT3	58 (11.2)	15 (3.6)	34 (36.6)	9 (69.2)	
Biopsy Gleason sum					
<=7	267 (51.6)	232 (56.4)	35 (37.6)	0 (0)	<0.0001
>7	250 (48.4)	179 (43.6)	58 (62.4)	13 (100)	
Specimen Gleason sum					
<=7	301 (58.2)	250 (60.8)	50 (53.8)	1 (7.7)	0.0004
>7	216 (41.8)	161 (39.2)	43 (46.2)	12 (92.3)	
Surgical margin					
R0	289 (55.9)	244 (59.4)	39 (41.9)	6 (46.2)	0.0072
R1	228 (44.1)	167 (40.6)	54 (58.1)	7 (53.8)	
Pathological stage					
pT2	150 (29.0)	134 (32.6)	14 (15.1)	2 (15.4)	0.0007
pT3	366 (70.8)	277 (67.4)	78 (83.9)	11 (84.6)	
pT4	1 (0.2)	0 (0)	1 (1.1)	0 (0)	
Lymph node involvement					
No	444 (87.6)	364 (90.8)	72 (77.4)	8 (61.5)	0.0001
Yes	63 (12.4)	37 (9.2)	21 (22.6)	5 (38.5)	

Data were stratified in three groups of risk factors

radiotherapy in 1.5 % of cases, androgen deprivation therapy in 2.1 % of cases, and RT combined with ADT in 1.7 % of cases. Salvage treatments (182 cases, 35.2 %) were salvage radiotherapy in 18 % of cases, androgen deprivation therapy in 11.8 %, RT combined with ADT in 0.8 % and chemotherapy in 4.5 %.

Overall, median follow-up was 25.2 months. The 2-year and 5-year RFS rate was 55.21 (49.80; 60.28) and 41.67 (35.35; 47.86) respectively.

The prognostic sub-stratification based on these 3 factors was significantly predictive for adverse pathologic features and for oncologic outcomes. BCR-free survival was, respectively, 56.4 % (50.0; 62.5), 27.06 % (16.4; 38.86) and 18.46 % (3.06; 30.33) for 1RF, 2RF and 3RF ($p < 0.0001$) (Fig. 1). However, no predominant negative criterion was however found.

In univariable analysis, predictors of oncologic outcomes were PSA, number of risk factor, postoperatively positive lymph node, surgical margin, pT stage (Table 2).

In multivariable analysis, no preoperative predictor was independently predictive for recurrence-free survival. Postoperative pT stage and positive lymph node status were independent predictors of recurrence-free survival (Table 3).

Figure 1 (Additional file 2: Figures S1 and S2) shows Kaplan-Meier curves depending Biochemical free recurrence rates according to number of risk factors (RF), SC disease, surgical margin, lymph node invasion and stage after RP (Additional files 1 and 2). The rate of BCR free recurrence was significantly improved with the number of risk factors (log-rank test, $p < 0.001$).

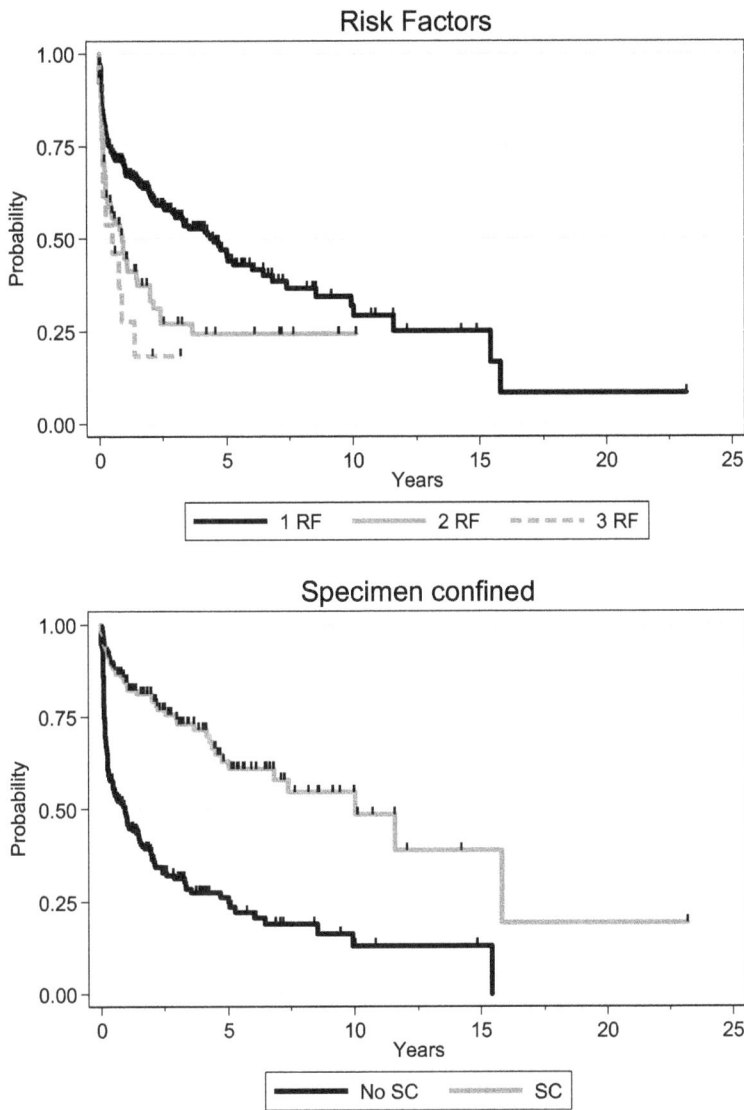

Fig. 1 Kaplan-Meier curves depending Biochemical free recurrence rates for 3 groups of risk factors (RF)

Discussion

In this current study, we demonstrated the different outcomes in high risk PCa according to the number of preoperative risk factors identified: the increasing number of RF was correlated with poorer BCR-free survival.

Indeed, at present, urologists face the dilemma of deciding which treatment is best adapted for hrPCa patients: ADT, radiotherapy, RP or a multimodality approach. When asked, most physicians commonly say they prefer ADT associated with radiotherapy [15]. Nevertheless, RP has, however, whether combined with or without multimodal therapies, produced good oncologic outcomes in the large multicentric series [11–13]. Post-surgery recurrence risk depends mainly on the pathological final assessment in RP specimens. But, an accurate preoperative patient selection is essential when choosing what initial treatment will be used in decision-making.

Preoperatively, the identification of high-risk PCa can be based on at least three well-defined predictors of the extent of the disease and the post treatment outcome as defined by d'Amico et al. [3]. Others studies and our own have shown that the D'Amico classification is a highly heterogeneous PCa risk subgroup. Because of a lack of uniform definition of hrPCa, there is an urgent need to classify hrPCa according to different prognosis groups. Indeed, the present study clearly identified 3 different populations with different oncologic outcomes, all of which depend on the number of risk factors.

Table 2 Univariate analysis of biochemical recurrence (BCR)

	Event (BCR)	Survival (%)	CI 95 %	p
Age				
<65y	115/285	48.54	40.88; 55.77	0.8
≥65y	94/232	50.84	42.09; 58.93	
Clinical stage				
≤cT2a-b	165/408	50.44	44.04; 56.50	0.91
≥cT2c-T3	44/109	45.20	31.83; 57.64	
Biopsy Gleason score				
≤7	107/267	50.58	42.59; 58.02	0.73
>7	102/250	48.66	40.35; 56.45	
PSA				
<20	75/240	61.21	52.20; 69.02	0.0001
≥20	134/277	40.00	32.79; 47.10	
Specimen confined				
No SC	159/291	31.30	24.61; 38.19	0.0001
SC	50/226	74.41	65.75; 81.19	
Margin				
R0	82/289	66.18	58.42; 72.83	0.0001
R1	127/228	28.64	21.32; 36.36	
Risk factors				
1	148/411	56.54	50.02; 62.55	0.0001
2	51/93	27.06	16.40; 38.86	
3	10/13	18.46	3.06; 44.09	
Positive lymph node				
N0	170/453	54.14	48.00; 59.87	0.0001
N1	39/63	9.95	1.15; 30.33	
Pathological stage				
pT2	28/150	79.63	69.84; 86.54	0.0001
pT3-pT4	181/367	37.78	31.27; 44.27	

Table 3 Multivariate analysis of biochemical recurrence BCR

	HR	95 % CI	p-value
PSA preoperative			
<20 ng/ml	1	(0.99; 1.81)	0.060
≥20 ng/ml	1.34		
SC			
No	1	(0.37; 1.00)	0.051
Yes	0.61		
Surgical margin			
M-	1	(0.97; 2.17)	0.068
M+	1.45		
Number of risk factors			
1	1	(0.86; 1.70)	0.27
2	1.21	(0.70; 2.74)	0.34
3	1.38		
Lymph node invasion			
No	1	(1.46; 3.20)	<0.001
Yes	2.16		
PT Stage			
pT2	1	(1.43; 3.48)	<0.001
pT3-4	2.23		

The first population identified, characterized by 1 risk factor and benefited the most from surgery because of favorable cancer control with good BCR-free survival rates. Similarly, prior studies have attempted to better stratify patients with hrPCa based on the number of risks factors [12, 16]. Joniau et al. and Spahn et al. showed more favorable outcomes (BCR-free survival, CSS and OS) when there is only one. Our study confirms these results.

Conversely, the risk of recurrence appears to be very high in patients with high-grade disease and who still have at least 2 risk factors despite radical surgery along with a great deal of adjuvant and salvage treatment strategies. Multimodal treatment strategies are probably warranted in those cases. Prospective trials on the timing of adjuvant or salvage ADT and RT will hopefully provide some answers.

In our study, the PSM rate was around forty percent and more then 70 % had pT3 disease, but only 1.5 % of the patients received adjuvant radiotherapy (ART). On the other hand, salvage treatments (35.2 %) were often proposed. Most of recommendation proposed RT after RP in cases of extracapsular extension, GS > 7, PSM because of a high risk of local recurrence. Currently, the question about the time of treatment is always open: immediate adjuvant RT or salvage RT after biological monitoring. 3 studies showed a benefit of immediate ART (SWOG 8794, ARO and EORTC 22911) in comparison with no adjuvant treatment. But the time of treatment is still discussed and we should wait the results of AFU-GETUG 17 trial. Some recent studies showed a better functional recovery if RT is not performed immediately after RP. For these two reasons, urologists in this study preferred salvage RT.

Finally, we have demonstrated that men with only one high risk factor had a better BCR-free survival rate than men with two or more.

Therefore, we identified a subgroup, for which RP led to favorable outcomes, corresponding to the ideal candidate for RP in high risk PCa. Recently, Fossati et al. showed an increased diagnosis of localized and less extensive high-grade prostate cancer was observed over the last two decades. In this context, patients with high-risk disease selected for radical prostatectomy had better cancer control over time [17].

The nomogram published by Briganti et al. has led to selection improvement for patients candidates for RP as a primary treatment for high risk PCa [18]. This predictive tool helps in predicting a specimen-confined (SC) disease in clinical high risk PCa (40 % in their study). This nomogram was recently externally validated by Roumiguié et al. who confirmed good oncologic outcomes in this heterogeneous subgroup of high risk PCa thanks to a large proportion of specimen-confined PCa, but with a decreased accuracy for intermediate risks requiring improvements in treatment decision-making by new parameters such as multiparametric MRI and biomarkers [19].

Our study is not without certain limitations. Firstly, though the study period frame was long, it featured (ranging from 1990 to 2013) and with only 523 patients, sub group analysis based on years of surgery was not statistically achievable. Secondly, the changes over time in pathology assessment (Gleason score grading), patient selection and operative techniques such as nerve-sparing procedures impacting the margin status, presented unavoidable biases. No centralized pathology was available between the two centres. Finally, because of the lack of key data, the final analysis only included 523 of the 814 patients identified.

In multivariate analysis, Gleason score and number of RF was not an independent factor as showed in other studies [12, 18]. We can explain this result by a number of "poor" high-risk patients in your study to small to show statistically differences.

Finally, it is surgery (RP) itself that provides the most accurate knowledge of the pathologic tumour and to adapt adjuvant therapies based on the risk of recurrence (pT stage and lymph node invasion).

Thus, the use of such a sub-stratification prognostic approach should improve the accuracy of predicting pathologic and oncologic results, thus optimizing the selection of patients for whom primary cancer control is possible. However, even when optimal predictions are made, those high-risk patients showing adverse pathologic outcomes should still be considered as candidates for a multimodal, combined approach. In these cases, cancer control after surgery should be optimized by either adjuvant RT, HT, or a combination of both treatments.

Conclusion

Finally, oncologic results after RP are heterogenous within the hrPCa risk group. Sub-stratification based on three well-defined criteria leads a better identification of the most aggressive cancers. In contrast, the presence of a single RF seems to be the most appropriate circumstance for RP. Such results may help urologists in scheduling post-operative monitoring and management.

Additional files

Additional file 1: Table S1. Different groups of risk factors (RF).

Additional file 2: Figures S1. Kaplan-Meier curves depending Biochemical free recurrence rates (independant factors (1)). Figure S2 Kaplan-Meier curves depending Biochemical free recurrence rates ((independant factors (2)).

Abbreviations
ADT, androgen deprivation therapy; BCR, biochemical recurrence; GS, Gleason score; hrPCa, high risk prostate cancer; HT, hormo; LNI, Lymph node involvement; PCa, Prostate cancer; PSA, prostate specific antigen; RF, risk factor; RP, radical prostatectomy; RT, radiation therapy; SC, specimen confined

Acknowledgements
None.

Funding
None.

Authors' contributions
JBB: Protocol/project development, Data collection or management, Data analysis, Manuscript writing/editing. MR: Data collection or management, Manuscript writing/editing. TF: Data analysis. TB: Data collection or management. ADLT: Protocol/project development. BM: Protocol/project development. LS: Data collection or management. MS: Protocol/project development. GP: Manuscript writing/editing, Protocol/project development. I confirm that all authors have read and approve of the final version of the manuscript.

Competing of interests
The authors declare that they have no competing interests.

Author details
[1]Department of Urology, Andrology and Renal Transplantation, CHU Rangueil, 1, av J Pouilhès, 31059 Toulouse, France. [2]Institut Claudius Regaud, IUCT-O, Toulouse F-31059, France. [3]Department of Urology, Andrology and Renal Transplantation, CHU Mondor, Créteil, France. [4]Department of Urology, Clinique St Jean du Languedoc, Toulouse, France.

References
1. Heidenreich A, Bellmunt J, Bolla M, et al. EAU guidelines on prostate cancer. Part 1: screening, diagnosis, and treatment of clinically localised disease. Eur Urol. 2011;59:61–71.
2. Bosetti C, Bertuccio P, Chatenoud L, Negri E, La Vecchia C, Levi F. Trends in mortality from urologic cancers in Europe, 1970–2008. Eur Urol. 2011;60:1–15.
3. D'Amico AV, Whittington R, Malkowicz SB, et al. Biochemical outcome after radical prostatectomy, external beam radiation therapy, or interstitial radiation therapy for clinically localized prostate cancer. JAMA. 1998;280: 969–74.
4. Garzotto M, Hung AY. Contemporary management of high-risk localized prostate cancer. Curr Urol Rep. 2010;11:159–64.
5. Gerber GS, Thisted RA, Chodak GW, et al. Results of radical prostatectomy in men with locally advanced prostate cancer: multi-institutional pooled analysis. Eur Urol. 1997;32:385–90.

6. Sooriakumaran P, Nyberg T, Akre O, et al. Comparative effectiveness of radical prostatectomy and radiotherapy in prostate cancer: observational study of mortality outcomes. BMJ. 2014;348:g1502.

7. Westover K, Chen MH, Moul J, et al. Radical prostatectomy vs radiation therapy and androgen-suppression therapy in high-risk prostate cancer. BJU Int. 2012;110:1116–21.

8. Abdollah F, Schmitges J, Sun M, et al. Comparison of mortality outcomes after radical prostatectomy versus radiotherapy in patients with localized prostate cancer: a population-based analysis. Int J Urol. 2012;19:836–44. author reply 844–835.

9. Wilt TJ, Brawer MK, Jones KM, et al. Radical prostatectomy versus observation for localized prostate cancer. N Engl J Med. 2012;367:203–13.

10. Bill-Axelson A, Holmberg L, Ruutu M, et al. Radical prostatectomy versus watchful waiting in early prostate cancer. N Engl J Med. 2011;364:1708–17.

11. Ploussard G, Masson-Lecomte A, Beauval JB, et al. Radical prostatectomy for high-risk prostate cancer defined by preoperative criteria: oncologic follow-up in national multicenter study in 813 patients and assessment of easy-to-use prognostic substratification. Urology. 2011;78:607–13.

12. Spahn M, Joniau S, Gontero P, et al. Outcome predictors of radical prostatectomy in patients with prostate-specific antigen greater than 20 ng/ml: a European multi-institutional study of 712 patients. Eur Urol. 2010;58:1–7. discussion 10–11.

13. Loeb S, Schaeffer EM, Trock BJ, Epstein JI, Humphreys EB, Walsh PC. What are the outcomes of radical prostatectomy for high-risk prostate cancer? Urology. 2010;76:710–4.

14. Walsh PC. Preservation of sexual function in the surgical treatment of prostatic cancer–an anatomic surgical approach. Important Adv Oncol. 1988;161–170.

15. Meng MV, Elkin EP, Latini DM, Duchane J, Carroll PR. Treatment of patients with high risk localized prostate cancer: results from cancer of the prostate strategic urological research endeavor (CaPSURE). J Urol. 2005;173:1557–61.

16. Joniau S, Briganti A, Gontero P, et al. Stratification of high-risk prostate cancer into prognostic categories: a European multi-institutional study. Eur Urol. 2015;67:157–64.

17. Fossati N, Passoni NM, Moschini M, et al. Impact of stage migration and practice changes on high-risk prostate cancer: results from patients treated with radical prostatectomy over the last two decades. BJU Int. 2015

18. Briganti A, Joniau S, Gontero P, et al. Identifying the best candidate for radical prostatectomy among patients with high-risk prostate cancer. Eur Urol. 2012;61:584–92.

19. Roumiguie M, Beauval JB, Filleron T, et al. External validation of the Briganti nomogram to estimate the probability of specimen-confined disease in patients with high-risk prostate cancer. BJU Int. 2014

8

Preserved micturition after intradetrusor onabotulinumtoxinA injection for treatment of neurogenic bladder dysfunction in Parkinson's disease

Stephanie C. Knüpfer[1*], Susanne A. Schneider[2], Mareike M. Averhoff[1], Carsten M. Naumann[1], Günther Deuschl[2], Klaus-Peter Jünemann[1] and Moritz F. Hamann[1]

Abstract

Background: To assess the efficacy and safety of intradetrusor onabotulinumtoxinA (OnabotA) injection treatment in patients with neurogenic lower urinary tract dysfunction (NLUTD), especially for patients with Parkinson disease (PD).

Methods: PD patients refractory to oral antimuscarinic participated in an off-label use study and were evaluated prior and after 200 IU OnabotA injection into detrusor muscle, including trigone. Changes due to treatment were evaluated using bladder diaries, urodynamics, and questionnaires. Statistical analysis comprised Wilcoxon rank-sum test. Values are presented as mean ± standard deviation.

Results: Ten PD patients (4 female and 6 male, mean age: 67.9 ± 5.36 years) with LUTD were enrolled. All patients tolerated the treatment. Bladder diary variables decreased significantly ($p \leq 0.011$) after OnabotA injection compared to variables prior injection. Desire to void and maximum bladder capacity increased significantly in urodynamics ($p \leq 0.05$). Maximum detrusor pressure during voiding phase normalised from 56.2 to 18.75 cm/H_2O. Detrusor overactivity was less often detectable. All patients voided spontaneously. Mean post void residual (PVR) volume was 77.0 ± 119.78 mL postoperatively. No urinary retention or side effects have been observed during/after treatment. Mean follow-up time was 4 months (range of 1–12). 4 patients requested repeated injection after a mean period of 10 months between first and second injection.

Conclusions: Our data confirm the efficacy and safety of 200 IU OnabotA injection in patients with neurogenic LUTD due to PD. The risk of urinary retention or high post-urinary residual volumes seems to be minor after OnabotA-injection. More research is needed with larger sample size to confirm the significance of these findings.

Keywords: Parkinson's disease, OnabotulinumtoxinA (OnabotA) injection, Neurogenic lower urinary tract dysfunction, International Consultation and Incontinence Questionnaire-Lower Urinary Tract Symptoms Quality of Life (ICIQ-UI)

Abbreviation: BPH, Benign prostate hyperplasia; FDV, First desire to void; FSFI, Female sexual function index; ICIQ, International consultation on incontinence questionnaire; ICIQ-LUT Sqol, International consultation and incontinence questionnaire-lower urinary tract symptoms quality of life; ICS, International continence society; IIEF, International index of erectile function; ISC, Intermittent self-catheterization; IU, International units; LUTD, Lower urinary tract dysfunction;

(Continued on next page)

* Correspondence: sknuepfer@paralab.balgrist.ch
[1]Department of Urology and Pediatric Urology, University Medical Centre Schleswig-Holstein, Arnold-Heller-Strasse 3, Campus Kiel 24105, Germany
Full list of author information is available at the end of the article

Background

Lower urinary tract dysfunction (LUTD) such as urinary urgency, frequency, and incontinence commonly occurs in neurological diseases, having a significant impact on quality of life, affecting emotional, social, sexual, occupational, and physical aspects of daily life [1]. Therapy of such neurogenic LUTD (NLUTD) is challenging, because all available treatment modalities (i.e. conservative, minimally invasive and surgical treatments) may fail or cause significant side effects.

Parkinson's disease (PD) is the second most common neurodegenerative disease following Alzheimer's disease, both associated with considerable socio-economic burden [2]. Epidemiological studies revealed that LUTD may be the most common non-motor manifestation affecting about 27–64 % of PD patients. Due to neurogenic detrusor overactivity, which challenges more the urinary storage phase than the voiding phase, those patients mainly suffer from urinary urgency, increased urinary frequency (both during the day-time and particularly at night-time) and incontinence.

Several factors may account for the prevalence and severity of LUTD among PD patients, including disease duration, gender, and urinary tract comorbidities such as benign prostate hyperplasia (BPH) and alterations in the LUT related to aging. However, to date a clear correlation between LUT symptoms (LUTS), disease duration, neurological impairment, and age in patients with PD has not been established. Thus, to determine presence and severity of LUTD in PD standard neuro-urological evaluation including urodynamic investigations and established questionnaires, such as the International Consultation on Incontinence Questionnaire (ICIQ) are essential to obtain a precise diagnosis of LUTD and to improve the choice and adjustment of treatments.

In general, the dopaminergic system plays an important role in physiological micturition [3, 4]. However, little is known about the mechanism inducing neurogenic bladder overactivity in this disease. Dopaminergic neurons project to the pontine micturition center [5]. There is increasing evidence that dopaminergic pathway influences micturition depending on the type of dopamine receptors that are activated [4]. It has been demonstrated in animals, that activation of D1-like dopamine receptors causes inhibition, whereas D2-like receptors are involved in facilitation of the micturition reflex [6].

In PD, the degeneration of dopaminergic neurons in the substantia nigra and the subsequent loss of striatal dopamine cause neurogenic detrusor overactivity, which might be attributed to the deactivation of the D1-mediated tonic inhibition [3, 7].

Besides dopaminergic agents, which have an effect on motor symptoms but only a slight effect on LUTD [8], antimuscarinics are generally used as a first-line treatment [9]. However, the treatment benefit is limited by central side effects (i.e. dry mouth, constipation, cognitive impairment), which occur in approximately 60 % of treated PD patients [3]. Moreover, simultaneous supplementation of antimuscarinics and PD medication is limited by the negative interaction [10]. Furthermore, antimuscarinics have yet not been evaluated in randomized multi-center trials, and should thus be prescribed with caution in PD patients.

Apart from deep brain stimulation, which seems to improve bladder capacity, to decrease detrusor overactivity, and to increase the volume at first desire to void [11] no second or third line therapy for LUTD in PD patients is approved to date. In most cases pads, intermittent self or indwelling catheters or even invasive surgical treatments (i.e. bladder augmentation or urinary diversions) remain when urinary frequency and subsequent urinary incontinence persists and/or patients become severely immobile. These options are related to significant long-term complications. Thus, enhanced treatment is urgently needed.

Intradetrusor OnabotA-injections have emerged as an effective, minimally invasive, well-tolerated and widely accepted treatment for refractory neurogenic detrusor overactivity incontinence [12]. Although the mechanism of action of OnabotA has not been clarified completely, it is assumed that OnabotA inhibits vesicular acetylcholine release into the neuromuscular junction and thus induces reversible denervation of extrafusal motor fibers, which weakens muscle contraction [13].

Recently, 100 IU intradetrusor OnabotA-injections were noted to effectively alleviate detrusor overactivity in patients with PD without causing urinary retention or increasing the post void residual (PVR) [14]. Drug treatment usually starts with low dosage and might be increased in the case of dissatisfied treatment success. According to the literature, there are four small studies exploring the effect of intradetrusor OnabotA injection for LUTD in patients suffering from PD (Table 1). To

Table 1 Review of literature with comparison of previous and present studies of OnabotA-injections in PD

Reference	Sample size	Age [yrs]	Gender	Disease duration [yrs]	Dosage/sites	Injection localisation	Outcome measure	Result	Follow-up
Giannantoni et al. [15]	4	72–83	F (4)	4–12	200 IU/20	Intradetrusor incl. Trigone	UDI bladder diary Pressure flow QoL	Urinary frequency (day-/nighttime) decreased No urgency/urge incontinence ICIQ/UDI improved PVR increased no side effects	1/3 months 5 months Telephone interview
Giannantoni et al. [22]	8	66 ± 3	F (7) M (1)	N/A	100 IU/10	Intradetrusor	UDI bladder diary	Urinary frequency (day-/nighttime) decreased ICIQ/UDI improved PVR increased PVR 250 mL –>ISC in 2 female patients	1/3/6 months
Anderson et al. [14]	20	71.5	F (8) M (12)	10.6	100 IU/10–20	Intradetrusor incl. Trigone	UDI bladder diary Pressure flow QoL (KHQ)	Urinary frequency (day-/nighttime) decreased PVR increased AUA Symptom score decreased	6 months
Kulaksizoglu et al. [21]	16	67.2 ± 5.1	F (10) M (6)	6	500 IU/30 Dysport®	Intradetrusor	bladder diary QoL (SEAPI)	Urinary frequency (day-/nighttime) decreased No incontinence in 27 % patients ICIQ VAS scale caregiver PVR increased no side effects	1 week 3/6/9/12 months
Present study	10	67.9 ± 5.3	F (4) M (6)	9.2 ± 8.2	200 IU/20	Intradetrusor incl. Trigone	UDI bladder diary QoL (ICIQ)	Urinary frequency (day-/nighttime) decreased UDI improved QoL (ICIQ) improved PVR increased no side effects	4 months

yrs years, *F* female, *M* male, *IU* international units, *ICIQ* international consultation on incontinence questionnaire, *UDI* urodynamic investigation, *PVR* post void residual, *ISC* internittend self-catheterization, *AUA* American urological association, *VAS* visual analog scale, *QoL* quality of life, *incl.* inclusive

our knowledge intradetrusor 200 IU OnabotA injection has only been systematically assessed in a series of 4 female patients [15]. Thus, there is still a lack of data, which elucidate the impact of intradetrusor 200 IU OnabotA-injections in male patients as well as in a larger sample size with PD.

The aim of the study was to investigate effectiveness and safety of intradetrusor 200 IU OnabotA injections in patients with LUTD due to PD. We hypothesized that 200 IU OnabotA injection would effectively alleviate the LUTD in the patient group and voluntary voiding would still be possible.

Methods

Ten patients (4 female and 6 male, mean age: 67.9 ± 5.36 years) diagnosed with PD and LUTD refractory to at least two different types oral antimuscarinics were enrolled and participated in this off-label use study limited to 10 patients. All patients gave informed written consent. Study inclusion criteria were refractory LUTD with concomittant PD, as documented by a bladder diary, with urgency frequency syndrome and/or urgency incontinence refractory to antimuscarinics (i.e. Fesoterodinfumarat 4 mg/8 mg, Solifenacin succinat or Trospium) for at least 4 weeks. Patients were studied while on their usual drug regimens for PD, which included levodopa and dopaminergic agonists. One PD patient had deep brain stimulation of the subthalamic nucleus. No patient suffered from diabetes mellitus. Voluntary voiding was preserved in all patients. Patients were informed about the possibility of some form of catheterization if necessary, preferably intermittent self-catheterization (ISC) after OnabotA treatment. None of the patients was on anticoagulant therapy. Study exclusion criteria were unstable neurological disease, LUT malignancy, previous OnabotA treatment, untreated LUT obstruction, and missing informed consent.

Prior (visit 1) and in general 4 months postoperatively (visit 2), all patients underwent neuro-urological evaluation consisting of medical history, clinical examination, urine analysis, urinary tract ultrasound, urodynamic investigation, and urethrocystoscopy [16]. Urodynamics were performed according to good urodynamic practices as recommended by the International Continence Society (ICS) [17]. Patients were investigated in a sitting position. The bladder was filled with a room temperature mixture of 0.9 % NaCL solution and contrast medium. The clinical examination included digital rectal examination, vaginal inspection, and transrectal sonography. Urodynamics indicated in three patients a mild obstruction due to BPH (mean prostate volume: 49.5 ± 17.77 mL, PVR <50 % of the total bladder capacity), which disappeared after photo-selective laser vaporization of the prostate (PVP) prior to OnabotA-injection.

Quality of life (QOL) of patients was assessed using validated and highly recommended [18] International Consultation and Incontinence Questionnaire-Lower Urinary Tract Symptoms Quality of Life (ICIQ-LUT Sqol). This questionnaire contains 19 items on various aspects of QOL, which might be affected by leakage and another 3 items related to personal relationship. Total scores range from 19 to 76 points, with higher values indicating greater impact. The procedure was performed under general (or spinal, $n = 3$) anaesthesia.

Injection technique

Intradetrusor OnabotA-injections were performed under cystoscopic guidance. A total of 200 IU OnabotA (Botox, Allergan Inc., Irvine, CA) diluted in 10 IU per/mL were injected using a flexible injection needle (BONEE Ch/Fr 05, 1.7 mm, Coloplast) into the detrusor muscle distributed among 16–17 submucosal/intradetrusor sites and 3–4 sites into the trigone due to the results of Abdel-Meguid et al. [19]. The injection was given gently and penetration of the detrusor muscle and thus injection into perivesical tissues was prevented. Currently, no other injection technique could demonstrate any significant advantage [20]. Thus, the standard intradetrusorial injection technique was used based on several published data [12, 29].

Postoperatively, in all patients bladder drainage (indwelling 16Ch Foley catheter) was maintained for at least 24 h to prevent complications (bladder bleeding, urethral and bladder neck edema). After the removal of the catheter and prior to patients discharge, spontaneous micturition and bladder emptying was verified based on PVR. Follow-up neuro-urological evaluation was done in general 4 month after OnabotA-injection.

Statistical analysis

Statistical analyses were performed using IBM SPSS Statistics 19 for Windows (IBM™ Illinois, USA). Analyses were performed using Wilcoxon signed rank test for paired samples, due to the not normal distribution of the data tested by Kolmogorov-Smirnov test. For all statistical analysis a significance level of $p < 0.05$ was used. All values are presented as mean ± standard deviation (SD).

Results

Ten patients (4 female and 6 male, mean age: 67.9 ± 5.36 years) diagnosed with PD (mean duration: 9.2 ± 8.2 years) and LUTD refractory to oral antimuscarinics participated in the study. The procedure was well tolerated. Epidemiological and clinical patients' characteristics are summarized in Table 2. Preoperatively all ten patients complained about increased daytime (mean: 12.0 ± 3.39 times per day) and night-time (mean: 4.3 ± 2.32 times per night) urinary frequency, and a high pad

Table 2 Patients characteristics

Diagnosis	n	Sex	Age [yrs]	Disease duration [yrs]	ICIQ		Day time frequency		Night time frequency		Pad consumption	
					Visit 1	Visit 2	Visit 1	Visit 2	Visit 1	Visit 2	Visit 1	Visit 2
PD	10	4 F, 6 M	67.9 ± 5.36	9.2 ± 8.2	16.63 ± 3.40	8.75 ± 3.99*	12.72 ± 3.39	5.50 ± 3.4**	4.30 ± 2.32	1.6 ± 0.97**	2.8 ± 2.35	1 ± 0.94*

Total mean (±SD) values of age (years), disease duration (years), bladder diary parameters, and ICIQ score from 10 patients suffering from Parkinson disease (PD) at baseline visit (Visit 1) and postoperative visit (Visit 2)

PD Parkinson disease, F female, M male, yrs years, ICIQ international consultation on incontinence questionnaire, significance level: $*p \leq 0.05$, $**p = 0.005$

consumption (mean: 2.8 ± 2.35 per day) due to urinary incontinence episode (Table 2). The mean ICIQ score was 16.63 ± 3.4 points (Table 2). All patients voided spontaneously, only 1 of 10 patients had a PVR greater than 150 mL. None of the patients performed the ISC. Preoperative urodynamic investigations showed detrusor overactivity in 9 of 10 patients, characterized by a low threshold desire to void, high detrusor pressure and decreased maximum cystometric capacity (MCC) (Table 3). Postoperatively, bladder diary data showed significant decreased urinary frequency (day-and nighttime; $p = 0.005$, Fig. 1) and in pad use ($p = 0.01$, Fig. 1) compared to the situation before OnabotA-injection, which is reflected in the significantly improved ICIQ score ($p = 0.018$, Fig. 1). Overall, urodynamic investigations confirmed an improvement (Table 3). Mean MCC increased significantly from 196.2 ± 88.29 mL preoperatively to 332.6 ± 135.45 mL postoperatively ($p = 0.005$, Fig. 2). Detrusor overactivity was observed on urodynamic in 9 patients before and in 2 patients after OnabotA-injection. Postoperatively, mean bladder volume increased significantly from 100 ± 51.51 mL to 202.38 ± 105.82 mL and from 151.3 ± 61.41 mL to 271.5 ± 94.07 mL ($p \leq 0.05$) at first desire to void (FDV) and strong desire to void (SDV), respectively (Fig. 2). In 8 patients the maximum detrusor pressure in the contraction period of micturition decreased significantly from a mean of 57.9 ± 33.1 cmH$_2$O preoperatively to 18 ± 16.55 cmH$_2$O postoperatively ($p = 0.018$). No significant differences was found between the maximum flow rate (Qmax) before and after OnabotA injection ($p = 0.212$). Although, PVR

increased from 61.28 ± 75.91 mL to 77.0 ± 119.78 mL postoperatively, a significant difference was not observed (Fig. 2). In 2 patients PVR increased beyond the upper normal limit of 100 ml, however, they remained clinically asymptomatic. In all patients the micturition was preserved after OnabotA-injection. Patients were discharged from hospital 24 h after catheter removal and confirmation of spontaneous voiding. No form of catheterization was needed.

During the 4-month's follow up no adverse advent included urinary tract infection or haematuria occurred. 4 of 10 patients received a re-injection due to declining effect after a mean period of 9.75 ± 4.85 months. Postoperatively, the antiparkinson medication remained unchanged in all patients.

Discussion

In line with previous studies [14, 15, 21, 22], we found in PD patients a significant improvement in urodynamic-, bladder diary parameters and consequently in the ICIQ score after 200 IU OnabotA injection with preserved micturition. The mean age of our patients was representative of the PD population.

The application of OnabotA injection in patients with NLUTD was pioneered by Schurch and colleagues [22]. After OnabotA injection (200 of 300 IU, Botox®, Allergan) in patients with spinal cord injury urodynamic-as well as bladder diary parameters improved significantly [23]. Since then, several studies, including randomized, placebo-controlled trials have approved the evidence of

Table 3 Urodynamic findings in the current study

Urodynamics	Mean ± SD Visit 1	Mean ± SD Visit 2	p Value
First Urge to Void (mL)	100 ± 51.51	202.38 ± 105.82	0.050
Strong Urge to Void (mL)	151.3 ± 61.41	271.5 ± 94.07	0.017
Maximal cystometric capacity (mL)	196.2 ± 88.29	332.6 ± 135.45	0.005
Maximum detrusor pressure during voiding phase [cm/H2O]	57.9 ± 33.1	18 ± 16.55	0.018
Bladder compliance [mL/cmH20]	18.65 ± 6.19	29.75 ± 28.79	0.123
Maximum flow rate [mL/s]	10.4 ± 3.14	13.03 ± 4.8	0.212
Voided volume [mL]	131.7 ± 96.56	246.8 ± 113.39	0.005
Post void residual [mL]	61.28 ± 75.91	77.0 ± 119.78	0.575

Total mean (±SD) values of urodynamic parameters from 10 patients suffering from Parkinson disease (PD) at baseline visit (Visit 1) and postoperative visit (Visit 2). Significance level of t-test is 0.05

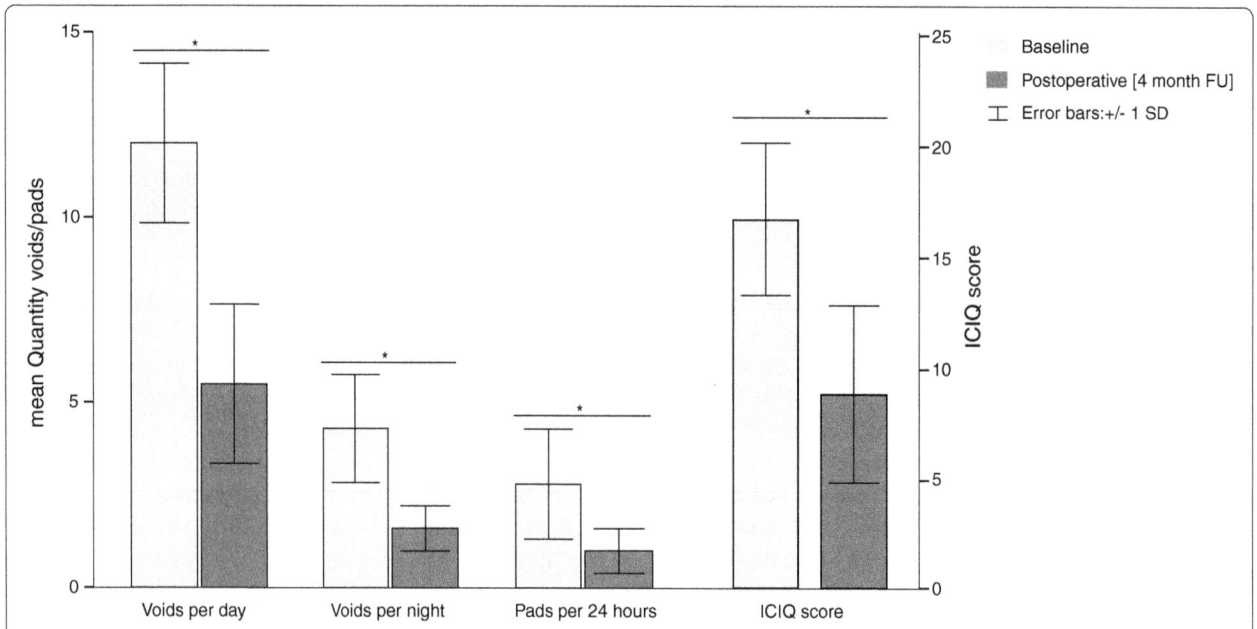

Fig. 1 Three day bladder diary results regarding day-time and night-time frequency and pad consumption and International Consultation and Incontinence Questionnaire-Lower Urinary Tract Symptoms Quality of Life (ICIQ-LUT Sqol) in all patients with PD at baseline visit (*light grey bars*) and postoperative visit (4 month follow up (FU), *dark grey bars*). Data presented as mean ± standard deviation (SD). Asterisk indicates $p \leq 0.05$. Significance level is 0.05

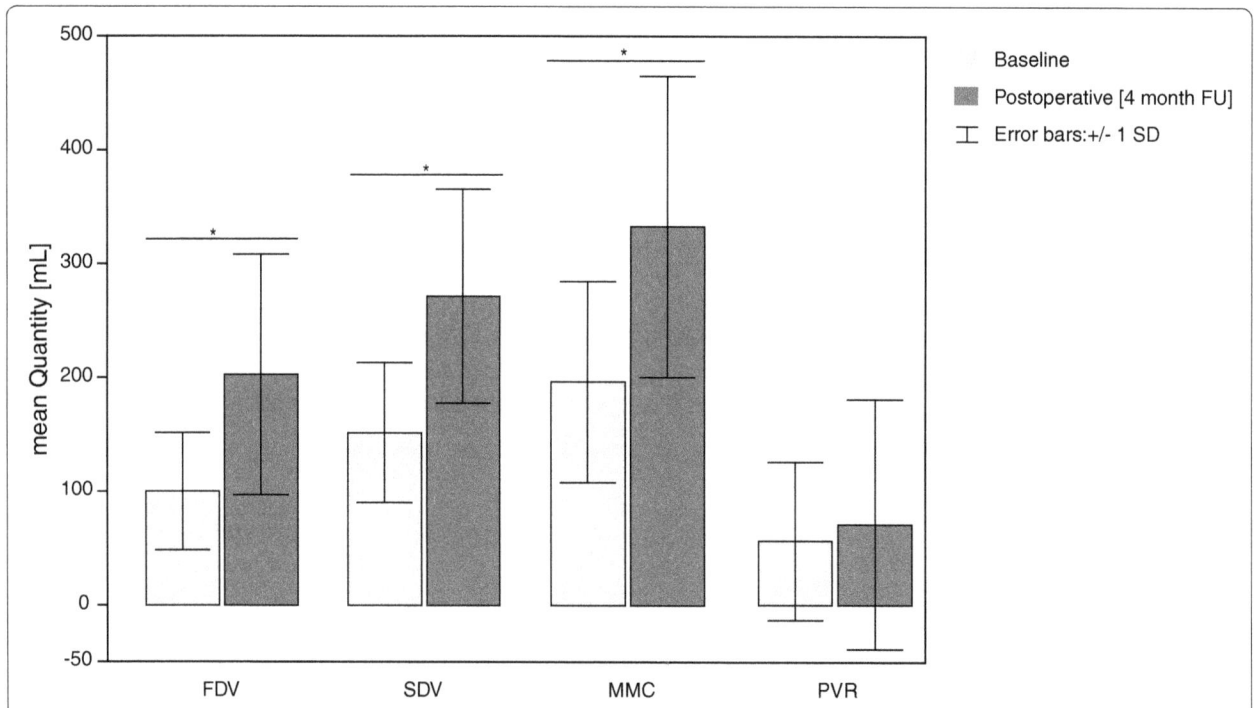

Fig. 2 Volume at first desire to void (FDV), strong desire to void (SDV), maximal cystometric capacity (MMC), and post void residual (PVR) at baseline visit (*light grey bars*) and postoperative visit (4 month follow up (FU), *dark grey bars*). Data presented as mean ± standard deviation (SD). Asterisk indicates $p \leq 0.05$. Significance level is 0.05

OnabotA injection in the treatment of neurogenic detrusor overactivity (NDO) using different study protocols [12, 24, 25].

Despite the fact that efficacy and safety of OnabotA injection has been studied in patients suffering from multiple sclerosis (MS) and spinal cord injury (SCI), there are only few data providing information on the impact of OnabotA injection on urodynamic-, bladder diary parameters, and ICIQ scores, including the specific dosage of 200 IU in PD patients. Currently, only 4 studies are available describing the effect of OnabotA injection in a PD population (Table 1).

Due to different study protocols used, the comparison of results from recent studies [14, 15, 21, 22] with our data is difficult. However, most parameters at the follow-up visits provided global improvement in urodynamic- and/or bladder diary parameters. With respect to decreased urinary frequency (day-and night time) results from the study by Anderson et al. [14] appear to be less pronounced than in the present study. Our data provide significant changes in the urinary frequency related to OnabotA-injection, which could be due to the elevated dosage of 200 IU. However, previous literature [22] also observed a significant improvement on urodynamic-and bladder diary parameters using 100 IU OnabotA-injection. Unfortunately, the latter findings mainly focused on female patients, and thus hamper a comparison with the present results.

Currently only two studies in PD patients [15, 21] are available describing the effects of an increased dosage exceeding 200 IU of intradetrusor OnabotA-injections. The first study, published by Giannantoni and colleagues [15] used OnabotA in a mixed population consisting of PD and multiple system atrophy. It demonstrated significant improvement in urodynamic-, bladder diary parameters as well as in the QoL. Our data confirm these effects in a considerably larger PD population. The second of these studies [21] used a different agent, Dysport ®, which may hamper an comparison due to particular pharmacodynamics.

Evidence concerning relevant PVR in patients treated with 200 IU OnabotA injection intravesically is controversial and sparse. Recently, published data showed an increased PVR and even urinary retention in patients with NLUTD, excluding PD [12, 26]. In contrast to these observations, White et al. [27] detected no PVR, when using 200 IU OnabotA-injections. Again, these controversial results might be attributed to the heterogeneity of patients' cohorts with clinical symptoms of idiopathic or neurogenic detrusor overactivity. In our PD group PVR increased after the injection of 200 IU OnabotA. The increase was not significant and no form of catheterization was needed. Physiologically, this might be attributed to the fact, that only few PD patients

demonstrate detrusor-sphincter dyssynergia [28] and thus voiding function remains unimpaired. On the other hand a dose dependent impact of OnabotA on detrusor contractility has to be taken into account. Although low dosage of OnabotA injection does not necessarily prevent the need for de novo ISC or even indwelling catheterization [22] the reduction of detrusor contractility in patients with NLUTD remains a relevant factor [12, 26]. Thus, independently of the dosage used, PD patients should be encouraged to learn ISC prior to OnabotA injection.

According to treatment technique, the injection into the bladder trigone is still under debate. The first reported injection techniques spared the trigone due to the potential complication of vesicourethral reflux (VUR) [29]. However, a recent prospective study evaluated the impact of trigonal OnabotA injection (300 IU) and observed no de novo VUR [19]. In addition, Lucioni et al. [30] observed no significant differences between the effects of sole trigonal and combined trigonal and intradetrusor OnabotA injection (300 IU). With regard to PD patients, the studies by Giannantoni [22], Anderson et al. [14] and the present study observed no treatment complication after trigonal OnabotA injection which might indicate a good eligibility of the technique in the selected patient group.

Impaired cognitive function is common in PD, affecting up to 30 % of patients, which might be aggravated by anaesthesia [31]. But to date, it is unclear how far general anaesthesia impairs cognitive performance of PD patients. In line with the literature [15, 22], we mainly performed OnabotA-injections under general anaesthesia. Giannantoni et al. [22] excluded patients with cognitive impairment. However, in none of our patients an extended distinctive cognitive impairment was noted within a period of up to 4 months postoperatively. In all treated patients orientation, memory, and attention was present. Noteworthy, Anderson [14] and Kulaksizoglu [21] performed OnabotA treatment under local anaesthesia with respect to comorbidities and possible interactions with other parkinsonian medications this approach seems to be favourable in PD patients.

To avoid obstructive problems studies by Giannantoni et al. [15, 22] focused on female cases: overall 12 cases included only one male. The present study investigates both sexes. In fact, three of our patients received a PVP 3 months prior to OnabotA injection due to a mild obstructive micturition which didn't change PVR and urinary urgency significantly (mean change in PVR 28.4 (±52.7), ml $p = 0.82$). This approach is in line with results of Kessler et al. that showed that TURP resolves urge symptoms in up to 70 % [32]. But, according to the non-significant change in PVR between mean values of preoperative and postoperative data, it is unlikely that only PVP is the cause of the global improvement in urodynamic-and/or bladder diary parameters. Especially the persistent urinary urgency after PVP in those patients are caused by urogenic pathogenesis rather than subvesical obstruction.

In the follow-up, patients demonstrated significant improvement for QoL. To evaluate the QoL we chose the short from of ICIQ-LUT Sqol questionnaire, recommended by the International Continence Society (ICS), to make the evaluation of QoL more practical, particularly with regard to existing tremor in the upper limb.

Although we demonstrated a preserved micturition after intradetrusor OnabotA injection (200 IU) for treatment of NLUTD in Parkinson's disease this study is limited by the small sample size, which is probably the cause of the high SD in some outcome parameters. Furthermore, it cannot be ruled out that comorbidities and their specific therapies do not affect in a limited extent the results of the bladder function. Nevertheless, our results, based on the largest published series are promising. All patients experienced significant benefit from OnabotA injection, which justify further prospective placebo-controlled investigations in this special patient group.

Conclusions

Patients with PD have a high prevalence of LUTD and most commonly suffer from storage but not voiding symptoms due to NDO. Although the exact mechanism of how OnabotA injection modulates NDO is not clear, OnabotA injection (200 IU) is an effective and safe treatment method in patients with PD due to the significantly improved of urodynamic-, bladder diary parameters, and QoL due to ICIQ. In contrast to the common apprehension based on observation in other neurogenic bladder dysfunctions, the risk of urinary retention or increased post void residual bladder volume seems to be a minimal in PD patients.

However, the number of investigated patients is low with high inter study heterogeneity and there is a lack of randomized controlled trials. Thus, well-designed, adequately powered studies are needed before more widespread use of OnabotA injection (200 IU) for neurogenic LUTD can be recommended.

Ethical and dissemination

This trial was performed in accordance with the World Medical Association Declaration of Helsinki [33], the guidelines for Good Clinical Practice [34]. This study was approved by the local ethics committee (Ethikkommision Kiel) and all patients gave written informed consent according to the Helsinki II declaration. Handling of all personal data will strictly comply with the Good Clinical Practice [34].

Acknowledgements
The authors would like to acknowledge Andrea Guerra of the Department of Urology and Pediatric Urology, University Medical Centre Schleswig-Holstein, Campus Kiel for her assistance with the urodynamic investigation. No external funding was obtained for this work.

Funding
No funding.

Authors' contributors
SCK, CMN, KPJ, and MFH created the study design. SCK and MFH drafted the manuscript. SAS, MA, CMN, GD, and KPJ critically reviewed the manuscript. All the authors read and approved the final manuscript.

Competing interests
All authors declare that they have no competing interests.

Ethics approval and consent to participate
This study has been approved by the local ethics committees (Ethikkommission Kiel AZ: D416/13) and all patients gave written informed consent according to the Helsinki II declaration.

Author details
[1]Department of Urology and Pediatric Urology, University Medical Centre Schleswig-Holstein, Arnold-Heller-Strasse 3, Campus Kiel 24105, Germany. [2]Department of Neurology, University Medical Centre Schleswig-Holstein, Campus Kiel, Germany.

References
1. Coyne KS, Wein AJ, Tubaro A, Sexton CC, Thompson CL, Kopp ZS, Aiyer LP. The burden of lower urinary tract symptoms: evaluating the effect of LUTS on health-related quality of life, anxiety and depression: EpiLUTS. BJU Int. 2009;103(3):4–11.
2. Chin-Chan M, Navarro-Yepes J, Quintanilla-Vega B. Environmental pollutants as risk factors for neurodegenerative disorders: Alzheimer and Parkinson diseases. Front Cell Neurosci. 2015;9:124.
3. Winge K, Fowler CJ. Bladder dysfunction in Parkinsonism: mechanisms, prevalence, symptoms, and management. Mov Disord. 2006;21(6):737–45.
4. Ogawa T, Seki S, Masuda H, Igawa Y, Nishizawa O, Kuno S, Chancellor MB, De Groat WC, Yoshimura N. Dopaminergic mechanisms controlling urethral function in rats. Neurourol Urodyn. 2006;25(5):480–9.
5. Yoshimura N, Mizuta E, Kuno S, Sasa M, Yoshida O. The dopamine D1 receptor agonist SKF 38393 suppresses detrusor hyperreflexia in the monkey with parkinsonism induced by 1-methyl-4-phenyl-1,2,3,6-tetrahydropyridine (MPTP). Neuropharmacology. 1993;32(4):315–21.
6. Seki S, Igawa Y, Kaidoh K, Ishizuka O, Nishizawa O, Andersson KE. Role of dopamine D1 and D2 receptors in the micturition reflex in conscious rats. Neurourol Urodyn. 2001;20(1):105–13.
7. Fowler CJ. Update on the neurology of Parkinson's disease. Neurourol Urodyn. 2007;26(1):103–9.
8. Winge K, Werdelin LM, Nielsen KK, Stimpel H. Effects of dopaminergic treatment on bladder function in Parkinson's disease. Neurourol Urodyn. 2004;23(7):689–96.
9. Pannek JBB, Castro-Diaz D, Del Popolo G, Groen J, Karsenty G, Kessler TM, Kramer G, Ströhrer M. EAU guidelines on neuro-urology. 2014.
10. Kay GG, Ebinger U. Preserving cognitive function for patients with overactive bladder: evidence for a differential effect with darifenacin. Int J Clin Pract. 2008;62(11):1792–800.
11. Seif C, Herzog J, van der Horst C, Schrader B, Volkmann J, Deuschl G, Juenemann KP, Braun PM. Effect of subthalamic deep brain stimulation on the function of the urinary bladder. Ann Neurol. 2004;55(1):118–20.
12. Ginsberg D, Gousse A, Keppenne V, Sievert KD, Thompson C, Lam W, Brin MF, Jenkins B, Haag-Molkenteller C. Phase 3 efficacy and tolerability study of

onabotulinumtoxinA for urinary incontinence from neurogenic detrusor overactivity. J Urol. 2012;187(6):2131–9.

13. A AGaB. Neurophysiological effects of otulinumtoxin type A. Neurotox Res. 2006;9:109–14.

14. Anderson RU, Orenberg EK, Glowe P. OnabotulinumtoxinA office treatment for neurogenic bladder incontinence in Parkinson's disease. Urology. 2014;83(1):22–7.

15. Giannantoni A, Rossi A, Mearini E, Del Zingaro M, Porena M, Berardelli A. Botulinum toxin A for overactive bladder and detrusor muscle overactivity in patients with Parkinson's disease and multiple system atrophy. J Urol. 2009;182(4):1453–7.

16. Blok B PJ, Castro Diaz D, del Popolo G, Groen J, Gross T, Hamid R, Karsenty D, Kessler TM, Schneider MP, 't Hoen L. EAU Guidelines on Neuro-Urology, 2015. [http://uroweb.org/wp-content/uploads/21-Neuro-Urology_LR2.pdf].

17. Abrams P, Cardozo L, Fall M, Griffiths D, Rosier P, Ulmsten U, Van Kerrebroeck P, Victor A, Wein A. The standardisation of terminology of lower urinary tract function: report from the Standardisation Sub-committee of the International Continence Society. Neurourol Urodyn. 2002;21(2):167–78.

18. Abrams P, Andersson KE, Birder L, Brubaker L, Cardozo L, Chapple C, Cottenden A, Davila W, De Ridder D, Dmochowski R, Drake M, Dubeau C, Fry C, Hanno P, Smith JH, Herschorn S, Hosker G, Kelleher C, Koelbl H, Khoury S, Madoff R, Milsom I, Moore K, Newman D, Nitti V, Norton C, Nygaard I, Payne C, Smith A, Staskin D, et al. Fourth International Consultation on Incontinence Recommendations of the International Scientific Committee: Evaluation and treatment of urinary incontinence, pelvic organ prolapse, and fecal incontinence. Neurourol Urodyn. 2010;29(1):213–40.

19. Abdel-Meguid T. Botulinum toxin A injections into neurogenic overactive bladder-to include or exclude the trigone? A prospective, randomized, controlled trial. J Urol. 2010;184(6):2423–8.

20. Samal V, Mecl J, Sram J. Submucosal Administration of OnabotulinumtoxinA in the treatment of Neurogenic Detrusor Overactivity: Pilot Single-Centre Experience and Comparison with standard injection into the Detrusor. Urology International. 2013;91:423–8.

21. Kulaksizoglu H, Parman Y. Use of botulinim toxin-A for the treatment of overactive bladder symptoms in patients with Parkinsons's disease. Parkinsonism Relat Disord. 2010;16(8):531–4.

22. Giannantoni A, Conte A, Proietti S, Giovannozzi S, Rossi A, Fabbrini G, Porena M, Berardelli A. Botulinum toxin type A in patients with Parkinson's disease and refractory overactive bladder. J Urol. 2011; 186(3):960–4.

23. Schurch B, Stohrer M, Kramer G, Schmid DM, Gaul G, Hauri D. Botulinum-A toxin for treating detrusor hyperreflexia in spinal cord injured patients: a new alternative to anticholinergic drugs? Preliminary results J Urol. 2000;164(1):692–7.

24. Mehnert U, Birzele J, Reuter K, Schurch B. The effect of botulinum toxin type a on overactive bladder symptoms in patients with multiple sclerosis: a pilot study. J Urol. 2010;184(3):1011–6.

25. Apostolidis A, Dasgupta P, Denys P, Elneil S, Fowler CJ, Giannantoni A, Karsenty G, Schulte-Baukloh H, Schurch B, Wyndaele JJ. Recommendations on the use of botulinum toxin in the treatment of lower urinary tract disorders and pelvic floor dysfunctions: a European consensus report. Eur Urol. 2009;55(1):100–19.

26. Cruz F, Herschorn S, Aliotta P, Brin M, Thompson C, Lam W, Daniell G, Heesakkers J, Haag-Molkenteller C. Efficacy and safety of onabotulinumtoxinA in patients with urinary incontinence due to neurogenic detrusor overactivity: a randomised, double-blind, placebo-controlled trial. Eur Urol. 2011;60(4):742–50.

27. White WM, Pickens RB, Doggweiler R, Klein FA. Short-term efficacy of botulinum toxin a for refractory overactive bladder in the elderly population. J Urol. 2008;180(6):2522–6.

28. Araki I, Kitahara M, Oida T, Kuno S. Voiding dysfunction and Parkinson's disease: urodynamic abnormalities and urinary symptoms. J Urol. 2000;164(5):1640–3.

29. Schurch B, Schmid DM, Stohrer M. Treatment of neurogenic incontinence with botulinum toxin A. N Engl J Med. 2000;342(9):665.

30. Lucioni A, Rapp DE, Gong EM, Fedunok P, Bales GT. Intravesical botulinum type A toxin injection in patients with overactive bladder: Trigone versus trigone-sparing injection. Can J Urol. 2006;13(5):3291–5.

31. Wüllner U, Standop J, Kaut O, Coenen V, Kalenka A, Wappler F. Parkinson's disease. Perioperative management and anesthesia. Anaesthesist. 2012;61(2):97–105.

32. Roth B, Studer UE, Fowler CJ, Kessler TM. Benign prostatic obstruction and parkinson's disease-should transurethral resection of the prostate be avoided? J Urol. 2009;181(5):2209–13.

33. Association WM. World Medical Association Declaration of Helsinki: ethical principles for medical research involving human subjects. JAMA. 2013; 310(20):2191–4.

34. International conference on harmonisation: Good clinical practice guideline. 1996 [http://www.ich.org/products/guidelines/efficacy/article/efficacy-guidelines]

9

Transvaginal rectocele repair with human dermal allograft interposition and bilateral sacrospinous fixation with a minimum eight-year follow-up

Serge P. Marinkovic*, Scott Hughes, Donghua Xie, Lisa M. Gillen and Christina M. Marinkovic

Abstract

Background: Human dermal allografts have been used for over a decade for interpositional repair of rectoceles. How do dermal allografts perform with regards to success rate and complications with 8 years' minimum follow-up?

Methods: We retrospectively reviewed 41 consecutive patients undergoing dermal allograft interposition procedures between October 2001 and December 2005 (Repliform, Boston Scientific, Natick, MA, USA) for stage two, three, and four International Continence Society (ICS) symptomatic rectocele repairs with bilateral sacrospinous fixation. Failure was defined as recurrent stage two International Continence Society prolapse (Ap $\geq$ −1 and/or Bp $\geq$ −1). All questionnaires were completed 1 week before surgery and at follow-up (September 2014 through December 2014).

Results: The mean preoperative and postoperative A(p) were $0.95 \pm 0.70, -1.90 \pm 0.52$ and B(p) $1.30 \pm 0.84, -2.13 \pm 0.51$ ($p < 0.001$). With a mean follow-up of 116.5 ± 18.9 months, a success rate of 73 % (30/41) was achieved, with anatomical reduction of prolapse. For splinting and digitations, an 82 % cure rate was realized. The Pelvic Floor Distress Inventory (PFDI) pre- and post-operative results showed significant improvement ($p < 0.001$). There were two incisional exposures (5 %). Seventy percent of patients were secondary repairs while 30 % were primary repairs (81 % success rate, $p < 0.36$). One patient experienced nerve entrapment and subsequent unilateral takedown. Patient satisfaction was 77 %.

Conclusions: Our retrospective study approaching long-term results demonstrated that symptomatic rectocele procedures with human dermal allograft interposition provide an effective anatomical and functional repair with acceptable complication rates.

Keywords: Rectocele repair, Sacrospinous fixation, Human dermal allograft

Background

Pelvic organ prolapse is a common surgical women's health care issue affecting over ten million American women, at a projected cost of two billion dollars (USD) each year [1]. Approximately 12 % of adult women will eventually require surgical therapy for their symptomatic prolapse [2]. Prolapse is the result of a multitude of molecular and physiological changes that cause weakening in one or more supportive structures in the pelvic compartment. Rectal protrusions are attributed to connective tissue defects in the rectovaginal fascia that are level two Delancey pelvic support mechanisms. The most commonly used surgical procedures for repair in this area involve suture ligation with native tissue plication [3]. Another method of rectocele repair is defect-specific reapproximation of the rectovaginal fascia without levator plication [4, 5]. This procedure results in less postoperative pain but not much improvement in reduced rectocele recurrence.

Practitioners have tended to agree that, in the instance of transvaginal organ prolapse repairs, patients' innate connective tissue defects can be repaired with the interposition of biologic human allograft dermal material [6, 7]

* Correspondence: urourogyn@yahoo.com
Department of Urology, Detroit Medical Center, Harper/Hutzel Hospital, Detroit, MI 48202, USA

or synthetic materials such as polypropylene [8]. Today, these biologic materials [9] abound, yet long-term studies are lacking. Available studies have multitudes of clinical criteria for evaluation and measurements for failure, making comparisons inaccurate and difficult to assess. Clinical assessments are often retrospective and include a variety of surgical approaches, so clear-cut evaluations and critiques regarding usefulness remain unclear.

Synthetic materials categorized via the Amid [10] (1997) five-material classification system have been applied to what was originally used for general surgeons' herniorrhaphy procedures and are now also applied to female pelvic prolapse surgeries (Table 1). Materials are separated into macroporous, microporous, or both, and include three well-studied materials: polypropylene, mersilene and polytetrafluoroethylene. In 2011, the Federal Drug Administration issued a stern warning against the transvaginal utilization of synthetic materials, prompting a voluntary removal of several pelvic floor reconstruction products from the market (i.e., Prolift, Gynecare, Somerset, New Jersey). As a result, surgeons were left with fewer options for transvaginal prolapse repairs. For more than 12 years, we have extensively used dermal allograft materials (Repliform, Boston Scientific, Natick, Massachusetts, USA) for symptomatic rectocele repairs with bilateral sacrospinous fixation [11–14] and now report our minimum eight-year follow-up experience with this human allograft product.

Methods

Between October 2001 and December 2005, we performed 41 consecutive symptomatic repairs with human dermal allograft interposition and bilateral sacrospinous fixation for stage two, three, or four International Continence Society rectoceles, with or without digitation and/or splinting. All rectoceles were performed with suture ligation of the new human dermal allograft fascia to the rectovaginal fascia with bilateral sacrospinous fixation. Surgeries were performed in their entirety by the first author. The Caprio device [11] (Boston Scientific, Natick, MA, USA) was used, with 0-polypropylene sutures (two sutures applied to the right sacrospinous ligament and another two to the left ligament). Failure was defined as recurrent International Continence Society stage two or more prolapses. All patients underwent a complete history and physical examination with International Continence Society prolapse (POP) scoring. Urodynamics were performed only if the patient was also undergoing a concomitant continence procedure performed with a tension-free vaginal tape (TVT, Gynecare, Somerset, New Jersey), tension-free vaginal tape obturator (TVTO, Gynecare, Somerset, New Jersey) or tension-free vaginal tape-Secur (Gynecare, Somerset, New Jersey, USA). Urodynamic results are not included in this study. All preoperative and postoperative data were collected between September 2014 and December 2014. Our research was performed in accordance with the Declaration of Helsinki and was approved by the Harper Hospital Institutional Review Board (Study #033512MP4E). The Pelvic Floor Distress Inventory-20 (PFDI) [15] and the 7 point Likert Visual Analogue Scale questionnaire were used to objectively determine patient satisfaction and improvement of symptoms following surgery. On the Likert Scale (Table 2), only levels of five, six and seven were recorded as satisfactory outcomes. Levels 1–4 were recorded as unsuccessful outcomes. All patients included their age, parity, body mass index, smoking status, menopausal, hormone therapy, and prior pelvic surgery. All exposures were treated the same, with two grams of topical estrogen thrice weekly for 6 weeks. Follow-up examinations were performed by an unaffiliated, board-certified gynecologist with 30 years of experience, who was well acquainted with POPQ staging and scoring. Statistical analyses were performed using the Statistical Package for Social Sciences, version 11.0 (SPSS, Chicago, Illinois). Analyses included simple means, medians, and chi square comparisons.

Results and discussion

The mean preoperative and postoperative A(p) were $0.95 \pm 0.70, -1.90 \pm 0.52$ and B(p) $1.30 \pm 0.84, -2.13 \pm 0.51$

Table 1 Classification of Synthetic Meshes (Amid, 1997)[10]

Type 1: Totally Macroporous (pore size > 75 μ)

- Prolene
- Gynemesh PS
- Gynecare TVT
- SPARC

Type 2: Totally Microporous (port size < 10 μ)

- Goretex

Type 3: Macroporous with Filaments or Microporous Components

- IVS
- Uratape
- Surgipro
- Mersilene
- Parietex

Type 4: Submicronic Pore Size (pore size < 1 μ)

Table 2 Likert Global Response Visual Analogue Scale for Rectocele Repair

Since having your rectocele repair, please rate your overall rectocele symptoms:

1.	Markedly Worse	1
2.	Moderately Worse	1
3.	Slightly worse	1
4.	Same	1
5.	Slightly improved	1
6.	Moderately improved	2
7.	Markedly improved	3

Table 3 Patient Demographics ($n = 41$)

Mean Age (yrs)	60.6 ± 16.3
Mean Follow-up (months)	116.5 ± 18.9
Mean Parity	2.6 ± 2.37
Mean Body Mass Index	34.4 ± 6.1
Smoker (percent)	34.1
Menopausal (percent)	65.3
Post-Hysterectomy (percent)	41.4
Hormone Replacement (percent)	40.9
Sexually active (percent)	24.1
Previous Pelvic Surgery (percent)	70.0
Mean Preoperative A (p)(centimeters)[a]	0.95 ± 0.70
Mean Postoperative A (p) (centimeters)[a]	−1.90 ± 0.52
Mean Preoperative B (p)(centimeters)[a]	1.30 ± 0.84
Mean Postoperative B (p)(centimeters)[a]	−2.13 ± 0.51
Mean PreOp PFDI-20 (/300)[a]	129.6 ± 26.7 (78–223)
Mean PostOp PFDI-20 (/300)[a]	60.9 ± 18.4 (32–108)
Biological erosion (percent)	7.3
De novo dyspareunia (percent)	17.0
Complication rate (percent)	12.1
Patient satisfaction (percent)[b]	77.0
Prolapse Failure Rate (percent)[c]	27.0
Time to Prolapse Failure (months)	24.7 ± 15.3

[a]Changes between pre- and postoperative Pelvic Floor Distress Inventory (PFDI-20, $n = 41$) and A(p) and B(p) were statistically significant at $p = <0.001$ at the time of patients' last follow-up
[b]A 7 point Likert Global Response Scale was used, whereby responses five, six and seven were deemed successful. Numbers 1–4 were judged as failures. The 77 % satisfaction rate includes only the former and not the latter
[c]Eleven prolapse failures: 7 Stage 2 (ICS), 3 Stage 3, and 1 Stage 4

($p < 0.001$) (Table 3). With a mean follow-up of 116.5 ± 18.9 months, a success rate of 73 % (30/41 patients) was achieved, with the anatomical reduction of prolapse to ICS Stage 2 or less (Ap ≥ −1 and/or Bp ≥ −1). For splinting and digitation elimination, an 82 % cure rate was realized (15/18). In the follow-up period, 13 % (3/23) of patients complained of de novo splinting. First-time repairs demonstrated an 81 % anatomical success rate while secondary repairs detailed a 70 % anatomical repair. Seventy percent were secondary repair, with a 70 % success rate while 30 % of the patients were primary repairs (81 % success rate) ($p < 0.36$). The Pelvic Floor Distress Inventory (PFDI) pre- and postoperative results showed significant improvement ($p < 0.001$). There were three incisional exposures (7 %) of the human dermal allograft, which responded to estrogen replacement therapy for 6 to 8 weeks. One patient experienced rectal outflow obstruction and another pelvic nerve entrapment, which caused left gluteal pain. Both required re-operative take down at two and twenty weeks after rectocele repair. Patient satisfaction was 77 % (Table 3). De novo dyspareunia was 17 %.

A review of rectocele repairs shows that, for a host of reasons, procedures without augmentation have not been successful. Pelvic floor remodeling of the supportive connective tissue continues to occur, with increased activity of collagenase and elastase enzymes [16, 17]. Elastase degradation leads to decreased connective tissue flexibility and expansion [18]. Together, these biologically enzyme processes lead to a potentially weaker pelvic floor infrastructure [18].

Native tissue amended with suture ligation and/or fixation to autologous ligaments or bone may lead to compromised clinical results because of the continual exposure to connective tissue remodeling [19–22]. Surgical treatment has seen the development of many transvaginal synthetic pelvic floor prolapse repair kits [23]. These kits have not fared as well as transvaginal stress incontinence instruments and materials, which are made of similar synthetic materials but with a more limited exposure area. [24] While stress incontinence kits are not exempt from failure or complications including exposure or erosion into the vagina or pelvic organ, in the past 5 years, prolapse repair kits have found themselves at the forefront of malpractice litigation. In the early 2000's several studies with the biological xenograft (porcine) product Pelvichol [25] (C.R. Bard, Inc. Murray Hill, New Jersey, USA) demonstrated hastened reabsorption by the body and left pelvic floor surgeons much less enthusiastic towards its use. However, experience with human dermal allograft in 2000 gave us adequate two-year and four-year data for rectocele repairs [5, 6] while we still used abdominal sacrocolpopexy for all multi-compartment prolapse repairs. Approaching 10 years' follow-up (116.5 ± 18.9 months), a good success rate can be attributed to a lasting biological material and augmentation of the posterior pelvic floor compartment with a concomitant bilateral sacrospinous fixation with permanent suture. Limitations of our study included two major complications: the unilateral takedown of the rectocele repair/augmentation because of rectal outflow obstruction, and pelvic nerve entrapment, which required a unilateral takedown. These complications combined with three vaginal exposures gave us a complication rate of 12 %. Both patients were morbidly obese, less than five feet tall, with body mass index scores of 40 and 41.

The 11 patients who failed their surgery had a mean time to failure of 24.7 ± 15.3 months. At the time of their sacrocolpopexy, we carefully examined the pelvic compartment for the human dermal allograft. Quantities of tissue were still found circumscribing the periphery of the rectovaginal fascia, but the attachment to the polypropylene suture had, in most cases, pulled through from the sacrospinous ligament and/or the tissue was tattered in appearance. Of these 11, eight elected to have surgery to repair their rectoceles, but because the prolapse now involved more than one compartment, six of the eight elected to undergo sacrocolpopexy with anterior and posterior polypropylene mesh interposition.

Encouraging factors for the utilization of human dermal allograft include its good anatomical reduction of the rectocele, as well as symptom improvement with a follow-up in many cases exceeding 10 years. This efficacy can be considered a driving force for its continued utilization in the posterior compartment symptomatic rectocele repair; however, Level 1 and/or Level 2–1 evidence studies should be conducted to better compare the efficacy and safety of human dermal allograft to other pelvic floor materials.

Conclusions
Our retrospective study demonstrated that rectocele repairs with biological augmentation and bilateral sacrospinous fixation with a minimum 8 years' follow-up provide a good anatomical and functional repair with an acceptable complication rate.

Brief summary
Human dermal allograft interposition repair of rectoceles can be used safely and successfully, with good patient satisfaction in follow-up periods approaching 10 years.

Competing interests
The authors declare that they have no competing interests and have not received any financial remuneration from any source.

Authors' contributions
The following authors (SPM, SH, DX, LMG, CMM) all contributed equally to this paper in its writing, statistical analyses, and formatting for publication. All authors read and approved the final manuscript.

Acknowledgements
There are no acknowledgements for this paper.

References
1. Subak LL, Waetjen LE, van den Eeden S, Thom DH, Vittinghoff E, Brown JS. Cost of pelvic organ prolapse surgery in the United States. Obstet Gynecol. 2001;98(4):646–651.
2. Maher C, Feiner B, Baessler K, Adams EJ, Hagen S, Glazener CM. Surgical management of pelvic organ prolapse in women. Cochrane Database Syst Rev. 2010;14(4):CD004014. doi:10.1002/14651858.CD004014.pub4.
3. Grimes CL, Tan-Kim J, Whitcomb EL, Lukacz ES, Menefee SA. Long-term outcomes after native tissue vs. biological graft-augmented repair in the posterior compartment. Int Urogynecol J. 2012;23(5):597–604.
4. Cruikshank SH, Muniz M. Outcomes study: a comparison of cure rates in 695 patients undergoing sacrospinous ligament fixation alone and with other site-specific procedures a 16-year study. Am J Obstet Gynecol. 2003;188(6):1509–12.
5. Biehl RC, Moore RD, Miklos JR, Kohli N, Anand IS, Mattox TF. Site-specific rectocele repair with dermal graft augmentation: comparison of procine dermal xenograft (Pelvicol) and human dermal allograft. Surg Technol Int. 2008;17:174–80.
6. Kohli N, Miklos JR. Dermal graft-augmented rectocele repair. Int Urogynecol J Pelvic Floor Dysfunct. 2003;14(2):146–9.
7. Miklos JR, Kohli N, Moore R. Levatorplasty release and reconstruction of rectovaginal septum using allogenic dermal graft. Int Urogynecol J Pelvic Floor Dysfunctionct. 2002; 13(1):44–46.
8. Lo TS, Horng SG, Huang HJ, Lee SJ, Liang CC. Repair of recurrent vaginal vault prolapse using sacrospinous ligament fixation with mesh interposition and reinforcement. Acta Obstet Gynecol Scand. 2005;84(10):992–5.
9. Yurteri-Kaplan LA, Gutman RE. The use of biological materials in urogynecologic reconstruction: a systematic review. Plast Reconstr Surg. 2012;130(5):242S–53S. doi: 10.1097/PRS.0b013e31826154e4.
10. Amid PK, Lichtenstein IL. Current assessment of Lichtenstein tension free hernia repair. Chirurg. 1997;68(10):959–64.
11. Maggiore ULR, Alessandi F, Remorgida V, Venturini PL, Ferrero S. Vaginal sacrospinous colpopexy using the Capio suture-capturing device versus traditional technique: feasibility and outcome. Arch Gynecol Obstet. 2013;287(2):267–74.
12. Halaska M, Maxova K, Sottner O, Svabik K, Mlcoch M, Kolarik D, Mala I, Krofta L, Halaska MJ. A multicenter, randomized, prospective, controlled study comparing sacrospinous fixation and transvaginal mesh in the treatment of posthysterectomy vaginal vault prolapse. Am J Obstet Gynecol. 2012;207(4):301e1–7. doi:10.1016/j.ajog.2012.08.016.
13. Paraiso MF, Barber MD, Muir TW, Walters MD. Rectocele repair: a randomized trial of three surgical techniques including graft augmentation. Am J Obstet Gynecol. 2006;195(6):1762–71.
14. Darai E, Coutant C, Rouzier R, Ballester M, David-Montefiore E, Apfelbaum D. Genital prolapse repair using porcine skin implant and bilateral sacrospinous fixation: midterm functional outcome and quality –of-life assessment. Urology. 2009;73(2):245–50.
15. Barber MD, Walters MD, Cundiff GW, Pessri trial group. Responsiveness of the pelvic floor distress inventory (PFDI) and pelvic floor impact questionnaire (PFIQ) in women undergoing vaginal surgery and pessary treatment for pelvic organ prolapse. Am J. Obstet Gynecol. 2006;194(5):1492–8.
16. Campeau L, Gorbachinsky I, Badlani GH, Andersson KE. Pelvic floor disorders: linking genetic risk factors to biochemical changes. BJU Int. 2011;108(8):1240–7.
17. Aboushwareb T, McKenzie P, Wezel F, Southgate J, Badlani GH. Is tissue engineering and biomaterials the future for lower urinary tract dysfunction (LUTD)/pelvic organ prolapse (POP)? Neurourol Urodyn. 2011;30(5):775–82.
18. Moon YJ, Choi JR, Jeon MJ, Kim SK, Bai SW. Alteration of elastin metabolism in women with pelvic floor prolapse. J Urol. 2011;185(5):1786–92. doi: 10.1016/j.juro.2010.12.040. Epub 2011 Mar 21.
19. Kolhoff DM, Cheng EY, Sharma AK. Urological applications of engineered tissue. Regen Med. 2011;6:757–65.
20. Liang CC, Huang HY, Chang SD. Gene expression and immunoreactivity of elastolytic enzymes in the uterosacral ligaments from women with uterine prolapse. Reprod Sci. 2012;19(4):354–9.
21. Ferrari MM, Rossi G, Biondi ML, Vigano P, Dell'utri C, Meschia M. Type 1 collagen and matrix metalloproteinase 1,3, and 9 gene polymorphisms in the predisposition to pelvic organ prolapse. Arch Gynecol Obstet. 2012;285(6):1581–6.
22. Chen B, Yeh J. Alterations in connective tissue metabolism in stress incontinence and prolapse. J Urol. 2011;186(5):1768–72.
23. Ellington DR, Richter HE. Indications, contraindications, and complications of mesh in surgical treatment of pelvic organ prolapse. Clin Obstet Gynecol. 2013;56(2):276–88.
24. Zoorob D, Karram M. Management of mesh complications and vaginal constriction: a urogynecology perspective. Urol Clin North Am. 2012;39(3):413–8.
25. Dahlgren E, Kjolhede P, RPOP-PELVICHOL study group. Long –term outcome of porcine skin graft in surgical treatment of recurrent pelvic organ prolapse. An open randomized controlled multicenter study. Acta Obstet Gynecol Scand. 2011;90(12):1393–401.

10

Quality-of-life outcomes and unmet needs between ileal conduit and orthotopic ileal neobladder after radical cystectomy in a Chinese population

Yi Huang[1,2†], Xiuwu Pan[1,3†], Qiwei Zhou[4†], Hai Huang[1], Lin Li[1,3], Xingang Cui[3*], Guodong Wang[5*], Ren Jizhong[1], Lei Yin[1], Danfeng Xu[1] and Yi Hong[1]

Abstract

Background: Health-related quality-of-life (HRQoL) is an important consideration after radical cystectomy (RC). Lack of effective ways to assess HRQoL after RC and unawareness of disease-specific problems related to ileal conduit (IC) and orthotopic ileal neobladder (OIN) are serious problems. The present study was to evaluate and compare morbidity and HRQoL between IC and OIN after RC, and examine their unmet needs in the two groups.

Methods: A retrospective analysis was made of 294 patients treated with RC in our hospital between 2007 and 2013. Matched pair analysis was used to determine the patients of IC and OIN groups. Patient HRQoL between IC and OIN groups was assessed using the bladder-specific bladder cancer index (BCI) and European Organization for Research and Treatment of Cancer Body Image scale (BIS) questionnaires. Unmet information of patients undergoing these two urinary diversions was recorded through individual interviews.

Results: Of the 117 included patients, 39 patients were treated with OIN and the other 78 matched patients with IC as controls for matched pair analysis. There was no significant difference in baseline characteristics between the two groups. OIN patients showed significantly better BIS scores in terms of HRQoL outcomes after RC at a short-term (<1 year) follow-up level, but there was no significant difference at a long-term (>1 year) follow-up level between the two groups. Interestingly, urinary bother (UB) and urinary function (UF) were poor in OIN patients at the one-year follow-up level, but there was no significant difference in UB between the two groups at the long term follow-up level. Unmet needs analysis showed that OIN patients had a more positive attitude towards treatment and participated in physical and social activities more positively, although they may have more urine leakage problems.

Conclusions: The mean BIS score in OIN group patients was significantly better than that in IC group patients at the one-year follow-up level, but there was no significant difference at the long-term follow-up level. Due attention should be paid to some particular unmet needs in individual patients in managing the two UD modalities.

Keywords: Bladder cancer, Laparoscopy, Radical cystectomy, Orthotopic Ileal, Neobladder, Ileal conduit, Quality-of-life

* Correspondence: xingangcui@126.com; louis_w@126.com
†Equal contributors
[3]Department of Urinary Surgery of Third Affiliated Hospital, Second Military Medical University, No. 700, Moyu Road, Jiading District, Shanghai 201805, China
[5]Department of Stomatology of Changzheng Hospital, Second Military Medical University, Shanghai, China
Full list of author information is available at the end of the article

Background

Radical cystectomy (RC) with bilateral pelvic lymphadenectomy is the standard treatment for muscle-invasive and high-risk non-muscle-invasive urothelial carcinoma of the bladder (UCB) [1]. There are numerous choices for urinary diversion (UD) after RC. Ileal conduit (IC) continues to be the most common form of UD, while orthotopic ileal neobladder (OIN) is the preferred continent UD in some patients owing to its functional and psychological advantages [2, 3], although it is contraindicated for patients with intraurethral tumors and urethral stricture.

In the past decade, health-related quality-of-life (HRQoL) is an important consideration after RC, because this traumatic event is often associated with significant changes in body image, urinary and sexual functions, interpersonal relationships, and psychosocial stress outcomes [4]. Although there is no convincing evidence to support the conclusion that OIN is superior to IC [5], most patients are likely to choose OIN at the individual level despite the informed risk of problematic orthotipic voiding.

Given the controversies over the choice of different UD options partly due to the lack of effective ways to assess HRQoL after RC and unawareness of disease-specific problems related to IC and OIN in most Chinese patients, the present study retrospectively compared the discrepancies in the HRQoL of patients treated with IC or OIN, in an attempt to better assess the two different UD by combined use of BIS and BCI questionnaires during the follow-up periods. In addition, specific unmet needs in patients of the two groups were also clarified.

Methods

Patient selection

Recruited in this study were patients who underwent RC at the Department of Urology of Shanghai Changzheng Hospital (Shanghai, China) between January 2007 and December 2013. Inclusion criteria were patients who underwent RC with OIN or IC and were able to fully understand the questionnaires and fill out the questionnaire forms. Exclusion criteria were 1) patients who had psychiatric disorders, histories of alcohol or substance abuse, cognitive morbidity such as Alzheimer's disease, or additional oncological disease; 2) patients whose follow-up duration was less than one year; and 3) patients who were lost to follow-up or experienced recurrences or died during the one-year follow-up period. Finally, 205 IC patients and 89 OIN patients were included in this study for analysis. This study was approved by the ethics board of Shanghai Changzheng Hospital in accordance with the Declaration of Helsinki, and all patients provided informed consent.

Surgical procedures

Most patients in our center underwent laparoscopic radical cystectomy (LRC) after RC, using the OIN reconstruction technique described by Hautmann et al. [6]. Contraindications for OIN were ASA score > 3, severe cardiac insufficiency, decompensated pulmonary function, impaired renal function (serum creatinine >2 mg/dL), the presence of intraurethral tumors and/or urethral stricture, a history of previous bowel resection, abnormal abdominal straining and extensive muscle-invasive UCB. The patient who has these contraindications for OIN chose IC reconstruction. The IC was constructed in a standard fashion by using the minimum amount of the ileum. However, some patients who did not have these contraindications for OIN chose between IC and OIN reconstruction after impartial counselling. Standard pelvic lymph node dissection (PLND) was performed in all patients.

Baseline patient characteristics

Data regarding preoperative, perioperative and pathologic characteristics were collected. Preoperative variables included age, sex, body mass index (BMI), ASA classification, comorbid conditions (previous abdominal/pelvic surgery, other malignancy, cardiovascular disease, pulmonary disease, hypertension and diabetes), and the smoking status. Perioperative variables were operative time (OT), estimated blood loss (EBL), the number of lymph nodes removed, transfusion, conversion to open surgery, and short-term complications classified according to the modified Clavien classification system [7]. Pathologic characteristics were histopathologic tumor type, grade and stage defined according to the TNM classification and the WHO System 2004.

Outcome evaluation

HRQoL outcomes were measured using the BIS [8] and BCI [9] questionnaires. All the questionnaire forms were filled out by patients personally and completed preoperatively and at 6-month intervals after surgery. The BIS published by Hopwood et al. [8] for assessing body image changes in patients with cancer is generally accepted as a brief patient self-report measure in conjunction with the EORTC-QOL Study group. It contains 10 items including affective, behavioral and cognitive aspects. Each item is scored on a 0–3 scale and the overall summary scores range from 0 to 30, with higher scores representing progression of the symptoms. The BCI initially created by Gilbert et al. [9] consists of 34 items within three primary domains assessing urinary, bowel and sexual functions. All these items are responded through the 5-point Likert scale. Each primary domain contains two parts (function and bother) and are standardized to the 0–100 scale, with higher scores representing better HRQoL. The unmet need information was retrospectively collected by another interview guide design by Mohamed et al. [10].

Peri-operative outcomes (OT, EBL, the number of lymph nodes removed, transfusion and conversion to open surgery) are shown in Additional file 1: Table S5. The simple outcomes following OIN including the daytime/continence rate, ISC rate, maximum neobladder volume (mL) and postvoid residual are shown in Additional file 2: Table S6.

Statistical analysis

Patients were selected for matched pair analysis (MPA) and blinded to outcomes. Exact matching was performed for the following primary factors potentially correlated to the poor preoperative QoL: age at operation (the allowed difference was less than 10 years), gender (needs to be identical), and ASA (needs to be identical). The matching process resulted in 117 patients involved.

All statistical analyses were performed using SAS software (v9.3, SAS Institute, Cary, NC). The results are presented as mean (range) values and percentages. The Chi-Square test and Wilcoxon rank-sum test were used to see whether there was a significant difference between the two UDs. The repeat measures of ANOVA (analysis of variance) were performed in the 1-year follow-up and the long-term follow-up periods (longer than 1 year), respectively. A P value <0.05 was considered statistically significant.

Results

A total of 294 patients underwent RC with pre- and postoperative follow-up data available. Pair matching identified 39 OIN and 78 IC patients suitable for inclusion in this analysis. The patient demographics and clinical characteristics are shown in Table 1 and Additional file 3: Table S1.

Figure 1 presents the mean BIS score for each UD over time. The mean BIS score in IC patients was lower than that in OIN patients in the one year follow-up period ($P = 0.003$). However, there was no significant difference between the two UD types at the long-term follow-up level ($P = 0.114$), suggesting that time had a positive effect on BIS of both groups ($P <0.001$). Figure 2a shows that urinary function (UF) based on BCI score was better in IC patients than that in OIN patients at both one-year follow-up and long-term follow-up levels ($P < 0.001$ and $P = 0.0074$). Interestingly, ANOVA analysis showed that with time prolonging, UF was improved in both groups as compared with their previous state ($P < 0.001$). Figure 2b shows that urinary bother (UB) in terms of BCI score favored IC group at the one-year follow-up level ($P = 0.004$), although the two UD types showed no significant difference ($P = 0.720$) at the 5-year follow-up

level. Similarly, UB in both groups was also improved over time ($P < 0.001$).

The unmet need at the time of diagnosis is shown in Additional file 4: Table S2. It was found that more IC patients focused on self-care following surgery as compared with OIN patients ($P = 0.001$), and in the themes of involvement in the treatment decision making more OIN patients made their own personal choice of treatment ($P = 0.020$). The Additional file 5: Table S3 presents the details of unmet needs following surgery, showing that IC patients had less difficulty with urine leakage ($P = 0.001$) and received more help from their family members or friends ($P = 0.004$). The Additional file 6: Table S4 shows the details of unmet needs following surgery during survivorship, indicating that IC patients had more limited physical and social activities ($P < 0.001$), although the OIN patients also had some worries about the future ($P = 0.011$).

Discussion

There are still some controversies over whether OIN is the most optimal form of UD after RC in terms of HRQoL. Although some studies [11–13] reported that OIN could provide marginally better HRQoL scores than IC, other studies [14–16] argued that there was no significant difference between them. However, there is significant selection bias in these studies in comparing HRQoL between OIN and IC patients, which may cause differences in the preoperative status between these studies. In addition, most of these studies neglected the disease-specific QoL in comparing HRQoL outcomes between the two UDs. For these reasons, we performed a match pair analysis in the present study. Based on the similar baseline characteristics, we evaluated the HRQoL from two aspects at regular intervals postoperatively: one is the change of body image change by using the BIS questionnaire [8], and the other is the disease-specific QoL by using BCI questionnaire [9]. To further understand the details of cancer trajectory, we also presented intermediate profiles by Interview Guide (IG) [10] about the unmet need information. It was found that OIN patients were better in body image, and IC patients were better in UF and UB at the one-year follow-up level. Surprisingly, there was no significant difference in BIS and UB between the two groups at the long-term follow-up level, although UF remained a problem in OIN patients. We also found some differences in unmet need at each time point of the illness trajectory.

It was found in our study that BIS in OIN patients was superior to that in IC patients within the one-year follow-up period. However, a previous study [17] showed no significant difference in BIS, and in their longitudinal model they found that age was correlated with the BIS, suggesting that older patients had slightly better scores.

Table 1 Demographics and clinical characteristics data after matched pair analysis

Characteristic	After MAP (1:2) 117		P
	OIN (39)	IC (78)	
Mean age, yr (range)	63.6 (51.5–76.0)	64.0 (52.0–74.8)	0.885[a]
Sex ratio (M/F)	34/5	68/10	match
Mean BMI, kg/m2 (range)	21.7 (18.7–24.4)	22.0 (18.8–25.4)	0.637[a]
ASA class, N (%)			Match
1	6 (15.4)	12 (15.4)	
2	24 (61.5)	48 (61.5)	
3	9 (23.1)	18 (23.1)	
Smoking history, N (%)	9 (23.1)	20 (25.6)	0.762[c]
Previous abdominal or pelvic surgery, N (%)	4 (10.3)	11 (14.1)	0.558[c]
Comorbidities, N (%)			
Cardiovascular disease	3 (7.7)	8 (10.3)	0.911[b]
Pulmonary disease	5 (12.8)	16 (20.5)	0.307[c]
Hypertension	9 (23.1)	28 (35.9)	0.160[c]
Diabetes	7 (17.9)	16 (20.5)	0.742[c]
Histological type, N (%)			0.890[b]
Pure TCC	36 (92.3)	74 (94.9)	
Other pathology	3 (7.7)	4 (5.1)	
Histological grade, N (%)			0.651[c]
Grade 1 and Grade 2	9 (23.1)	15 (19.2)	
Grade 3	28 (71.8)	58 (74.4)	
Pathologic T stage, N (%)			0.476[a]
Organ-confined: ≤pT2, pN0	33 (84.6)	62 (79.5)	
Non-organ-confined: pT3-pT4, pN0	6 (15.4)	14 (17.9)	
Lymph node-positive: pN+	0	2 (2.6)	
Highest grade of complication, N (%)			0.562[a]
I	4 (10.3)	8 (10.3)	
II	4 (10.3)	7 (9.0)	
III	3 (7.7)	3 (3.8)	
IV	0	0	
V	0	0	

[a]Wilcoxon rank-sum test
[b]Pearson chi-squared test with continuity correction
[c]Chi-Square

To overcome this shortage, we also performed an MPA in our study in term of age, gender and ASA, score so that the baseline characteristics of these two groups were more comparable. It is worth to mention that there was no significant difference in BIS between the two groups at the long-term follow-up level ($P = 0.1136$), which may be directly related to the positive effect of time, as was the case with that reported in previous studies [17–19], although it needs a relatively long time.

In addition, OIN patients had poorer UF than IC patients, which is consistent with the conclusion of Gilbert et al. [9] who originally designed the BCI questionnaire related to UF, saying that OIN patients had more voiding problems as compared with IC patients. The long-term follow-up results obtained at 12, 24 and 36 months showed that urination always remained a problem in OIN patients, but it tended to be stable after 12 months, which is similar to the conclusion of Hedgepeth et al. [17]. It is generally considered that urinary leakage in OIN patients may result from the loss of reflex micturition and injury to the urethral sphincter. In order to reduce the adverse effects due to urinary dysfunction, patients need to form a new habit of urination and on the other hand the doctor's instructions about functional

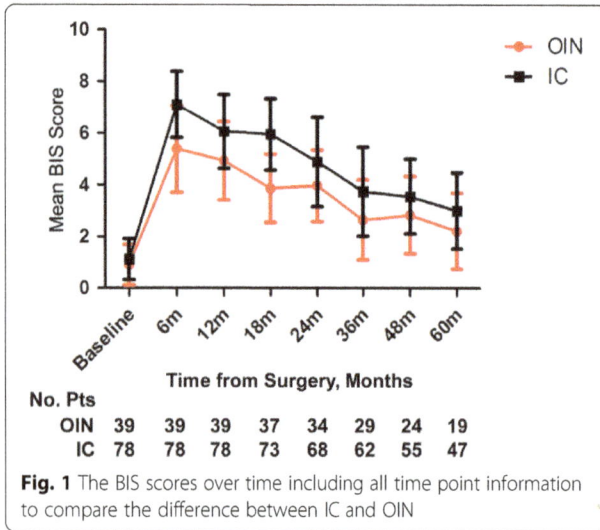

Fig. 1 The BIS scores over time including all time point information to compare the difference between IC and OIN

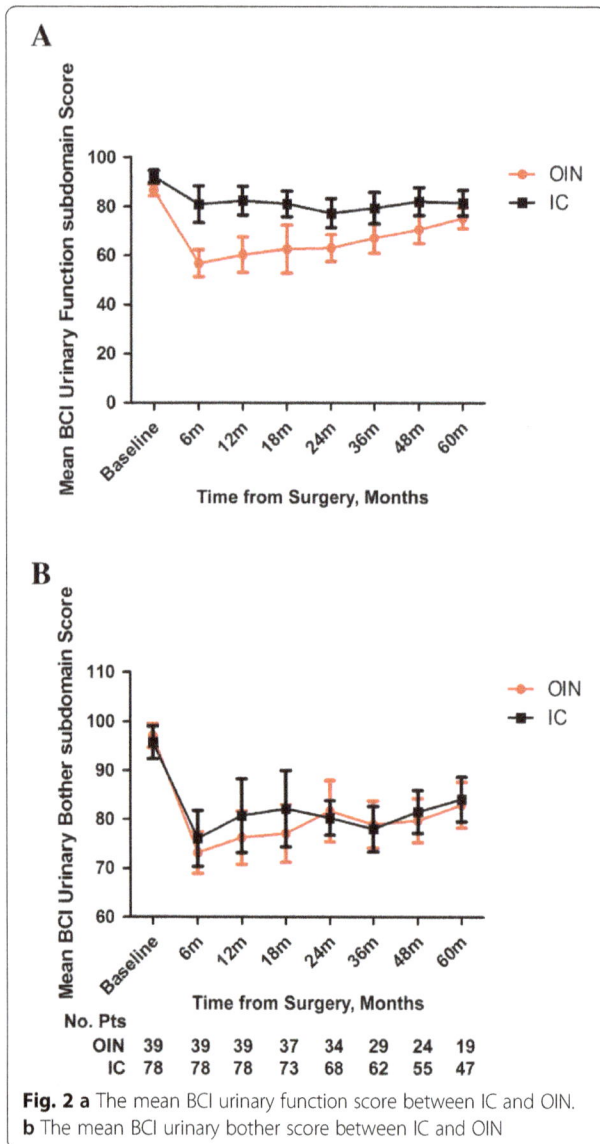

Fig. 2 a The mean BCI urinary function score between IC and OIN. **b** The mean BCI urinary bother score between IC and OIN

training such as Kegel Exercise may help to reinforce the function of the urethral sphincter of patients. As shown in Fig. 2a, the UF was improved markedly at 12 months. However, IC patients had to face the problem of peristomal urinary leak from the pouch, which can only be overcome by good self-care or with the assistance of care providers. We also found that this problem was improved satisfactorily after 12 months. Figure 2b shows that OIN patients had more UB than did IC patients within a year, while there was no significant difference between the two groups in a longer follow-up duration. However, Hedgepeth et al. [17] reported no significant difference in UB between OIN and IC groups, probably because of the difference in baseline UB between the two groups. We consider that poorer UB within a year in OIN group may be due to the UF, because our long-term follow-up observation showed that UB was improved with the improved UF (Fig. 2b). Moreover, UB did not deteriorate significantly compared with that before surgery in IC patients. To some extent, it may be due to the fact that patients always had the UB at the diagnostic phase with the anxiety of caring about malignant tumor for the occurrence of hematuria and urine frequency. Most postoperative patients were bothered by problems of peristomal urinary leakage, foul urine odor and wearing of urine ostomy pouches, which can be improved or adapt. Based on previous studies and our present study, neither of the two UDs shows absolute advantage. Therefore, in the clinical practice, we not only need to make an optimal decision upon surgical options, but also make every endeavor to improve the postoperative HRQoL of special patients.

The measures that we used to assess HRQoL in patients with muscle invasive bladder cancer (MIBC) were unable to distinguish between health related problems and the patient desire or need to receive professional attention or care for these problems. it was imperative to identify and address the unmet needs of patients with MIBC at each time point of the illness trajectory. To optimize the quality of provided health care and gain more comprehensive understanding about potential changes in patient needs and challenges, the responsible physician may be more helpful to the patients to achieve better quality of life. Firstly, more IC patients were concerned about their postoperative self-care problems during the diagnostic phase, presumably because of the apprehension about the postoperative use of urine ostomy pouches. OIN patients without the above worries can make an autonomous choice to live a normal life as ordinary people. Secondly, at the time of following after surgery, OIN patients met with more problems with urine leakage during the short-term postoperative phase, which is consistent with the conclusion of previous studies [17]. However, most of these patients did not seek help from their family members or other care providers, suggesting that urine leakage did not bring them intolerable inconvenience. Thirdly, we found that IC patients had mild physical and social relationship problems during the long-term follow-up phase, which is consistent with a previous perspective study [11]. These problems may be related to the use or leakage of urinary ostomy pouches.

The present study has some limitations. Firstly, the information about the unmet needs in each patient was collected retrospectively, which may run potential risk of recall bias. Secondly, the number of female patients with bladder cancer is relatively small, accounting for about 10 % of all bladder cancer cases in the Chinese population [20, 21]. Thirdly, as nerve-sparing RC was not performed in our included patients, sexual life was lost completely in part of these patients. But as most of our patients were too shy to talk about their sexual life to doctors and other unfamiliar relations, it was difficult for us to make an evaluation on this problem. Fourthly, the number of OIN patients is relatively small. One reason is due to the preference of surgery on the part of the doctor, and the other is due to the consideration on the part of the patient. Fifthly, there is a deviation in our groups' complication rates according to previous studies, two reasons may affect the complication rate in our study: (1) some patients who had high-grade complications were unwilling to participate in our follow-up questionnaire; (2) some high-grade complications related to radical cystectomy were avoided successfully due to the skilled surgical technique and rich experience of our department.

Conclusion

BIS scores were significantly better in OIN patients during the short-term (<1 year) follow-up period, while there was no significant difference between IC and OIN groups during the long-term (>1 year) follow-up periods. Urine function remains a problem in OIN patients as compared with IC patients during both short- and long-term follow-up periods. Due attention should be paid to some particular unmet needs in individual patients in managing the two UD modalities.

Additional files

Additional file 1: Table S5. Peri-operative outcomes.
Additional file 2: Table S6. Continence outcomes following OIN.

Additional file 3: Table S1. Demographics and clinical characteristics data before matched pair analysis.
Additional file 4: Table S2. Unmet informational and supportive care needs at the time of diagnosis.

Additional file 5: Table S3. Unmet informational and supportive care needs following surgery.
Additional file 6: Table S4. Unmet informational and support needs during survivorship.

Abbreviations
ASA: American society of anesthesiologists; BCI: Bladder-specific bladder cancer index; BMI: Body mass index; BSI: European organization for research and treatment of cancer body image scale; CUD: Continent urinary diversion; EBL: Estimated blood loss; EORTC-QLQ-C30: European organization for research and treatment of cancer quality-of-life core questionnaire; FACT-G: Functional assessment of cancer therapy-general; HRQoL: Health-related quality-of-life; IC: Ileal conduit; LRC: Laparoscopic radical cystectomy; MIBC: Muscle invasive bladder cancer; MPA: Matched pair analysis; OIN: Ileal neobladder; OT: Operative time; PLND: Pelvic lymph node dissection; RC: Radical cystectomy; UB: Urinary bother; UF: Urinary function; UCB: Urothelial carcinoma of the bladder.

Competing interest
The authors declare that they have no competing interests.

Authors' contributions
YH (Huang), XP and QZ designed the study. YH (Huang), XP, QZ, HH, LL, JR, LY, DX and YH (Hong) acquired the data. YH (Huang), XP and QZ did the statistical analysis of the data. YH (Huang), XP, QZ, HH and LL interpreted the data. YH (Huang), XP, QZ drafted the manuscript. XC and GW provided a critical revision of the manuscript. All authors read and approved the final manuscript.

Acknowledgments
This work was supported by grants from Shanghai Municipal Education Commission for Innovative Research Project (No. 14zz084); the Military Health Care Special Subjects (No. 13BJZ29); the National Natural Science Foundation of China (No. 30973006, 81170637); and Shanghai Municipal Committee of Science and Technology General Programs for Medicine (No. 11JC1402302).

Author details
[1]Department of Urinary Surgery of Changzheng Hospital, Second Military Medical University, No. 415, Fengyang Road, Huangpu District, Shanghai 200003, China. [2]Department of Urinary Surgery of Navy Hospital of Xiamen, No. 23, Zhenhai Road, Siming District, Xiamen 361000, China. [3]Department of Urinary Surgery of Third Affiliated Hospital, Second Military Medical University, No. 700, Moyu Road, Jiading District, Shanghai 201805, China. [4]Department of Urinary Surgery of No. 313 Hospital of PLA, No. 50, Haibinnan Road, Longgang District, Huludao City, Liaoning 125000, China. [5]Department of Stomatology of Changzheng Hospital, Second Military Medical University, Shanghai, China.

References
1. Witjes JA, Comperat E, Cowan NC, De Santis M, Gakis G, Lebret T, et al. EAU guidelines on muscle-invasive and metastatic bladder cancer: summary of the 2013 guidelines. Eur Urol. 2014;65:778–92.
2. Sullivan LD, Chow VD, Ko DS, Wright JE, McLoughlin MG. An evaluation of quality of life in patients with continent urinary diversions after cystectomy. Br J Urol. 1998;81:699–704.
3. Hautmann RE. Complications and results after cystectomy in male and female patients with locally invasive bladder cancer. Eur Urol. 1998;33:23–4.
4. Ali AS, Hayes MC, Birch B, Dudderidge T, Somani BK. Health related quality of life (HRQoL) after cystectomy: Comparison between orthotopic neobladder and ileal conduit diversion. Eur J Surg Oncol. 2015;41:295-9.
5. Hautmann RE, Abol-Enein H, Davidsson T, Gudjonsson S, Hautmann SH, Holm HV, et al. ICUD-EAU international consultation on bladder cancer 2012: urinary diversion. Eur Urol. 2013;63:67–80.
6. Hautmann RE, Egghart G, Frohneberg D, Miller K. The ileal neobladder. J Urol. 1988;139:39–42.

7.   Shabsigh A, Korets R, Vora KC, Brooks CM, Cronin AM, Savage C, et al. Defining early morbidity of radical cystectomy for patients with bladder cancer using a standardized reporting methodology. Eur Urol. 2009;55:164–74.

8.   Gilbert SM, Wood DP, Dunn RL, et al. Measuring health-related quality of life outcomes in bladder cancer patients using the Bladder Cancer Index (BCI). Cancer. 2007;109:1756–62.

9.   Mohamed NE, Chaoprang HP, Hudson S, Revenson TA, Lee CT, Quale DZ, et al. Muscle invasive bladder cancer: examining survivor burden and unmet needs. J Urol. 2014;191:48–53.

10. Hopwood P, Fletcher I, Lee A, Al Ghazal S. A body image scale for use with cancer patients. Eur J Cancer. 2001;37:189–97.

11. Singh V, Yadav R, Sinha RJ, Gupta DK. Prospective comparison of quality-of-life outcomes between ileal conduit urinary diversion and orthotopic neobladder reconstruction after radical cystectomy: a statistical model. BJU Int. 2014;113:726–32.

12. Philip J, Manikandan R, Venugopal S, Desouza J, Javlé PM. Orthotopic neobladder versus ileal conduit urinary diversion after cystectomy–a quality-of-life based comparison. Ann R Coll Surg Engl. 2009;91:565–9.

13. Erber B, Schrader M, Miller K, Schostak M, Baumunk D, Lingnau A, et al. Morbidity and quality of life in bladder cancer patients following cystectomy and urinary diversion: a single-institution comparison of ileal conduit versus orthotopic neobladder. ISRN Urol. 2012. 2012: doi: 10.5402/2012/342796.

14. Fujisawa M, Isotani S, Gotoh A, Okada H, Arakawa S, Kamidono S. Health-related quality of life with orthotopic neobladder versus ileal conduit according to the SF-36 survey. Urology. 2000;55:862–5.

15. Hara I, Miyake H, Hara S, Gotoh A, Nakamura I, Okada H, et al. Health-related quality of life after radical cystectomy for bladder cancer: a comparison of ileal conduit and orthotopic bladder replacement. BJU Int. 2002;89:10–3.

16. Autorino R, Quarto G, Di LG, De Sio M, Perdonà S, Giannarini G, et al. Health related quality of life after radical cystectomy: comparison of ileal conduit to continent orthotopic neobladder. Eur J Surg Oncol. 2009;35:858–64.

17. Hedgepeth RC, Gilbert SM, He C, Lee CT, Wood DP Jr. Body image and bladder cancer specific quality of life in patients with ileal conduit and neobladder urinary diversions. Urology. 2010;76:671–5.

18. Poch MA, Stegemann AP, Rehman S, Sharif MA, Hussain A, Consiglio JD, et al. Short-term patient reported health-related quality of life (HRQL) outcomes after robot-assisted radical cystectomy (RARC). BJU Int. 2014;113:260–5.

19. Aboumohamed AA, Raza SJ, Al-Daghmin A, Tallman C, Creighton T, Crossley H, et al. Health-related quality of life outcomes after robot-assisted and open radical cystectomy using a validated bladder-specific instrument: a multi-institutional study. Urology. 2014;83:1300–8.

20. Huang J, Lin T, Liu H, Xu K, Zhang C, Jiang C, et al. Laparoscopic radical cystectomy with orthotopic ileal neobladder for bladder cancer: oncologic results of 171 cases with a median 3-year follow-up. Eur Urol. 2010;58:442–9.

21. Zeng S, Zhang Z, Yu X, Song R, Wei R, Zhao J, et al. Laparoscopic versus open radical cystectomy for elderly patients over 75-year-old: a single center comparative analysis. PLoS One. 2014;9:e98950.

11

Defining competency in flexible cystoscopy: a novel approach using cumulative Sum analysis

Kenneth R. MacKenzie* and Jonathan Aning

Abstract

Background: Flexible cystoscopy (FC) is one of the most frequently performed urological intervention. Cumulative sum analysis (CUSUM) allows objective assessment of a proceduralist's performance to ensure acceptable outcomes. This study investigated the application of CUSUM to assess a trainee's learning curve and maintenance of competence in performing FC.

Methods: A single urology trainee, with no previous experience of FC, performed FCs between August 2013 and February 2014. For assessment FC was divided into 5 steps. Each step was assigned a CUSUM completion score. The primary outcome measure was successful performance of a complete FC. Prospective data were collected and analysed using CUSUM.

Results: In total, 419 FCs were performed. Acceptable performance of FC was achieved by the 122nd procedure. Complete assessment of the ureteric orifices and trigone was the most difficult step of FC to achieve consistently. Competence for complete FC was achieved following 289 procedures.

Conclusion: CUSUM analysis objectively assesses acquisition of competence in flexible cystoscopy. Recommended indicative numbers may underestimate the number of FCs trainees require to achieve, and maintain, competency. Validation of CUSUM method in a larger cohort of trainees should be considered.

Keywords: Flexible cystoscopy, Cumulative sum, CUSUM analysis, Learning curve

Background

Flexible cystoscopy (FC) is a vital diagnostic and therapeutic urological procedure, which enables immediate visual assessment of both the urethra and bladder.

FC comprises multiple steps, each of which require varying degrees of endoscopic skill. It is often assumed that competence in performing FC is achieved in the early years of urological training or within a limited number of procedures. Guidance informing assessment of competency in performing FC is limited. In 2000, a working party of the British Association of Urological Surgeons (BAUS) recommended that a minimum of 60 FCs should be performed under supervision to achieve technical competence [1]. This number has not been validated. It is now recog- nised that individuals training to perform a procedure, acquire skills at different rates [2]. Indicative numbers are a weak method of assessing competence and fail to identify or aid struggling trainees. There is a need for a more objective method to assess competency and guide training.

Cumulative Sum (CUSUM) analysis is a statistical tool that can be used to evaluate the development of competence in defined tasks [3]. CUSUM analysis has previously been used to chart learning curves and maintaining competency in surgical techniques, but not in FC, in vivo [3].

The aim of this study was to prospectively define the learning curve in FC of a surgical trainee with no previous FC experience and to evaluate the role of CUSUM as an objective measure of achieving and maintaining competency.

* Correspondence: Kenneth.r.mackenzie@gmail.com
Department of Urology, The Newcastle upon Tyne Hospitals NHS Foundation Trust, Freeman Hospital, Newcastle-Upon-Tyne NE7 7DN, UK

Methods

Setting

From August 2013 to February 2014 a Trust Grade in Urology, 2 years post qualification, with no previous experience in FC or endoscopy maintained a prospective database of all FCs performed at Weston General Hospital, North Somerset. The trainee intended to pursue a career in Urology and observed ten FCs prior to starting to perform FC. All FCs were performed using a flexible video cystoscope (Karl Storz, Germany). A senior Specialty Trainee competent in performing FC, or a consultant, provided supervision during each procedure.

Outcome measures

FC was deconstructed into five key components for the purpose of assessment; these were defined prior to starting the project. The components were based on FC steps recommended by the Intercollegiate Surgical Curriculum Programme (ISCP) and the British Association of Urology Nurses for training and assessment (Table 1) [4–6].

CUSUM analysis requires an acceptable and unacceptable failure rate to define success and competence. Consultant Urologists in the South West of England were emailed a link to an online questionnaire describing the study. In the questionnaire consultants were asked to allocate acceptable failure rates for each flexible cystoscopy step. Of 65 invited to participate, 13 consultants completed the questionnaire. Each step has a different acceptable and unacceptable failure rate to take into account more challenging steps of the procedure (Table 1).

Data analysis

The Type I and Type II error rates for CUSUM analysis were set at 0.10, as a standard. [7, 8] The acceptable and unacceptable failure rates varied with each step, however, were critical for the derivation of a CUSUM score. The CUSUM score (S) was calculated for each step (Additional file 1). For each success, a decrement of (S)

is applied and each failure, an increase of $(1 - S)$ is applied. The total score is cumulative and the total score is plotted as a continual plotted line.

Horizontal control lines are plotted at regular intervals on the y-axis. The spacing between control lines is calculated using a standardised equation (Additional file 1).

Graph interpretation

The CUSUM value is plotted on the y-axis against the number of procedures on the x-axis. The CUSUM plotted line is a running sum of increments (1- S) and decrements (S).

Therefore, if the plotted line crosses the control line in an upward trend, performance is deemed unacceptable. If the control line is crossed in a downward trend then performance is deemed acceptable. If performance is maintained between two control lines then acceptable performance is being maintained. Competence is declared when 2 consecutive control lines are crossed in a downward fashion [9, 10].

Results

Four hundred nineteen FCs were performed under local anaesthesia during the study period in 251 Males and 168 Females, median age 70 years (range 16–96). Indications for FC are detailed in Table 2.

Each of the five steps has been evaluated individually and is presented in the order FC is performed. For each step, a number of procedures were excluded due to pathology preventing complete examination. The pathologies excluded were: urethral stricture, gross haematuria, obscuring malignancy and bladder stones.

1. Atraumatic passage of cystoscope via urethra
   Figure 1 shows the CUSUM score plotted against the number of procedures. It can be seen that the unacceptable control line [crossing the horizontal control line on the y-axis in an upwards fashion

Table 1 Five components of endoscopic assessment

	Area of assessment	Steps included	UFR	AFR
1.	Atraumatic passage of the cystoscope into the Bladder	Insertion of instillagel Insertion under direct vision Insertion of cystoscope into the bladder	3 %	1 %
2.	Examination of body and dome of bladder	Examine the dome, right and left lateral wall and posterior wall	3 %	1 %
3.	Examination of trigone and ureteric orifice		15 %	5 %
4.	Examination of bladder neck	Performed by inverting the cystoscope	3 %	1 %
5.	Performance of the full procedure		15 %	5 %

UFR unacceptable failure rate, *AFR* acceptable failure rate

Table 2 Indications for flexible cystoscopy

Indication	Number of patients ($n = 417$)
Haematuria	226 (54 %)
Surveillance for Bladder Cancer	149 (36 %)
Recurrent Urinary Tract Infections	16 (4 %)
To identify a stricture	9 (2 %)
Lower Urinary Tract Pain	6 (1 %)
Bladder stones	4 (1 %)
Neobladder surveillance	3 (1 %)
Lower Urinary Tract Symptoms	2 (<1 %)
Suspected fistula	1 (<1 %)
Surveillance follow Ureteric Cancer	1 (<1 %)

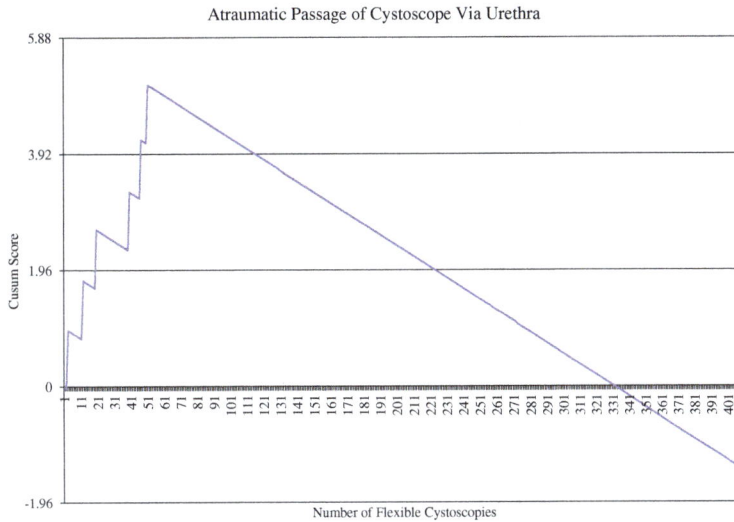

Fig. 1 Cumulative Sum (CUSUM) score for atraumatic passage of cystoscope via urethra (n = 409). Acceptable failure rate at 0.01 and unacceptable failure rate at 0.03. Type I and II error rate 0.1. Each horizontal line on the y-axis represents a control line (h = 1.96). Filled arrow identifies when competence is achieved

(positive gradient)] is first crossed at attempt 19 and again at attempt 47. During the first 51 attempts (Maximal point) there was a failure rate of 12 %. Performance begins to improve (no further unacceptable control lines crossed) and acceptable performance can be first concluded following attempt 117 when the acceptable control line is crossed [crossing the horizontal grid line from above to below (negative gradient)] [8]. Performance continues to improve crossing two further control lines following attempt 224 and 332. This component

successfully completed by 117 procedures and competence following 224 procedures.

2. Assessment of Body and Dome of Bladder
   Figure 2 shows the unacceptable control line (horizontal line crossed in an upwards fashion) is first crossed following attempt 3. The maximal point is achieved following 4 procedures and no further unacceptable control lines are crossed. Acceptable performance can be concluded following attempt 59 when the acceptable control line is crossed (crossing the horizontal line in a

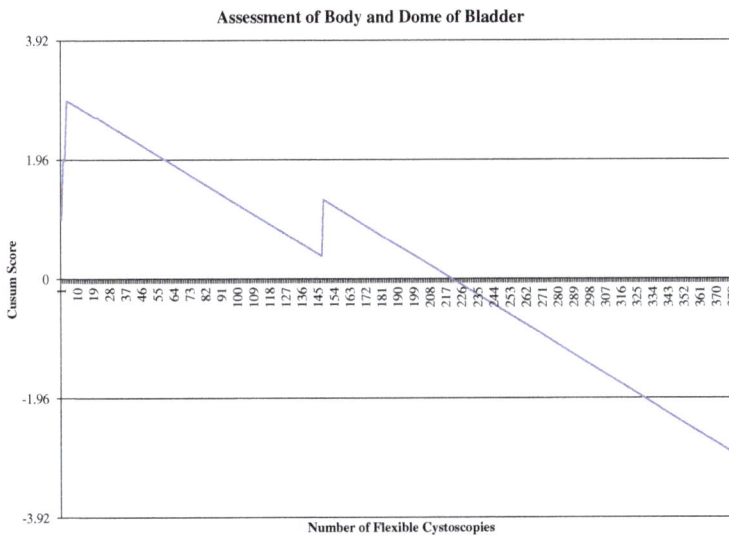

Fig. 2 Cumulative Sum (CUSUM) for assessment of body and dome of bladder (n = 384). Acceptable failure rate at 0.01 and unacceptable failure rate at 0.03. Type I and II error rate 0.1. Each horizontal line on the y-axis represents a control line (h = 1.96)

downwards fashion). No further failures occur and performance continues to improve, crossing two further control lines following attempt 221 and 330.

This component successfully completed by 59 procedures and competence following 221 procedures.

3. Identification of Trigone and Ureteric Orifices

Figure 3 shows the unacceptable control line (horizontal line crossed in an upwards fashion) is first crossed following the 3rd attempt with a further 15 unacceptable control lines continually crossed. Although the first acceptable control line is crossed following the 74th attempt, the overall trend continues upwards until attempt 136. From attempt 136 to 257 satisfactory performance is evident as no further unacceptable control lines are crossed. Three acceptable control lines are crossed following 258th to 301st procedure, although the unacceptable control line is crossed following 302nd procedure. No further unacceptable control lines are crossed in the final 81 procedures. Competence achieved following 279 procedures.

Due to the large number of acceptable and unacceptable control lines being crossed during CUSUM score, the average failure rate was calculated with the number of procedures being divided into thirds. The initial failure rate for the first 128 attempts was 34 %. Between the 128th and 254th procedures the failure rate improved to 9 % then continued to improve further with a failure rate of 5 % between the 254th and 383rd procedure.

4. Examination of the bladder neck

Figure 4 shows the unacceptable control line (horizontal line crossed in an upwards fashion) is first crossed following attempt 2 and again following attempt 4, 11 and 23. The maximal point is reached following the 23rd procedure. Acceptable performance can be concluded following the 65th procedure when the acceptable control line is crossed (crossing the horizontal line in a downwards fashion). However, failure following the 103rd procedure leads to an unacceptable control line being crossed. No further unacceptable control lines are crossed following this procedure, with the acceptable control line being crossed following the 121st, 229th and 338th procedure.

This component successfully completed by 103 procedures and competence following 229 procedures.

5. Performance of full procedure

Figure 5 shows the unacceptable control line first crossed following the 2nd attempt with a further 19 unacceptable control lines continually crossed. Acceptable performance is first achieved when the control line is crossed following the 118th procedure. However, acceptable performance is not maintained with multiple unacceptable control lines crossed. The maximal point was reached following 257th procedure with a sustained period of acceptable performance following this, crossing 2 consequence acceptable control lines following the 286th procedure. Competence achieved following 286 procedures.

Due to the large number of acceptable and unacceptable control lines being crossed, the average

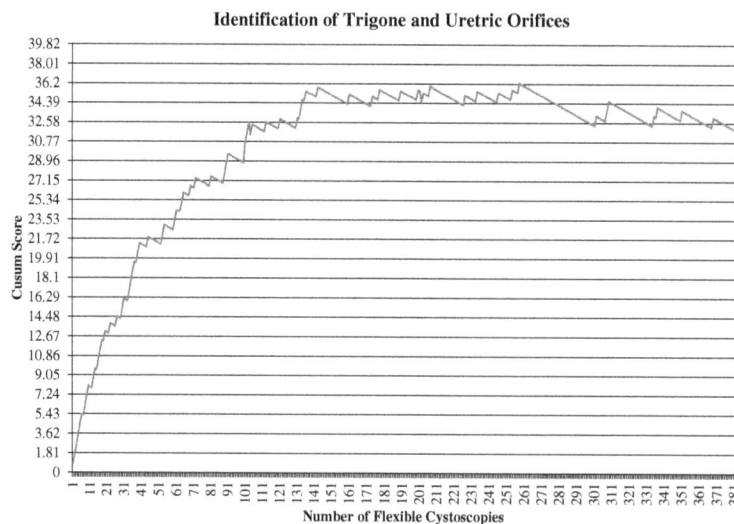

Fig. 3 Cumulative Sum (CUSUM) for identification of trigone and ureteric orifices (*n* = 383). Acceptable failure rate set at 0.05 and unacceptable failure rate at 0.15. Type I and II error rates 0.10. Each horizontal line on the y-axis represents a control line (h = 1.81)

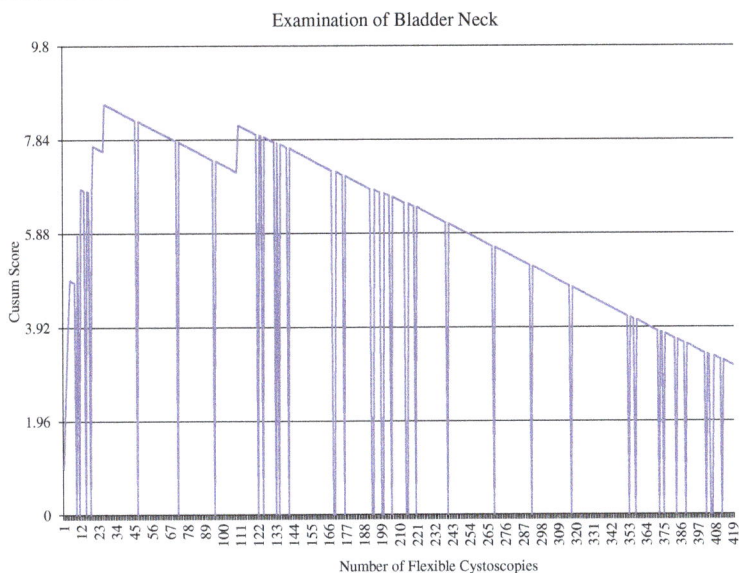

Fig. 4 Cumulative Sum (CUSUM) for examination of the bladder neck ($n = 383$). Acceptable failure rate set at 0.01 and unacceptable failure rate set at 0.03. Type I and II error rate 0.1. Each horizontal line on the y-axis represents a control line (h = 1.96)

failure rate was calculated with the number of procedures being divided into thirds. The failure rate of the first 128 procedures was 38 %. The failure rate between 128th and 256th procedure was 13 %. Improvement continued with a failure rate of 6 % between 257th and 383rd procedure.

Discussion

This study describes the learning curve to competency in FC of a trainee with no previous experience in endoscopy under supervision. In an era of quality assurance and credentialing the results provide further evidence that CUSUM analysis is an objective technique, which can be used to evaluate progression to competence.

The prospective data in the current study demonstrate that CUSUM is a relatively simple and sensitive method to apply practically to self assessment in surgical training. CUSUM was able to highlight areas for improvement, guiding further training in addition to defining competence. In this study, the trainee took longer to achieve, and maintain, competency than suggested indicative numbers [1].

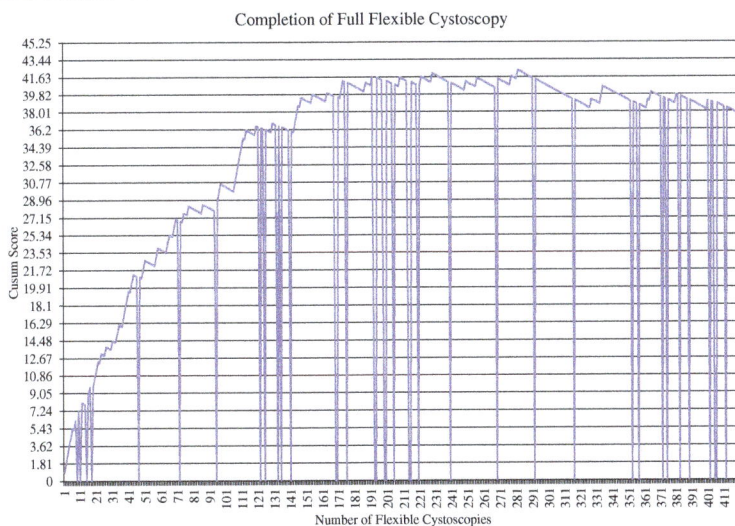

Fig. 5 Cumulative Sum (CUSUM) score for completion of full flexible cystoscopy ($n = 383$). Acceptable failure rate set at 0.05 and unacceptable failure rate at 0.15. Type I and II error rates 0.10. Each horizontal line on the y-axis represents a control line (h = 1.81)

The utility of CUSUM was that it was able to define the specific aspects of the procedure which the trainee found most difficult. For three out of five of the components, acceptable performance was maintained following the 122nd procedure. Competence in examination of the ureteric orifices and trigone was a FC step which took substantially longer to acquire, being achieved by the 280th procedure. CUSUM highlighted this as an area for targeted tuition in this trainee.

Even if it is assumed that performing a minimum number of procedures will result in competence the number of FCs required to attain competence has never been validated. BAUS recommended a minimum of 60 procedures in 2000 [1]. In 2014 the Speciality Advisory committee in Urology (SAC) stipulated that the indicative number of FCs which must be performed for the award of a Certificate of Completed Training (CCT) in Urology should be 300. Prior to this, a review of logbook data from trainees applying for CCT between 2010 and 2012 revealed that only 42 % had recorded flexible cystoscopy activity [11]. This wide range of recommendations and trainee activity highlights the need for an alternative method, such as CUSUM, to be introduced as a more robust modality for determining competence.

CUSUM analysis has not previously been used to assess skill acquisition in FC. Studies, using virtual reality simulators to assess skill acquisition for FC, have developed a five-point Global Rating Score (GRS). Although this has been of value in evaluating technical and non-technical skills, it may be limited by inter assessor variability [12, 13]. Such variability does not occur with CUSUM analysis due to each defined task having a binary outcome. In addition CUSUM has the advantage of being suitable for both self-assessment and supervisor assessment. As a result, CUSUM analysis has the potential to be incorporated into the trainee's curriculum with the plotted graphs providing readily visualised, accurate, comparable evidence of progression and competence rather than the current implicit logbook approach.

While ideally CUSUM could be used as a tool for assessing skill acquisition, and its maintenance, in trainees and consultants a significant issue is that the statistical calculations are detailed and time intensive. This may be one of the reasons why, to date, CUSUM has not been widely adopted. A possible development would be creation of software to facilitate the data entry and analysis.

The present study has limitations; CUSUM was demonstrated to be an objective technique however the authors acknowledge that only one trainee's performance was assessed. Maguire et al. used CUSUM analysis for the evaluation of a group of trainees performing retropubic mid-urethral sling procedures [14]. In keeping with that study, our study found the number of procedures required to acquire, and maintain, competence in performing the procedure was significantly more than expected [14]. Furthermore, Maguire at al. identified considerable variability in the number of procedures each trainee needed to achieve competence [14]. For CUSUM to be used for FC assessment routinely its applicability would have to be evaluated in a larger trainee cohort where similar inter-trainee variability is likely be identified. The very least that such a study would achieve would be a more accurate estimate of the range of indicative numbers which a trainee requires to achieve, and maintain, competence.

A key element in CUSUM analysis is the determination of the acceptable and unacceptable failure rates of the FC procedure. Another possible limitation of this study is that these rates were based on a relatively small sample of thirteen consultants. Despite the sample being representative of the centres involved in training in the South West of England it would be desirable to increase this sample size in future studies.

Patient experience and complication rates are important outcome measures, which are integral to true competence. Currently these measures are not incorporated into UK urology trainees' assessments. These factors were not assessed in this study as part of the CUSUM analysis because the focus was on FC performance. It would be appropriate in future studies to incorporate patient experience into CUSUM and a parallel audit to accurately capture complications.

Conclusion

This study demonstrates the successful use of CUSUM analysis in the assessment of surgical competence for FC. The method is one, which could be used to assess, and monitor competence, in surgical trainees, however, validation of the process, using a larger trainee cohort, is required.

Additional files

Additional file 1: CUSUM Equation. Additional file 1 is the mathematical equation used to calculate the value to increase or decrease the CUSUM score along with the equation used to establish the interval between control lines for each graph.

Additional file 2: NHS health research authority approval. Additional file 2 is the outcome of the online assessment by the NHS health research authority and the MRC of the study design.

Abbreviations

BAUS, British Association of Urological Surgeons; CCT, certificate of completed training; CUSUM, cumulative sum; FC, flexible cystoscopy; GRS, global rating score; ISCP, Intercollegiate Surgical Curriculum Programme; MRC, medical research council; NHS, National Health Service; SAC, Surgical Advisory Committee

Acknowledgements
We would like to thank Professor Kenneth MacKenzie for his assistance and guidance in this research.

Funding
No funding obtained.

Authors' contributions
KM researched the literature, conceived the study, obtained and analysed the data. KM & JA wrote the first draft. Both authors reviewed and edited the manuscript and approved the final draft of the manuscript.

Authors' information
KM MBChB, MRCS (Ed), Core Surgical Trainee Year 2, Northern Deanery.
JA BMBS, BMedSci, DM, FRCS (Urol), Consultant Urologist and Associate clinical lecturer, Newcastle Upton Tyne NHS Trust and University of Newcastle.

Competing interests
The authors declare no conflict of interest

References
1. Shah J, Darzi A. Validation of a flexible cystoscopy course. BJU Int. 2002; 90(9):833–5.
2. Vassiliou MC, Kaneva PA, Poulouse BK, et al. How should we establish the clinical case numbers required to achieve proficiency in flexible endoscopy? Am J Surg. 2010;199:121–5.
3. Sharp JF, Cozens N, Robinson I. Assessment of surgical competence in parotid surgery using a CUSUM assessment tool. Clin Otolaryngol Allied Sci. 2003;28(3):248–51.
4. Flexible Cystoscopy: Training and Assessment Guideline. British Association of Urological Nurses (BAUN) and British Association Urological Surgeons (BAUS). http://www.baus.org.uk/professionals/baus_business/publications/15/flexible_cystoscopy_guidelines__assessment. Accessed 3 Aug 2013.
5. Flexible Cystoscopy: Performance Criteria, Training & Assessment Logbook. British Association of Urological Nurses (BAUN) and British Association Urological Surgeons (BAUS). www.baus.org.uk/Updates/publications-new/flexi-cystoscpy. Accessed 3 Aug 2013.
6. Flexible Cystoscopy (Local Anaesthetic/Male and Female), Intercollegiate Surgical Curriculum Programme (ISCP). http://www.iscp.ac.uk. Accessed 3 Aug 2013.
7. Bolsin S, Colson M. The use of the CUSUM technique in the assessment of trainee competence in new procedures. Int J Qual Health Care. 2000; 12(5):433–8.
8. Waller HM, Connor SJ. Cumulative sum (CUSUM) analysis provides an objective measure of competency during training in endoscopic retrograde cholangio-pancreatography (ERCP). HPB (Oxford). 2009;11(7):565–9.
9. Weerasinghe S, Mirghani H, Revel A, Abu-Sidan FM. Cumulative Sum (CUSUM) analysis in the assessment of trainee competence in fetal biometry measurement. Ultrasound Obstet Gynecol. 2006;28(2):199–203.
10. Naik VN, Devito I, Halpern SH. Cusum analysis is a useful tool to assess resident proficiency at insertion of labour epidurals. Can J Anaesth. 2003; 50(7):694–8.
11. Robinson R, O'Flynn K. Indicative operative numbers in urology training in the UK and Ireland. J Clin Urol. 2015;8(3):188–95.
12. Schout BM, Muijtjens AM, Hendrix AJ, et al. Acquisition of flexible cystoscopy skills on a virtual reality simulator by experts and novices. BJU Int. 2010;105(2):234–9.
13. Schout B, Ananias H, Bemelmans B, et al. Transfer of cysto-urethroscopy skills from a virtual-reality simulator to the operating room: a randomized controlled trial. BJU Int. 2010;106(2):226–31.
14. Maguire T, Mayne CJ, Terry T, Tincello DG. Analysis of the surgical learning curve using the cumulative sum (CUSUM) method. Neurourol Urodyn. 2013;32(7):964–7.

12

Lymphovascular invasion status at transurethral resection of bladder tumors may predict subsequent poor response of T1 tumors to bacillus Calmette-Guérin

Keishiro Fukumoto[1], Eiji Kikuchi[1*], Shuji Mikami[2], Akira Miyajima[1] and Mototsugu Oya[1]

Abstract

Background: Lymphovascular invasion (LVI) is an important step in the process of tumor dissemination and metastasis outside the primary organ, but the relationship between LVI and the prognosis of T1 non-muscle invasive bladder cancer (NMIBC) has not been fully evaluated. Accordingly, the present study was performed to evaluate whether LVI had an impact on the clinical outcome in patients with T1 NMIBC.

Methods: A total of 116 consecutive patients were diagnosed with T1 NMIBC from 1994 to 2013 at Keio University Hospital. All cases were reviewed by a single uro-pathologist. The prognostic significance of LVI was assessed in relation to recurrence and stage progression.

Results: The median follow-up period was 53 months. LVI was histologically confirmed in 30 patients (25.9%). There were no significant differences of clinical features between the patients with and without LVI. In T1 patients, univariate analysis demonstrated that LVI positivity was associated with stage progression ($p = 0.003$), but not with tumor recurrence ($p = 0.192$). Multivariate analysis confirmed that LVI was independently associated with stage progression ($p = 0.006$, hazard ratio = 4.00). In 85 patients who received BCG instillation, LVI was independently associated with both tumor recurrence and stage progression ($p = 0.036$ and 0.024, hazard ratio = 2.19 and 3.76).

Conclusions: LVI is a strong indicator of an increased risk of recurrence and progression in BCG-treated patients with T1 NMIBC. This information might assist clinicians to develop appropriate management and counseling strategies for these patients.

Keywords: Urinary bladder neoplasms, Carcinoma, Transitional cell, Lymphatic metastasis, Recurrence, Disease progression

Background

The optimum management and therapeutic strategy for T1 non-muscle invasive bladder cancer (NMIBC) are still being debated. As T1 NMIBC has a higher risk of recurrence and higher progression rate, current guidelines recommend adjuvant therapy with bacillus Calmette-Guérin (BCG) after transurethral resection of bladder tumor (TURBT) [1]. However, recurrence affects about half of all patients with T1 NMIBC who receive BCG therapy and 17 %–23 % show progression to muscle invasive tumors [2, 3]. Patients with a very high risk of recurrence and stage progression should receive more aggressive therapy such as immediate total cystectomy [4]. The clinical outcome of immediate cystectomy for T1 NMIBC is good, with the 10-year disease-specific survival rate being approximately 80 % [5, 6], but not all T1 patients need radical surgery, which has a relatively high morbidity rate and reduces the quality of life [7]. One of the major issues regarding management of T1 NMIBC is the lack of appropriate tools for identifying patients with a very high risk of stage progression. Various prognostic factors that predict a poor outcome of

* Correspondence: eiji-k@kb3.so-net.ne.jp
[1]Department of Urology, Keio University School of Medicine, 35 Shinanomachi, Shinjuku-ku, Tokyo 160-0016, Japan
Full list of author information is available at the end of the article

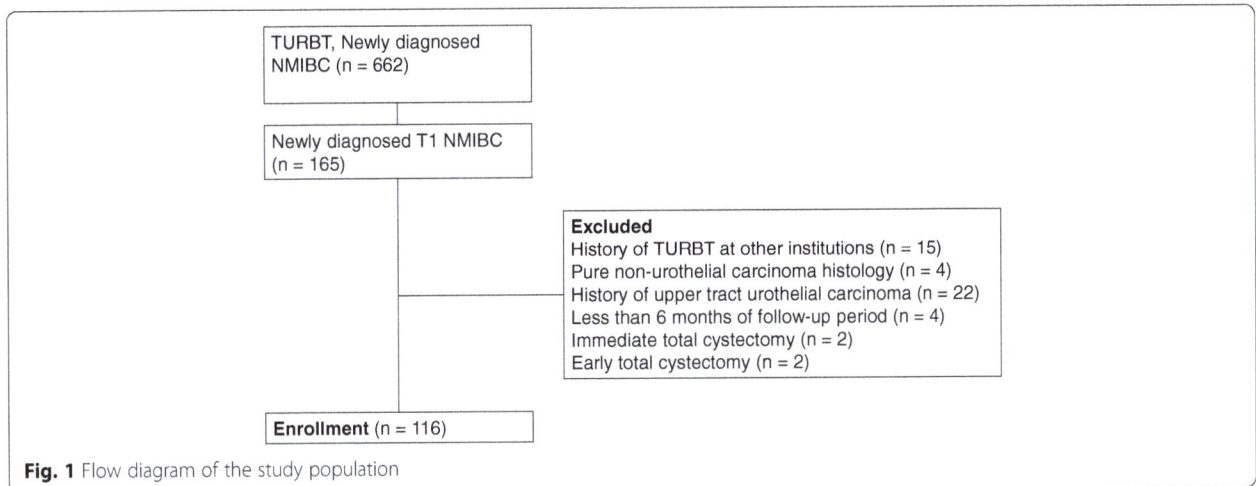

Fig. 1 Flow diagram of the study population

Flow diagram contents:

- TURBT, Newly diagnosed NMIBC (n = 662)
- Newly diagnosed T1 NMIBC (n = 165)

Excluded
History of TURBT at other institutions (n = 15)
Pure non-urothelial carcinoma histology (n = 4)
History of upper tract urothelial carcinoma (n = 22)
Less than 6 months of follow-up period (n = 4)
Immediate total cystectomy (n = 2)
Early total cystectomy (n = 2)

Enrollment (n = 116)

Ta/T1 NMIBC have been reported, including the sex [3], age [8, 9], tumor diameter [10], multifocality [8, 10], concomitant carcinoma in situ (CIS) [10, 11], CIS in the prostatic urethra [3], histological grade [8], and molecular grade determined by fluorescence in situ hybridization [12]. Lymphovascular invasion (LVI) is considered to be the most important step in the initiation of tumor dissemination/metastasis, and it has been identified as a strong indicator of a poor prognosis for various cancers, including carcinoma of the lung [13], breast [14], colon [15], kidney [16], and prostate [17], as well as urothelial carcinoma of the upper urinary tract [18, 19]. In patients with clinical stage I nonseminomatous testicular tumors, information on LVI status was reported to be important for making a decision about whether or not to provide adjuvant chemotherapy [20]. In patients with muscle invasive bladder cancer treated by total cystectomy, LVI is a strong indicator of poor survival, since the 10-year cancer-specific survival rate is 31.0 %–39.3 % for LVI-positive patients versus 72.0 %–73.6 % for LVI-negative patients [21, 22]. A few investigators have evaluated the influence of LVI in TURBT specimens of NMIBC patients, but conflicting results have been reported [23–26]. Therefore, we investigated the association of LVI status reviewed by a dedicated uro-pathologist with clinical background factors in T1 NMIBC patients and evaluated whether LVI was useful for identifying a higher risk of stage progression.

Methods
Patients
A total of 662 patients with newly diagnosed NMIBC were treated from January 1994 to December 2013 at Keio University Hospital and 165 patients had T1 NMIBC (Fig. 1). Fifteen patients who received TURBT at other institutions were excluded. Patients with pure non-urothelial carcinoma (e.g., squamous cell carcinoma

or adenocarcinoma), a history of upper tract urothelial carcinoma, and follow-up for less than 6 months were also excluded (4, 22, and 4 patients, respectively). Furthermore, we excluded 4 patients who had undergone total cystectomy without confirmation of progression. Two of them had received immediate total cystectomy, which meant that it was performed soon after TURBT without further intravesical therapy. The other 2 patients had received early total cystectomy, which was performed after recurrence but before stage progression. Finally, 116 subjects were included in this analysis, among whom 85 had received instillation of BCG after TURBT.

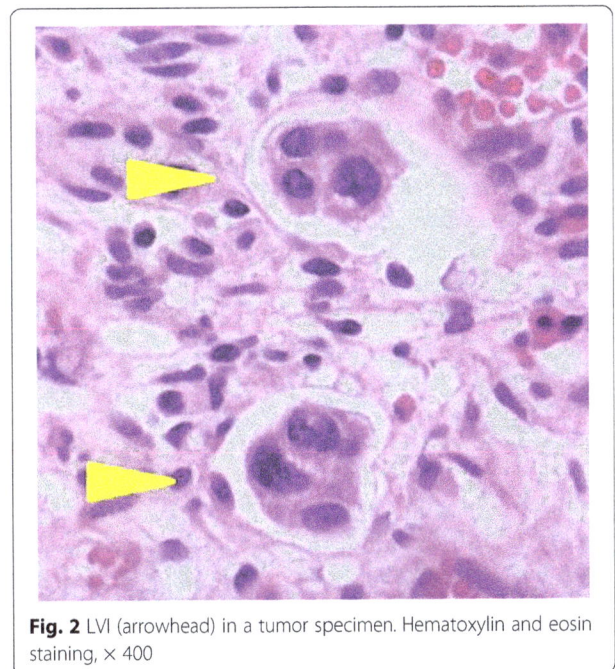

Fig. 2 LVI (arrowhead) in a tumor specimen. Hematoxylin and eosin staining, × 400

Table 1 Clinicopathological characteristics of 116 patients stratified according to LVI status

Characteristic	Total		LVI positive		LVI negative		p value
No. of patients	116		30		86		
Age							0.073
<70 years	55	(47.4 %)	10	(33.3 %)	45	(52.3 %)	
≥70 years	61	(52.6 %)	20	(66.7 %)	41	(47.7 %)	
Sex							0.256
Male	98	(84.5 %)	27	(90.0 %)	71	(82.6 %)	
Female	18	(15.5 %)	3	(10.0 %)	15	(17.4 %)	
Tumor grade							0.115
G1/2	7	(6.0 %)	0	(0.0%)	7	(8.1 %)	
G3	109	(94.0 %)	30	(100.0%)	79	(91.9 %)	
Concomitant CIS							0.247
Positive	26	(22.4 %)	9	(30.0 %)	17	(19.8 %)	
Negative	90	(77.6 %)	21	(70.0 %)	69	(80.2 %)	
Multifocality							0.638
Multiple	85	(73.3 %)	21	(70.0 %)	64	(74.4 %)	
Solitary	31	(26.7 %)	9	(30.0 %)	22	(25.6 %)	
BCG instillation							0.334
Yes	85	(73.3 %)	24	(80.0 %)	61	(70.9 %)	
No	31	(26.7 %)	6	(20.0 %)	25	(29.1 %)	
Intravesical chemotherapy							0.601
Yes	16	(13.8 %)	4	(13.3 %)	12	(14.0 %)	
No	100	(86.2 %)	26	(86.7%)	74	(86.0 %)	
History of Ta NMIBC							0.418
Recurrence	7	(6.0 %)	1	(3.3 %)	6	(7.0 %)	
Primary	109	(94.0 %)	29	(96.7 %)	80	(93.0 %)	

LVI Lymphovascular invasion, *CIS* Carcinoma in situ, *BCG* Bacillus Calmette-Guérin, *NMIBC* Non-muscle invasive bladder cancer

Evaluation of resected specimens

All specimens were reviewed by a dedicated uropathologist who was unaware of the clinical outcome. Based on examination of hematoxylin and eosin stained sections, LVI was considered to be present when tumor cells were unequivocally noted within or attached to the walls of a vascular or lymphatic space (Fig. 2). Multiple serial sections were viewed and immunohistochemical markers for lymphatic channels (D2-40) and endothelial cells (CD31/34) were used in equivocal cases.

Treatment

Intravesical BCG therapy was generally performed for intermediate or high risk NMIBC according to the current clinical guidelines [1]. However, the attending physician and/or patient sometimes decided against treatment with BCG because of side effects. Instillation of BCG was begun 4 to 5 weeks after TURBT and was continued at weekly intervals for 6 to 8 weeks at a dose of 80 mg (Tokyo 172 strain) or 81 mg (Connaught strain). Patients were followed postoperatively with cystoscopy and urinary cytology every 3 months for 2 years, every 6 months for the next 3 years, and annually thereafter. Excretory urography and/or computed tomography were performed to evaluate the upper urinary tract every year for 5 years after treatment.

Endpoints

We defined tumor recurrence as any evidence of disease on follow-up evaluation, while progression was defined as muscle invasion or metastasis. Recurrence-free survival time was calculated as the interval between TURBT and the date of tumor recurrence, while progression-free survival was determined from the date of TURBT to progression. Cancer-specific survival and overall survival were based on death from bladder cancer and death from any cause, respectively.

Statistical analysis

Variables were compared between different groups by using the χ2 test. Recurrence-and progression-free survival rates were estimated by the Kaplan-Meier method.

Table 2 Results of univariate and multivariate analyses

Characteristic	Recurrence-free survival			Progression-free survival		
	Univariate	Multivariate		Univariate	Multivariate	
	p value	HR (95 % CI)	p value	p value	HR (95 % CI)	p value
Age	0.133			0.775		
<70 years						
≥70 years						
Sex	0.166			0.861		
Male						
Female						
Tumor grade	0.916			0.289		
G1/2						
G3						
Concomitant CIS	0.653			0.925		
Positive						
Negative						
Multifocality	0.063			0.344		
Single						
Multiple						
BCG instillation	0.005		0.007	0.953		
Yes		0.44 (0.24–0.80)				
No						
Intravesical chemotherapy	0.007			0.631		
Yes						
No						
History of Ta NMIBC	0.735			0.245		
Recurrence						
Primary						
Lymphovascular invasion	0.192			0.003		0.006
Positive					4.00 (1.49–10.75)	
Negative						

Survival curves were compared with the log-rank test. Univariate and multivariate analyses of tumor recurrence and stage progression were done using the Cox proportional hazards model with stepwise forward regression. The independent variables included in survival analysis were patient age (<70 vs. ≥70 years), sex, tumor grade (G1/2 vs. G3), concomitant CIS, multifocality, intravesical BCG therapy, intravesical chemotherapy, a history of Ta NMIBC, and LVI status (positive or negative). Differences between groups were regarded as significant at $P < 0.05$. All analyses were performed with the SPSS v. 21.0 statistical software package (IBM Corp., Somers, NY).

Ethics and consent

This study was conducted subject to the guidelines of the Declaration of Helsinki and approved by our ethical committee. The reference number is 20130101. The ethical committee exempted obtaining informed consent because our study design was done by a retrospective fashion. Data were obtained from medical chart and patient identifying information was anonymized before analysis.

Results

Clinicopathological characteristics of the 116 patients

The median age of the patients was 70.6 years (range: 40 to 89 years). Men accounted for 84.5% of the patients ($n = 98$) and women for 15.5% ($n = 18$). LVI was histologically confirmed in 30 patients (25.9%). Table 1 presents the association between clinicopathological characteristics and LVI status in the 116 patients. There were no significant differences of clinical features between the LVI-positive and LVI-negative

Table 3 Clinicopathological characteristics of 85 BCG-treated patients stratified according to LVI status

Characteristic	Total		LVI positive		LVI negative		P value
No. of patients	85		24		61		
Age							0.074
<70 years	45	(52.9%)	9	(37.5%)	36	(59.0%)	
≥70 years	40	(47.1%)	15	(62.5%)	25	(41.0%)	
Sex							0.174
Male	71	(83.5%)	22	(91.7%)	49	(80.3%)	
Female	14	(16.5%)	2	(8.3%)	12	(19.7%)	
Tumor grade							0.258
G1/2	4	(4.7%)	0	(0.0%)	4	(6.6%)	
G3	81	(95.3%)	24	(100.0%)	57	(93.4%)	
Concomitant CIS							0.969
Positive	21	(24.7%)	6	(25.0%)	15	(24.6%)	
Negative	64	(75.3%)	18	(75.0%)	46	(75.4%)	
Multifocality							0.905
Multiple	61	(71.8%)	17	(70.8%)	44	(72.1%)	
Solitary	24	(28.2%)	7	(29.2%)	17	(27.9%)	
History of Ta NMIBC							0.563
Recurrence	5	(5.9%)	1	(4.2%)	4	(6.6%)	
Primary	80	(94.1%)	23	(95.8%)	57	(93.4%)	

patients. During the median follow-up period of 53 months (range: 6–239 months), 47 of 116 patients (40.5%) experienced recurrence and 16 patients (13.8%) showed stage progression. Of the 16 patients with stage progressions, one had distant metastasis. Fourteen patients died (12.1%) and 7 patients (6.0%) died of their disease.

Predictors of recurrence and stage progression in all patients

Univariate and multivariate analyses were performed to determine the predictors of tumor recurrence and stage progression (Table 2). Recurrence was noted in 16 patients (53.3%) from the LVI-positive group and 31 patients (36.0%) from the LVI-negative group. Treatment with BCG ($p = 0.005$) and intravesical chemotherapy ($p = 0.007$) had a significant influence on tumor recurrence according to univariate analysis. Multivariate Cox regression analysis showed that BCG therapy was an independent determinant of a lower risk of tumor recurrence ($p = 0.007$, hazard ratio (HR) = 0.44).

Nine patients (30.0%) with LVI demonstrated stage progression, as did 7 patients (8.1%) without LVI. Kaplan-Meier analysis showed that patients in the LVI-positive group had a higher risk of stage progression, with the 5-year progression-free survival rate being 61.8% in LVI-positive patients and 90.4% in LVI-negative

patients ($p = 0.003$). Multivariate analysis demonstrated that LVI had an independent influence on progression-free survival ($p = 0.006$, HR = 4.00).

Predictors of recurrence and stage progression in patients treated with BCG

We performed a subgroup analysis of the 85 patients who received BCG therapy. Their clinicopathological characteristics are listed in Table 3. There were no significant differences of clinical features between the LVI-positive and LVI-negative patients. We investigated whether LVI had a prognostic impact on tumor recurrence and stage progression (Table 4). Among the 85 patients, LVI was confirmed in 24 patients (28.2%). In the LVI-positive group, 13 patients (54.2%) experienced recurrence and 7 patients (29.2%) showed stage progression, while the corresponding numbers in the LVI-negative group were 16 (26.2%) and 5 (8.2%), respectively. Kaplan-Meier analysis revealed that the 5-year recurrence-free and progression-free survival rates of LVI-positive patients were 39.5% and 65.9%, respectively, which were significantly lower than those of LVI-negative patients (71.2% and 90.8%, $p = 0.032$ and 0.015, respectively; Figs. 3 and 4). Multivariate analysis confirmed that LVI had an independent influence on recurrence-free and progression-free survival in T1 NMIBC patients treated with BCG ($p = 0.036$ and 0.024, HR = 2.19 and 3.76, respectively).

Association of LVI status with cancer-specific survival and overall survival

Among 16 patients with stage progression, 7 underwent total cystectomy, 3 were treated with radiation therapy, and 1 received systemic chemotherapy. Five patients received no treatment at their request. The 5-year cancer-specific survival rate of LVI-negative patients was 96.3%, which was marginally higher than that of LVI-positive patients (79.8%, $p = 0.07$). The 5-year overall survival rate of LVI-negative patients was 89.4%, which was not significantly different from that of LVI-positive patients (71.8%, $p = 0.185$). In the patients treated with BCG, LVI status was not associated with either cancer-specific survival or overall survival ($p = 0.143$ and 0.235, respectively).

Discussion

Our study of 116 patients with T1 NMIBC revealed that LVI was significantly associated with stage progression after TURBT. In addition, we confirmed that LVI positivity was an independent risk factor for tumor recurrence and progression in T1 NMIBC patients treated with intravesical BCG instillation. To the best of our knowledge, this is the first report that LVI in TURBT specimens is significantly associated with recurrence and

Table 4 Results of univariate and multivariate analyses in patients treated with BCG after TURBT

Characteristic	Recurrence-free survival			Progression-free survival		
	Univariate	Multivariate		Univariate	Multivariate	
	p value	HR (95% CI)	p value	p value	HR (95% CI)	p value
Age	0.095			0.523		
<70 years						
≥70 years						
Sex	0.677			0.491		
Male						
Female						
Tumor grade	0.593			0.424		
G1/2						
G3						
Concomitant CIS	0.728			0.943		
Positive						
Negative						
Multifocality	0.064			0.250		
Single						
Multiple						
History of Ta NMIBC	0.694			0.079		
Recurrence						
Primary						
Lymphovascular invasion	0.032		0.036	0.015		0.024
Positive		2.19 (1.05–4.55)			3.76 (1.19–11.90)	
Negative						

stage progression of T1 NMIBC after treatment with BCG.

T1 NMIBC has a high potential for recurrence, and some patients experience stage progression that requires more aggressive therapy such as total cystectomy. Therefore, it is critical to identify the subset of T1 NMIBC patients whose tumors are highly malignant and have the potential to progress to muscle invasive disease. Various biological markers (such as p16, pRb, p53, MIB-1, and HSP90) have been studied for identifying aggressive T1 tumors [27–29], but these are relatively expensive and require additional procedures for histopathological analysis. In contrast, LVI can easily be investigated during standard histopathological evaluation.

Several investigators have already investigated whether the LVI status of TURBT specimens was a prognostic factor in patients with NMIBC. Lopez et al. [23] reported an LVI positivity rate of 10% (17/170 T1 NMIBC patients) in their series and found that the LVI status was associated with overall survival. However, their patients were collected from 1983 to 1990 and were treated by adjuvant intravesical chemotherapy (mitomycin C or Adriamycin). Also, they did not determine the predictive value of LVI status for recurrence or stage

progression by multivariate analysis. Andius et al. [24] analyzed 121 patients with T1 NMIBC, and found an association between LVI status and stage progression as well as cancer-specific survival. The same pathologist reviewed all histopathological material, as was done in our study, and LVI was confirmed in 12 patients (10%). In multivariate analysis, LVI was associated with both stage progression and cancer-specific survival. However, TURBT was performed between 1987 and 1988 in their study, and only one patient received adjuvant BCG instillation. Conflicting results with regard to the predictive value of LVI status for a poor clinical outcome have been reported in the era when BCG was established as standard adjuvant therapy for T1 NMIBC. Cho et al. [25] reviewed 118 patients with T1 NMIBC who underwent TURBT between 2001 and 2007, and evaluated the impact of LVI on tumor recurrence, stage progression, and metastasis. Two independent uro-pathologists reviewed the slides and found 33 LVI-positive patients (28%). Their multivariate analysis showed that LVI was significantly associated with tumor recurrence and stage progression, but the study population had a low rate of BCG instillation (22.9%). Branchereau et al. [26] assessed the prognostic value of LVI in 108 patients with high

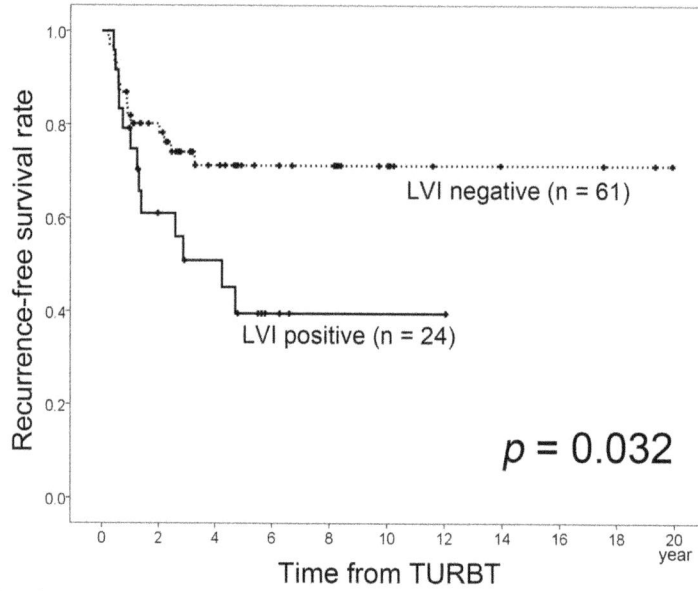

Fig. 3 Recurrence-free survival rate according to LVI status in patients treated with BCG

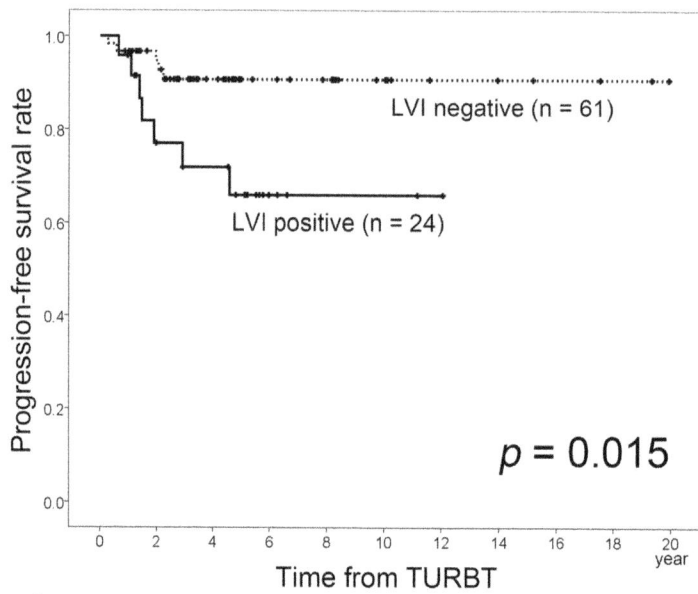

Fig. 4 Progression-free survival rate according to LVI status in patients treated with BCG

grade T1 NMIBC, including 60 patients (57%) who received adjuvant BCG therapy after TURBT. They reported that LVI was not associated with tumor recurrence, stage progression, cancer-specific survival, or overall survival. In contrast, we clearly demonstrated that LVI status could independently predict recurrence and stage progression in T1 NMIBC patients receiving BCG therapy and that evaluation of LVI in tumor specimens could provide useful information planning the appropriate management strategy and patient counseling.

In the present series, the LVI status was only described for 54 patients (46.6%) in the original pathology reports. Among the remaining 62 patients (53.4%), a further 13 LVI-positive cases were found after review by our uro-pathologist. At our institution, some pathologists routinely evaluate LVI, while others do not mention the LVI status. One of the reasons for this difference might be that the predictive role of LVI status in TURBT specimens has not been established clinically, especially for T1 NMIBC. Berman et al. evaluated 2802 patients with muscle invasive bladder tumors treated by total cystectomy using the Ontario cancer registry dataset and found that pathology reports failed to address LVI status in 25%, with LVI reporting rates being significantly higher at the high volume centers for total cystectomy [30]. They concluded that assessment of LVI status in a standardized manner across all bladder specimens by pathologists is essential to improve the diagnostic and therapeutic strategies for this cancer. Our findings indicated that urologists and pathologists should share information concerning the prognostic significance of LVI, even in T1 NMIBC, emphasizing the importance of assessing and reporting LVI.

The present study had several limitations, including a small number of patients initially diagnosed with T1 bladder cancer and the long study period of 20 years, which was likely to have led to the low repeat TURBT rate (18.1%). Furthermore, we did not routinely perform maintenance BCG therapy in patients initially diagnosed with T1 bladder cancer and treatment after TURBT was not uniform. While 85 patients (73.3%) were treated with BCG, others received intravesical chemotherapy (13.8%) or no adjuvant therapy (12.9%). Therefore, we performed a subgroup analysis of the patients who received BCG therapy, which revealed that LVI status was an independent predictor of recurrence and stage progression in these patients. Since this study was retrospective, we cannot exclude the possibility of unknown biases, but we believe that consistent pathological data was obtained because the same uro-pathologist reviewed all of the specimens.

Conclusions

The presence of LVI is a strong risk factor for tumor recurrence and stage progression in T1 NMIBC patients treated with BCG. This finding might assist in the development of appropriate management and counseling strategies for T1 NMIBC patients. Urologists and pathologists should be aware of the prognostic significance of LVI in T1 disease.

Abbreviations
NMIBC: Non-muscle invasive bladder cancer; BCG: Bacillus Calmette-Guérin; CIS: Carcinoma in situ; TURBT: Transurethral resection of bladder tumor; LVI: Lymphovascular invasion; HR: Hazard ratio.

Competing interests
The authors declare that they have no competing interests.

Authors' contributions
KF formulated the database, performed the analyses, and drafted the first manuscript. SM reviewed all TURBT specimens and revised the manuscript for pathological content. EK conceived the study, participated in its design and coordination, and helped to draft the manuscript. MA and OM assisted in the analysis and interpretation of data, and helped to draft the manuscript. All authors read and approved the final manuscript.

Acknowledgements
The authors are grateful to the staff of the Department of Urology and the Division of Diagnostic Pathology at Keio University School of Medicine. This work was supported by Japan Society for the Promotion of Science [KAKENHI Grant Number 15K20107].

Author details
[1]Department of Urology, Keio University School of Medicine, 35 Shinanomachi, Shinjuku-ku, Tokyo 160-0016, Japan. [2]Division of Diagnostic Pathology, Keio University School of Medicine, Tokyo, Japan.

References
1. Babjuk M, Burger M, Zigeuner R, Shariat SF, van Rhijn BW, Comperat E, et al. EAU guidelines on non-muscle-invasive urothelial carcinoma of the bladder: update 2013. Eur Urol. 2013;64(4):639–53.
2. Hemdan T, Johansson R, Jahnson S, Hellstrom P, Tasdemir I, Malmstrom PU, et al. 5-Year outcome of a randomized prospective study comparing bacillus Calmette-Guerin with epirubicin and interferon-alpha2b in patients with T1 bladder cancer. J Urol. 2014;191(5):1244–9.
3. Palou J, Sylvester RJ, Faba OR, Parada R, Pena JA, Algaba F, et al. Female gender and carcinoma in situ in the prostatic urethra are prognostic factors for recurrence, progression, and disease-specific mortality in T1G3 bladder cancer patients treated with bacillus Calmette-Guerin. Eur Urol. 2012;62(1):118–25.
4. Lebret T, Neuzillet Y. Indication and timing of cystectomy in high-risk bladder cancer. Curr Opin Urol. 2012;22(5):427–31.
5. Hautmann RE, Volkmer BG, Gust K. Quantification of the survival benefit of early versus deferred cystectomy in high-risk non-muscle invasive bladder cancer (T1 G3). World J Urol. 2009;27(3):347–51.
6. Denzinger S, Fritsche HM, Otto W, Blana A, Wieland WF, Burger M. Early versus deferred cystectomy for initial high-risk pT1G3 urothelial carcinoma of the bladder: do risk factors define feasibility of bladder-sparing approach? Eur Urol. 2008;53(1):146–52.
7. Roghmann F, Trinh QD, Braun K, von Bodman C, Brock M, Noldus J, et al. Standardized assessment of complications in a contemporary series of European patients undergoing radical cystectomy. Int J Urol. 2014;21(2):143–9.
8. Fernandez-Gomez J, Solsona E, Unda M, Martinez-Pineiro L, Gonzalez M, Hernandez R, et al. Prognostic factors in patients with non-muscle-invasive bladder cancer treated with bacillus Calmette-Guerin: multivariate analysis of data from four randomized CUETO trials. Eur Urol. 2008;53(5):992–1001.

9.   Joudi FN, Smith BJ, O'Donnell MA, Konety BR. The impact of age on the response of patients with superficial bladder cancer to intravesical immunotherapy. J Urol. 2006;175(5):1634–40.

10. Denzinger S, Otto W, Fritsche HM, Roessler W, Wieland WF, Hartmann A, et al. Bladder sparing approach for initial T1G3 bladder cancer: do multifocality, size of tumor or concomitant carcinoma in situ matter? A long-term analysis of 132 patients. Int J Urol. 2007;14(11):995–9.

11. Kakiashvili DM, van Rhijn BW, Trottier G, Jewett MA, Fleshner NE, Finelli A, et al. Long-term follow-up of T1 high-grade bladder cancer after intravesical bacille Calmette-Guerin treatment. BJU Int. 2011;107(4):540–6.

12. Lodde M, Mian C, Mayr R, Comploj E, Trenti E, Melotti R, et al. Recurrence and progression in patients with non-muscle invasive bladder cancer: Prognostic models including multicolor fluorescence in situ hybridization molecular grading. Int J Urol. 2014;21(10):968–72.

13. Mollberg NM, Bennette C, Howell E, Backhus L, Devine B, Ferguson MK. Lymphovascular invasion as a prognostic indicator in stage I non-small cell lung cancer: a systematic review and meta-analysis. Ann Thorac Surg. 2014; 97(3):965–71.

14. Rakha EA, Martin S, Lee AH, Morgan D, Pharoah PD, Hodi Z, et al. The prognostic significance of lymphovascular invasion in invasive breast carcinoma. Cancer. 2012;118(15):3670–80.

15. Lim SB, Yu CS, Jang SJ, Kim TW, Kim JH, Kim JC. Prognostic significance of lymphovascular invasion in sporadic colorectal cancer. Dis Colon Rectum. 2010;53(4):377–84.

16. Kim SH, Yang HK, Moon KC, Lee ES. Localized non-conventional renal cell carcinoma: prediction of clinical outcome according to histology. Int J Urol. 2014;21(4):359–64.

17. Cheng L, Jones TD, Lin H, Eble JN, Zeng G, Carr MD, et al. Lymphovascular invasion is an independent prognostic factor in prostatic adenocarcinoma. J Urol. 2005;174(6):2181–5.

18. Fujita K, Tanigawa G, Imamura R, Nakagawa M, Hayashi T, Kishimoto N, et al. Preoperative serum sodium is associated with cancer-specific survival in patients with upper urinary tract urothelial carcinoma treated by nephroureterectomy. Int J Urol. 2013;20(6):594–601.

19. Seisen T, Colin P, Hupertan V, Yates DR, Xylinas E, Nison L, et al. Post-operative nomogram to predict cancer-specific survival after radical nephroureterectomy in patients with localized and/or locally advanced upper tract urothelial carcinoma without metastasis. BJU Int. 2014;114(5):733–40.

20. Albers P, Albrecht W, Algaba F, Bokemeyer C, Cohn-Cedermark G, Fizazi K, et al. EAU guidelines on testicular cancer: 2011 update. Eur Urol. 2011;60(2): 304–19.

21. Shariat SF, Karakiewicz PI, Palapattu GS, Lotan Y, Rogers CG, Amiel GE, et al. Outcomes of radical cystectomy for transitional cell carcinoma of the bladder: a contemporary series from the Bladder Cancer Research Consortium. J Urol. 2006;176(6 Pt 1):2414–22.

22. Shariat SF, Svatek RS, Tilki D, Skinner E, Karakiewicz PI, Capitanio U, et al. International validation of the prognostic value of lymphovascular invasion in patients treated with radical cystectomy. BJU Int. 2010;105(10):1402–12.

23. Lopez JI, Angulo JC. The prognostic significance of vascular invasion in stage T1 bladder cancer. Histopathology. 1995;27(1):27–33.

24. Andius P, Johansson SL, Holmang S. Prognostic factors in stage T1 bladder cancer: tumor pattern (solid or papillary) and vascular invasion more important than depth of invasion. Urology. 2007;70(4):758–62.

25. Cho KS, Seo HK, Joung JY, Park WS, Ro JY, Han KS, et al. Lymphovascular invasion in transurethral resection specimens as predictor of progression and metastasis in patients with newly diagnosed T1 bladder urothelial cancer. J Urol. 2009;182(6):2625–30.

26. Branchereau J, Larue S, Vayleux B, Karam G, Bouchot O, Rigaud J. Prognostic value of the lymphovascular invasion in high-grade stage pT1 bladder cancer. Clin Genitourin Cancer. 2013;11(2):182–8.

27. Sato M, Yanai H, Morito T, Oda W, Shin-no Y, Yamadori I, et al. Association between the expression pattern of p16, pRb and p53 and the response to intravesical bacillus Calmette-Guerin therapy in patients with urothelial carcinoma in situ of the urinary bladder. Pathol Int. 2011;61(8):456–60.

28. Lebret T, Becette V, Herve JM, Molinie V, Barre P, Lugagne PM, et al. Prognostic value of MIB-1 antibody labeling index to predict response to Bacillus Calmette-Guerin therapy in a high-risk selected population of patients with stage T1 grade G3 bladder cancer. Eur Urol. 2000;37(6):654–9.

29. Lebret T, Watson RW, Molinie V, Poulain JE, O'Neill A, Fitzpatrick JM, et al. HSP90 expression: a new predictive factor for BCG response in stage Ta-T1 grade 3 bladder tumours. Eur Urol. 2007;51(1):161–6.

30. Berman DM, Kawashima A, Peng Y, Mackillop WJ, Siemens DR, Booth CM. Reporting trends and prognostic significance of lymphovascular invasion in muscle-invasive urothelial carcinoma: a population-based study. Int J Urol. 2014;22(2):163–70.

13

Multi-disciplinary surgical approach to the management of patients with renal cell carcinoma with venous tumor thrombus

Bishoy A. Gayed[1†], Ramy Youssef[1†], Oussama Darwish[1], Payal Kapur[2], Aditya Bagrodia[1], James Brugarolas[3], Ganesh Raj[1], J. Michael DiMaio[4], Arthur Sagalowsky[1] and Vitaly Margulis[1*]

Abstract

Background: The management of patients with renal cell carcinoma (RCC) with venous tumor thrombus (VTT) is challenging. We report our 15 year experience in the management of patients with RCC with VTT utilizing a multidisciplinary team approach, highlighting improved total and specifically Clavien III-V complication rates.

Methods: We reviewed the records of 146 consecutive patients who underwent radical nephrectomy with venous thrombectomy between 1998 and 2012. Data on patient history, staging, surgical techniques, morbidity, and survival were analyzed. Additionally, complication rates between two surgical eras, 1998–2006 and 2006–2012, were assessed.

Results: The study included 146 patients, 97 males (66 %), and a median age of 61 years (range, 24–83). Overall complications rate was 53 %, high grade complications (Clavien III -V) occurred in 10 % of patients. Most importantly, there was a lower incidence of overall and high grade complications (45 % and 8 %, respectively) in the last 6 years compared to the earlier surgeries included in the study (67 % and 13 % respectively) [$p = .008$ and .03, respectively). 30 day postoperative mortality was 2.7 %. 5 year overall survival (5Y- OS) and 5 year cancer specific survival (5Y- CSS) were 51 % and 40 %, respectively. Metastasis was the only independent predictor factor for CSS (HR 3.8, CI 1.9-7.6 and $p < .001$) and OS (HR 2.6, CI 1.5-4.7 and $p = .001$) in all patients.

Conclusions: Our data suggest that patients with RCC and VTT can be treated safely utilizing a multidisciplinary team approach leading to a decrease in complication rates.

Key words: Renal cell carcinoma, IVC thrombus, Outcomes

Background

In 2015, there will be nearly 62000 newly diagnosed cases of RCC and 14000 deaths due to RCC [1]. RCC has the propensity to extend into the renal vein, inferior vena cava (IVC) and up to the right atrium in up to 23 %, 10 %, and 1 % of cases, respectively [2, 3]. Refinements in clinical imaging, with CT and MRI, have improved accurate evaluation of primary tumors and the level of venous tumor thrombus (VTT) [2, 4]. Radical nephrectomy (RN) and IVC thrombectomy (IVCT) is challenging, particularly with a high VTT level [3–5].

Throughout the course of our experience, we have continued to improve our technique employing several modifications. We believe the most important modification we have made has been constantly ensuring we have the same urologic oncologists, cardiac anesthesia team, cardiac surgeons, and a dedicated cardiac scrub team at all cases. This brings familiarity to these challenging cases, which helps better manage both intraoperative and postoperative complications. Additionally, we have deferred from preforming sternotomies for high level 3 cases to avoid the morbidity of a sternotomy. With effective liver mobilization and use of pericardial windows

* Correspondence: vitaly.margulis@utsouthwestern.edu
†Equal contributors
[1]Department of Urology, University of Texas Southwestern Medical Center, 5323 Harry Hines Blvd., Dallas, TX 75390-9110, USA
Full list of author information is available at the end of the article

extirpation of high level 3 is facilitated both safely and effectively. This has equated to improved patient recovery in the postoperative setting.

Herein, we review the management of RCC with VTT in the last 15 years, aiming to outline prognostic factors, outcomes, and complication rates in the context of a dedicated multidisciplinary surgical team.

Methods
Patient selection
Clinical data from electronic medical records of patients treated by radical nephrectomy (RN) for RCC with renal vein or IVC thrombus at our institution from January 1998 to June 2012 were retrospectively analyzed and placed into a UT Southwestern Medical Center IRB approved database. Research was carried out in compliance with the Helsinki Declaration. We did not obtain informed consent from patients, as this was a retrospective study. Relevant clinical data, pathological features, surgical techniques, hospital stay, perioperative morbidity and mortality, follow up and survival data were collected.

Preoperative evaluation and surgical techniques
The tumors were routinely staged by using abdominal and chest CT scans and chest radiography. MRI was used for better evaluation of VTT level at the discretion of the treating physician. Bone scans were used selectively when clinically indicated. Tumor thrombus extension was classified into 4 levels: level I, extension into the renal vein; level II, extension into the infrahepatic IVC; level III, IVC extension to the level of hepatic veins but below the diaphragm; and level IV, IVC extension above the diaphragm [6].

Preoperative renal artery angioembolization was performed at the discretion of the surgeon to facilitate arterial vascular control in patients with bulky tumor thrombus, hilar adenopathy, or hypervascularity. Surgeries were managed by a multidisciplinary team which included an experienced urologic oncology surgeon, cardiothoracic surgeon and cardiac anesthesiologist, and cardiac scrub team. Trans-esophageal echocardiography was used intraoperatively by the anesthesiologist to verify the cephalad extent of the thrombus, to monitor for tumor emboli, to confirm the complete removal of VTT, and to assess hemodynamic stability. Data regarding the duration of surgery, estimated blood loss and intraoperative complications were recorded.

Pathologic evaluation
Pathologic staging was assigned according to the 2010 TNM staging system [7]. Grading of the tumors was evaluated according to Fuhrman classification [8]. Additionally, pathological tumor size, adrenal involvement, regional lymph node (LN) involvement, tumor necrosis, histopathological cell type and the presence of sarcomatoid differentiation were recorded.

Outcome evaluation and statistical analysis
Perioperative morbidity and mortality within the first 30 and 90 days were recorded and graded according to the Clavien-Dindo grading system [9]. Patients without metastases were routinely followed after surgery every 3 months in the first year, every 6 months in the second year and then annually. Follow up included history, physical examination, metabolic panel, liver function tests, chest x-ray and an abdominal CT scan. Bone scan, chest CT, positron emission tomography or MRI were performed when clinically indicated.

Survival time was calculated from the date of the operation to the date of last follow up or date of death. Disease recurrence was defined as local failure in the RN bed or regional LNs, or distant metastasis. Disease-free survival (DFS) was defined as the time between the date of surgery and the development of local recurrence or distant metastasis. Censored survival values represent patients who were alive without clinical evidence of disease at the last follow up. Cancer-specific survival (CSS) and overall survival (OS) were defined as the time between the date of surgery and death due to cancer (CSS) or due to any cause (OS). The following factors that could potentially affect outcomes were analyzed: age, gender, body mass index and performance status; T stage, VTT level, pathological tumor size, nodal involvement, metastasis at presentation, grade, sarcomatoid differentiation, histological subtype, fat invasion, adrenal involvement and tumor necrosis. Endpoints were CSS and OS. DFS was analyzed only in M0 patients. Finally, independent predictors of disease recurrence and cancer specific mortality were determined using multivariate Cox Regression analyses including only factors significant in univariate analyses. Statistically significant difference was set at $p < .05$. All statistical tests were performed with SPSS version 19.0.

Results
Clinico-pathological features
Patient demographics and clinical characteristics of the 146 patients included in the study are shown in Table 1. Hematuria and flank pain were the most common presenting symptoms (46 % and 38 % respectively). Overall, 42 (29 %) presented with distant metastases (M+), 29 patients (20 %) had LN+. and there was no significant relation between the VTT level and presence of M+ or LN+ disease ($p = 0.3$). Metastatic sites included: lungs (11 patients), liver (5 patients), bone (5 patients), adrenal (5 patients; 4 in the ipsilateral and 1 in the contralateral adrenal) and multiple sites (5 patients).

Table 1 Patient demographics and clinical characteristics

	All (%)	Era 1 (%)	Era 2 (%)
All patients (%)	146 (100)	64 (44)	82 (56)
Age, median (range) y	61 ± 12	57 ± 12	64 ± 11
	(24–82)	(35–83)	(24–82)
Sex			
Male	97 (66)	42 (66)	55 (67)
Female	49 (34)	22 (34)	27 (33)
Side			
Right	82 (56)	34 (53)	48 (59)
Left	64 (44)	30 (47)	34 (41)
Race or ethnic group			
Caucasian	96 (66)	41 (64)	55 (67)
Hispanic	25 (17)	15 (23)	10 (12)
Black	15 (10)	4 (6)	11 (13)
Other	10 (7)	4 (6)	6 (7)
Presenting symptoms			
Asymptomatic	22 (15)	7 (11)	15 (18)
Flank pain	56 (38)	27 (42)	29 (35)
Hematuria	67 (46)	34 (53)	33 (40)
Weight loss	43 (30)	16 (25)	27 (33)
Lower extremity swelling	13 (9)	6 (9)	7 (9)
Change in appetite	13 (9)	4 (6)	9 (11)
Feeling of fullness	9 (6)	4 (6)	5 (6)
Distended subcutaneous veins	2 (1)	0 (0)	2 (2)
DVT/PE	8 (6)	4 (6)	4 (5)
Smoking	51 (35)	14 (22)	37 (45)
BMI median	28 ± 5.6	28 ± 4.9	26 ± 6.0
(range)	(17–56)	(19–46)	(17–56)
Obese (BMI ≥ 30)	34 (23)	17 (27)	17 (21)
ECOG			
0	27 (18)	17 (27)	10 (12)
1	93 (64)	43 (67)	50 (61)
2	20 (14)	2 (3)	18 (22)
3	6 (4)	2 (3)	4 (5)
ASA			
2	51 (35)	24 (38)	27 (33)
3	73 (50)	32 (50)	41 (50)
4	22 (15)	8 (12)	14 (17)

MRI was performed in 95 (65 %) patients for better determination of VTT level. Patients with IVC thrombus had a 26 % incidence of LN+ disease versus 14 % in those with RV only thrombus (p = .07). The mean number of removed and positive LNs were 5 (range, 0–33) and 1 (range, 1–22); respectively. Detailed pathological features are shown in Table 2.

Surgical intervention

Surgical parameters and postoperative hospital stay data are included in the Additional file 1: Table S1. Preoperative renal artery angioembolization was performed in 27.4 % of all patients with any venous thrombus, and in 49.3 % of patients with level 2–4 thrombi. Chevron incision was the most common approach and was performed in all patients with level III and IV VTT (with midline strenotomy in cases where cardio-pulmonary bypass was needed). IVC clamping was used in most cases of level II and III VTT. Suprahepatic control of the IVC and control of porta hepatis were gained in level III VTT. More aggressive cardiothoracic procedures were reserved for patients with level IV and 3 patients with level III VTT who were hemodynamically unstable during the initial cross-clamping of the IVC. Right heart venovenous bypass was used to assist in removal of VTT in these 3 patients. Cardio-pulmonary bypass was needed in 5 patients with level IV VTT with mean bypass, aortic cross clamping and circulatory arrest times of 124, 59 and 25 min respectively.

Mean estimated blood loss was 1.5 L and blood loss was greatest in patients with level IV VTT. The mean operative time was around 5 h and it was correlated to level of thrombus (5.5, 6 and 6.5 h in level II, III and IV; respectively). Mean hospital stay was 8.8 days (range, 1–63) and mean ICU stay was 3 days (range, 0–51). Three patients had a complicated postoperative course and required longer care.

Peri-operative morbidity and mortality

Out of 146 patients, 4 (2.7 %) and 5 (3.4 %) patients died within 30 and 90 days after surgery, respectively. The causes of death included: pulmonary embolism, coagulopathy, bleeding and pneumonia. Complications occurred in 77 (53 %) of patients and only 15 patients (10 %) had high grade (Clavien III-V) complications (Tables 3 and 4). The most common perioperative complication was prolonged ileus (12 %). The occurrence of complications did not correlate with VTT level or other clinical parameters including patient age, performance status, smoking and preoperative renal artery embolization (p > 0.05). However, correlation was seen with duration of surgery (p = 0.04) and intraoperative blood loss (p = 0.016). Most importantly, there was a lower incidence of overall and high grade complications (45 % and 8 %, respectively) in the last 6 years compared to the earlier surgeries included in the study (67 % and 13 % respectively) (p = .008 and .03, respectively) (Table 5).

Oncological outcomes

Patients were followed up after RN for a median of 16 months (mean 26, range 0–163 months). At the time of the analysis, overall mortality was 44 % with a median

Table 2 Pathological Features of Entire Cohort

Characteristic	Total (%)	Level I (%)	Level II (%)	Level III (%)	Level IV (%)	P value
	146 (100)	77 (53)	48 (33)	12 (8)	9 (6)	
T stage						<0.001
T3a	75 (51)	75 (97)	0	0	0	
T3b	51 (35)	0	40 (83)	11 (92)	0	
T3c	8 (6)	0	0	0	8 (89)	
T4	12 (8)	2 (3)	8 (17)	1 (8)	1 (11)	
Grade						0.015
1	1 (1)	0	0	1 (8)	0	
2	24 (16)	17 (22)	5 (10)	1 (8)	1 (11)	
3	86 (59)	39 (51)	32 (67)	10 (84)	5 (56)	
4	35 (24)	21 (27)	1 (23)	0	3 (33)	
Path tumor size (cm)	10.2 ± 4.5	9.2 ± 4.3	11.7 ± 4.6	10 ± 2.9	12 ± 6.3	0.02
	(2–25)	(2–23)	(3.5-25)	(5.5-15)	(5–22)	
Metastasis						0.3
Absent	104 (71)	56 (73)	31 (65)	11 (92)	6 (67)	
Present	42 (29)	21 (27)	17 (35)	1 (8)	3 (33)	
LN						0.01
N0	69 (47)	30 (39)	29 (60)	5 (42)	5 (56)	
Nx	48 (33)	36 (47)	6 (13)	4 (33)	2 (22)	
N+	29 (20)	11 (14)	13 (27)	3 (25)	2 (22)	
Sarcomatoid Differentiation						0.3
Absent	127 (87)	68 (88)	39 (81)	12 (100)	8 (89)	
Present	19 (13)	9 (1)	9 (19)	0	1 (11)	
Adrenal Involvement						0.08
Absent	128 (88)	72 (94)	38 (79)	11 (92)	7 (78)	
Present	18 (12)	5 (6)	10 (21)	1 (8)	2 (22)	
Tumor Necrosis						0.4
Absent	52 (36)	32 (42)	15 (31)	3 (25)	2 (22)	
Present	94 (64)	45 (58)	33 (69)	9 (75)	7 (78)	
Fat Invasion						0.3
Absent	28 (19)	18 (23)	7 (15)	3 (25)	0 (0)	
Present	118 (81)	59 (77)	41 (85)	9 (75)	9 (100)	
Histological Subtype						0.7
Non clear cell	11 (8)	5 (6)	5 (10)	1 (8)	0 (0)	
Clear cell	135 (92)	72 (94)	43 (90)	11 (92)	9 (100)	

survival of 47 ± 4 months (range 38–56 months) and 34 % cancer specific mortality with a median CSS of 62 ± 17 months (range 29–94 months). Kaplan-Meier Survival analysis showed CSS at 2,3 and 5 years to be 70 %, 62 % and 51 %; OS at 2, 3 and 5 years to be 64 %, 57 % and 40 %; respectively (Fig. 1a). There was no significant difference in survival comparing the last 6 years to an earlier period with 3Y- CSS 62 % in both eras.

Prognostic factors

Kaplan-Meier survival analysis (Fig. 1b) demonstrated a significant difference between CSS rates in M0 and M+ patients (5Y-CSS was 68 % and 17 % in M0 and M+ patients; respectively, $p < 0.001$). Median CSS was 11 ± 4 months for M+ patients, while it was not yet reached for M0 patients. Multivariate Cox regression analyses (data not shown) demonstrated that M+ was the only

Table 3 Overall complications and grading according to Clavien-Dindo system

	Total (%)	Level I (%)	Level II (%)	Level III (%)	Level IV (%)	P value
	146 (100)	77 (52.7)	48 (32.9)	12 (8.2)	9 (6.2)	
Overall Complications	77 (53)	38 (49)	27 (56)	7 (58)	5 (56)	.86
Ileus/bowel	18 (12)	10 (13)	4 (8)	4 (33)	0 (0)	.07
DVT	5 (3)	1 (1)	1 (2)	2 (17)	1 (11)	.03
Pleural effusion	8 (6)	3 (4)	5 (10)	0	0 (0)	.4
Acute renal failure	7 (5)	4 (5)	2 (4)	0	1 (11)	.7
Coagulopathy	5 (3)	1 (1)	3 (6)	0	1 (11)	.2
PE	10 (7)	2 (3)	1 (2)	4 (33)	3 (33)	.001
Pneumonia	2 (1)	1 (1)	1 (2)	0	0 (0)	.9
Perioperative mortality	11 (8)	3 (4)	7(15)	0	1 (11)	0.1
Clavien I-II	63 (43)	33 (43)	21 (44)	7 (58)	2 (22)	.02
Clavien III-V	15 (10)	5 (6)	6 (13)	0	4 (44)	

independent predictor factor for CSS (HR 3.8, CI 1.9-7.6 and $p < .001$) and OS (HR 2.6, CI 1.5-4.7 and $p = .001$). LN+ was associated with a trend toward a poor CSS (HR 1.9, CI .97-3.6 and $p = .06$). In M+ patients, LN+ was the only factor significantly associated with poor oncological outcomes as shown from CSS analysis (HR 2.3, CI 1–5 and $P = .03$), and in OS analysis (HR 2, CI .96 – 4.3 and $P = .06$). In M0 patients, high VTT level (III and IV compared to I and II) was among the independent predictors of disease recurrence (HR 4.4, CI 2.1-9.4 and $P < .001$) and cancer specific mortality (HR 6.5, CI 2–21.2; $p = .002$) in multivariate Cox regression analysis. Other independent predictors of poor oncological outcomes included larger tumor size (>13 cm) and sarcomatoid differentiation (data not shown).

Discussion

Aggressive surgical resection is indicated in RCC with VTT as nephrectomy alone is associated with dismal

Table 4 Overall complications and grading according to Clavien-Dindo system by Era

	Total (%)	Era I (%)	Era II (%)	P value
	146 (100)	64 (44)	82 (56)	
Overall Complications	77 (53)	43 (67)	34 (42)	.002
Ileus/bowel	18 (12)	10 (16)	8 (10)	.3
DVT	5 (3)	2 (3)	3 (4)	.9
Pleural effusion	8 (6)	3 (5)	5 (6)	.7
Acute renal failure	7 (5)	4 (6)	3 (4)	.5
Coagulopathy	5 (3)	5 (8)	0 (0)	.01
PE	10 (7)	1 (2)	9 (11)	.025
Pneumonia	2 (1)	1 (2)	1 (1)	.9
Perioperative mortality	11 (8)	2 (3)	9 (11)	0.08
Clavien I-II	63 (43)	35 (55)	28 (34)	.02
Clavien III-V	15(10)	8 (13)	7 (8)	

prognosis [10]. Through an experienced team, consisting of a urologic oncology surgeon, cardiothoracic surgeon, cardiac anesthesiologist, and cardiac scrub team we were able to achieve satisfactory surgical and oncological outcomes and decrease the incidence of complications.

We noticed a significant reduction in the rate of overall and high grade complications (45 % and 8 %, respectively) in the last 6 years compared to the earlier surgeries included in the study (67 % and 13 % respectively) [$p = .008$ and .03, respectively]. We believe this reduction may be due to our multidisciplinary team approach, which provides uniform and consistent management of patients with VTT. The team approach further supports meticulous perioperative and postoperative planning and delivery of care, refinement of surgical technique, and improved anesthesia.

In terms of oncological outcomes, metastasis was found to be the strongest independent predictor of survival. Patients with M+ had a 3.8 times risk of cancer specific mortality compared to M0 patients ($p < .001$). While M0 patients had 5-Y CSS of 68 % and median survival that was not reached yet, M+ patients had a 17 % 5-Y CSS and 11 months median survival. Our survival rates were superior to those reported in the literature for M0 patients [3–5, 11–24] but they were similarly poor in M+ patients who were reported to have 4-30 % 5Y-CSS and 11–20 months median survival [3–5, 11–18, 21]. In this study, 29 % of patients had metastasis at presentation. This incidence was even higher in other series [14, 16]. Surgery might be indicated not only to improve oncological

Table 5 Overall High Grade Complication Rate by ERA

	Surgery Era	1998-2006	2006-2012	p value
Overall Complication Rate		67 %	45 %	.008
High Grade Complications Clavien III - V		13 %	8 %	.030

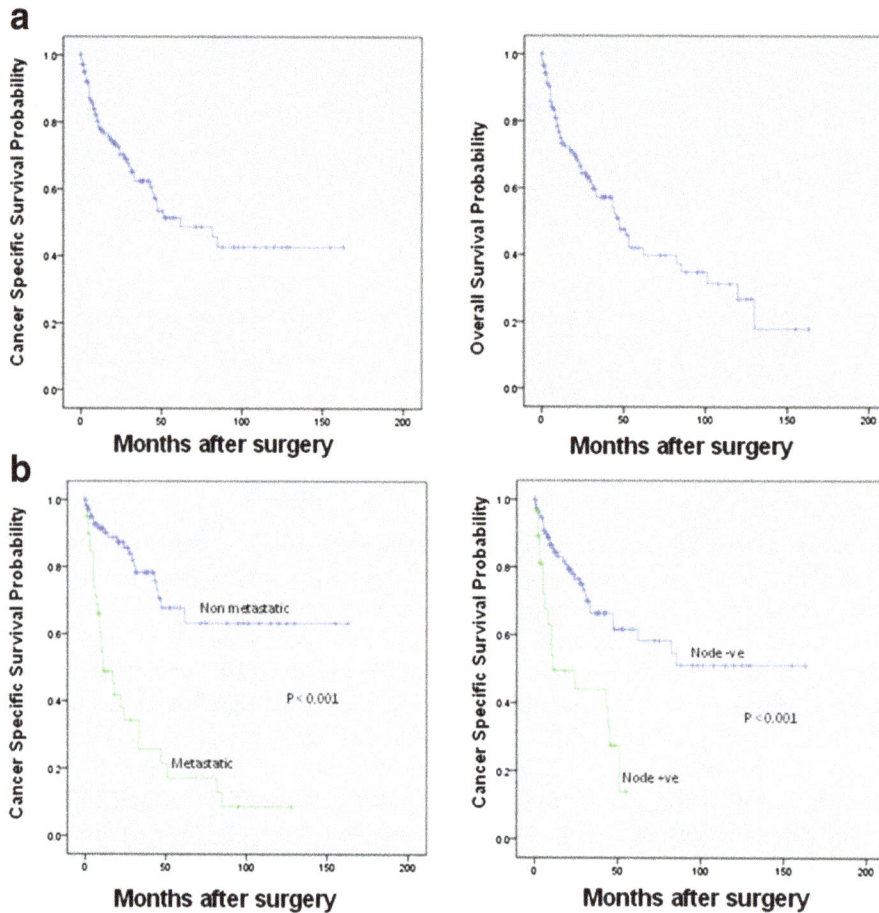

Fig. 1 a) Kaplan-Meier estimates of cancer-specific survival and overall survival for 146 patients after radical nephrectomy and venous thrombectomy. **b**) Kaplan-Meier estimates of cancer-specific survival stratified by presence of metastasis at presentation and LN status for 146 patients after radical nephrectomy and venous thrombectomy

outcomes but also to relieve symptoms and provide better quality of life. However, performance status and associated comorbidities should be considered [10].

Overall, LN+ showed a trend toward poor CSS (HR 1.9, CI and p = .06) and achieved prognostic significance only in M+ patients (HR 2.3 and p = .03). Perhaps, statistical significance, in the analysis involving all patients, would be reached if the sample size was larger and/or follow up was longer. The independent prognostic role of LN+ was reported in other RN and IVCT series [12, 14, 21, 24]. Previous studies support the role of aggressive debulking of regional nodal disease at the time of cytoreductive RN for metastatic RCC [2, 25, 26].

There has been wide variation in reporting different prognostic factors and the prognostic value of VTT level has been debated. Our prognostic factors were similar to those reported in the largest European study that included 1192 patients from 13 European centers [12] and the US based analysis including 1875 patients with RCC and VTT from the SEER database [27]. In both studies, metastasis was the most important independent predictor of worse survival.

Interestingly, analysis of data for all patients showed that metastasis was the only independent predictor of oncological outcomes. However, in M0 patients, features associated with aggressive tumor behavior (high level VTT, large tumor size, and sarcomatoid differentiation) had an independent prognostic role. The size of the tumor has been implicated in staging of RCC. Large tumor size was among the strongest predictors of worse survival in the international RCC-VTT consortium that included 1215 RN and IVCT from 11 American and European institutions [21] as well as in a population based analysis including 1875 patients with RCC and VTT from the SEER database [27]. Sarcomatoid differentiation was reported with an incidence of 9 % and was among the independent predictors of worse survival in RN and IVCT series [3, 14, 20]. We found sarcomatoid differentiation in 13 % of tumors and it did not correlate with higher VTT levels, as 95 % of tumors with sarcomatoid differentiation had level I or II VTT.

We acknowledge several limitations in this review. First, is the retrospective design with its inherited bias. Second, while our multidisciplinary approach has lead to a decrease in the rate of complications, other factors may have also lead to improved outcomes. Improvement in surgical technique, enhanced understanding of the biology of the disease, and improved delivery of medical care throughout the course of the study may have also lead to improved patient outcomes. Lastly, the impact of venous wall invasion by thrombus could not be evaluated, as it was not reported by consistent pathologic criteria over the period under review.

Conclusions

RN and VTT is a challenging surgery and while, improvements in surgical techniques and perioperative care have decreased surgical morbidity and mortality, we strongly advocate for management of these patients with an experienced multidisciplinary team. Our approach has resulted in improved overall complications and most importantly, high grade complications. A strong working relationship between all team members helps develop meticulous perioperative and postoperative planning and delivery of care, refinement of surgical technique, and improved anesthesia.

Abbreviations
IVC, Inferior vena cava; IVCT, Radical nephrectomy (RN) and IVC thrombectomy; LN, Lymph node; RCC, Renal Cell Carcinoma; RN, Radical nephrectomy; VTT, Renal Cell Carcinoma (RCC) with venous tumor thrombus

Acknowledgements
None.

Funding
No funding was obtained for this study.

Authors' contributions
BG conception and design, acquisition of data, analysis and interpretation of data; drafting of manuscript. RY conception and design, acquisition of data, or analysis and interpretation of data; drafting of manuscript. OD conception and design, acquisition of data, analysis and interpretation of data; drafting of manuscript. PK acquisition of data, analysis and interpretation of data. AB conception and design, acquisition of data, analysis and interpretation of data. JB conception and design, analysis and interpretation of data. GR conception and design, acquisition of data, analysis and interpretation of data. MD conception and design, acquisition of data, analysis and interpretation of data. AS conception and design, acquisition of data, analysis and interpretation of data. VM conception and design, acquisition of data, analysis and interpretation of data; drafting of manuscript. All authors have read and approved the final version of this manuscript.

Competing interests
None of the authors have any financial interests or conflicts of interests to disclose.

Author details
[1]Department of Urology, University of Texas Southwestern Medical Center, 5323 Harry Hines Blvd., Dallas, TX 75390-9110, USA. [2]Departments of Pathology, University of Texas Southwestern Medical Center, Dallas, TX, USA. [3]Departments of Medicine and Developmental Biology, University of Texas Southwestern Medical Center, Dallas, TX, USA. [4]Departments of Cardiothoracic Surgery, University of Texas Southwestern Medical Center, Dallas, TX, USA.

References
1. Siegel RL, Miller KD, Jemal A. Cancer statistics, 2015. CA Cancer J Clin. 2015; 65(1):5–29.
2. Margulis V, Master VA, Cost NG, et al. International consultation on urologic diseases and the European Association of Urology international consultation on locally advanced renal cell carcinoma. Eur Urol. 2011;60(4):673–83.
3. Karnes RJ, Blute ML. Surgery insight: management of renal cell carcinoma with associated inferior vena cava thrombus. Nat Clin Pract Urol. 2008;5(6): 329–39.
4. Gonzalez J. Update on surgical management of renal cell carcinoma with venous extension. Curr Urol Rep. 2012;13(1):8–15.
5. Pouliot F, Shuch B, Larochelle JC, Pantuck A, Belldegrun AS. Contemporary management of renal tumors with venous tumor thrombus. J Urol. 2010; 184(3):833–41. quiz 1235.
6. Neves RJ, Zincke H. Surgical treatment of renal cancer with vena cava extension. Br J Urol. 1987;59(5):390–5.
7. Edge SB, Compton CC. The American Joint Committee on Cancer: the 7th edition of the AJCC cancer staging manual and the future of TNM. Ann Surg Oncol. 2010;17(6):1471–4.
8. Fuhrman SA, Lasky LC, Limas C. Prognostic significance of morphologic parameters in renal cell carcinoma. Am J Surg Pathol. 1982;6(7):655–63.
9. Dindo D, Demartines N, Clavien PA. Classification of surgical complications: a new proposal with evaluation in a cohort of 6336 patients and results of a survey. Ann Surg. 2004;240(2):205–13.
10. Kirkali Z, Van Poppel H. A critical analysis of surgery for kidney cancer with vena cava invasion. Eur Urol. 2007;52(3):658–62.
11. Ciancio G, Manoharan M, Katkoori D, De Los SR, Soloway MS. Long-term survival in patients undergoing radical nephrectomy and inferior vena cava thrombectomy: single-center experience. Eur Urol. 2010;57(4):667–72.
12. Wagner B, Patard JJ, Mejean A, et al. Prognostic value of renal vein and inferior vena cava involvement in renal cell carcinoma. Eur Urol. 2009;55(2):452–9.
13. Lambert EH, Pierorazio PM, Shabsigh A, Olsson CA, Benson MC, McKiernan JM. Prognostic risk stratification and clinical outcomes in patients undergoing surgical treatment for renal cell carcinoma with vascular tumor thrombus. Urology. 2007;69(6):1054–8.
14. Klatte T, Pantuck AJ, Riggs SB, et al. Prognostic factors for renal cell carcinoma with tumor thrombus extension. J Urol. 2007;178(4 Pt 1):1189–95. discussion 95.
15. Haferkamp A, Bastian PJ, Jakobi H, et al. Renal cell carcinoma with tumor thrombus extension into the vena cava: prospective long-term followup. J Urol. 2007;177(5):1703–8.
16. Moinzadeh A, Libertino JA. Prognostic significance of tumor thrombus level in patients with renal cell carcinoma and venous tumor thrombus extension. Is all T3b the same? J Urol. 2004;171(2 Pt 1):598–601.
17. Sweeney P, Wood CG, Pisters LL, et al. Surgical management of renal cell carcinoma associated with complex inferior vena caval thrombi. Urol Oncol. 2003;21(5):327–33.

18. Ali AS, Vasdev N, Shanmuganathan S, et al. The surgical management and prognosis of renal cell cancer with IVC tumor thrombus: 15-years of experience using a multi-specialty approach at a single UK referral center. Urol Oncol. 2013;31(7):1298–304.

19. Parekh DJ, Cookson MS, Chapman W, et al. Renal cell carcinoma with renal vein and inferior vena caval involvement: clinicopathological features, surgical techniques and outcomes. J Urol. 2005;173(6):1897–902.

20. Blute ML, Leibovich BC, Lohse CM, Cheville JC, Zincke H. The Mayo Clinic experience with surgical management, complications and outcome for patients with renal cell carcinoma and venous tumour thrombus. BJU Int. 2004;94(1):33–41.

21. Martinez-Salamanca JI, Huang WC, Millan I, et al. Prognostic impact of the 2009 UICC/AJCC TNM staging system for renal cell carcinoma with venous extension. Eur Urol. 2011;59(1):120–7.

22. Al Otaibi M, Abou Youssif T, Alkhaldi A, et al. Renal cell carcinoma with inferior vena caval extention: impact of tumour extent on surgical outcome. BJU Int. 2009;104(10):1467–70.

23. Glazer AA, Novick AC. Long-term followup after surgical treatment for renal cell carcinoma extending into the right atrium. J Urol. 1996;155(2):448–50.

24. Vergho DC, Loeser A, Kocot A, Spahn M, Riedmiller H. Tumor thrombus of inferior vena cava in patients with renal cell carcinoma - clinical and oncological outcome of 50 patients after surgery. BMC Res Notes. 2012;5(1):264.

25. Pantuck AJ, Zisman A, Dorey F, et al. Renal cell carcinoma with retroperitoneal lymph nodes: role of lymph node dissection. J Urol. 2003; 169(6):2076–83.

26. Vasselli JR, Yang JC, Linehan WM, White DE, Rosenberg SA, Walther MM. Lack of retroperitoneal lymphadenopathy predicts survival of patients with metastatic renal cell carcinoma. J Urol. 2001;166(1):68–72.

27. Whitson JM, Reese AC, Meng MV. Population based analysis of survival in patients with renal cell carcinoma and venous tumor thrombus. Urol Oncol. 2013;31(2):259–63.

14

Flexible and rigid ureteroscopy in outpatient surgery

Abeni Oitchayomi, Arnaud Doerfler, Sophie Le Gal, Charles Chawhan and Xavier Tillou*

Abstract

Background: Outpatient surgery is critical to improve health care costs. The aim of the study was to prospectively evaluate the results of outpatient treatment of upper tract urinary stones by rigid or flexible ureteroscopy in a routine care setting.

Methods: A database was created at the creation of the outpatient surgery department. 87 patients underwent 100 ureteroscopic procedures for urinary lithiasis from June 2013 to March 2015.

Results: Most of our patients were male with 53 men (sex ratio M/F 1.13), with a mean age of 52.9 ± 15 years old (23.4–82.4). 44 % of ureteroscopies performed were flexible ureteroscopies, 31 % rigid ureteroscopies and 25 % associated rigid and flexible ureteroscopies. The average stone load was 10.1 ± 5.7 mm (2–30) The mean operating time was 58.3 ± 21.1 min (20–150). 82.9 % of patients had a single urinary stone and 17.1 % ($n = 14$) had 2 or more. 114 stones were treated, 57,1 % intrarenal. There were 6 (6 %) postoperative complications: three Clavien stage 2 infections; three Clavien stage 3b complications (two renal colics requiring ureteral stenting 48 h after discharge and 1 symptomatic perirenal urinoma 48 h after discharge). There was one intraoperative complication (1 %): a ureteral wound with contrast leakage. The rate of transfer to conventional hospitalization was 2.2 %. Stone size influenced the stone-free status ($p < 0.0001$) and the need for more than one session. There was a significant correlation between operative time and stone size above 10 mm ($p < 0.0001$).

Conclusions: Flexible and rigid ureteroscopy are safe and efficient procedures for upper urinary tract stones and can be carried out in an outpatient department. Stone size had an impact on postoperative stone-free status and operative time.

Keywords: Outpatient surgery, Ureteroscopy, Urinary lithiasis

Background

Ambulatory surgery is performed with admission and discharge of the patient on the same day, with a hospital stay of less than 12 h (no overnight stay). This management is much used in France, which is still lagging behind other countries such as the United States. Ambulatory surgery activity increased by 21 % between 2007 and 2010 in France [1, 2]. Urinary stone disease is common, affecting 3 men to 1 woman, with a peak incidence at between 40 and 50 years of age. Ureteroscopy can handle urinary stones of the ureter as well as in the kidney, being thus a serious alternative to percutaneous nephrolithotomy [3]. Endoscopic treatment of stones is a procedure with low morbidity, between 5 and 10 % [4] and thus it is a procedure performed increasingly in ambulatory surgery in many institutions with patients meeting the outpatient surgery criteria. Data for flexible ureteroscopy (FURS) in ambulatory surgery are few in the literature. Only one study described results of 33 FURS in day-case surgery [5]. FURS is indicated in the treatment of renal kidney stones below 2 cm, in overweight patients, patients with anticoagulants or antiplatelet therapy, urinary stone density greater than 1000 UH, cystine stones, inferior calyx position or if the patient has a particular kidney anatomy such as horseshoe kidney. Rigid ureteroscopy (RURS) is indicated in the treatment of ureteral stones, especially if greater than 1 cm. It can be performed on an emergency basis outside of an infectious episode. [2] The objective of this study was to

---

* Correspondence: xavtillou@gmail.com
Urology and Transplantation Department, University Hospital of Caen, CHU Cote de Nacre, Avenue de Cote de Nacre, 14033 Caen, France

show that all types of ureteroscopy are an efficient and safe procedure in outpatient surgery.

Methods

Design of the study

We collected prospectively the results of rigid and flexible ureteroscopy procedures for urinary stones performed in ambulatory surgery at our University Hospital from June 2013 to February 2015. Ureteroscopy in ambulatory surgery had already been performed as an outpatient modality for several years in our center. At our center, extracorporeal shock wave lithotripsy (ESWL) had not been available for many years. A prospectively maintained database was created at the same time as the opening of our dedicated outpatient surgery department in June 2013. In all there were 103 procedures performed during the study period. The aim of the study was to analyze every day clinical practice. The primary objective was to study the morbidity and early and late conversion rate to conventional hospitalization. The secondary objective was to investigate the efficacy of endoscopic procedures based on the stone-free status assessed by the surgical report or postoperative radiological exam (Ultrasonography or CT-scan) screening for stones under 3 mm in the upper urinary tract. Patients were seen at a postoperative control consultation between 1 and 3 months. Three patients were lost to follow-up because they completed it in another region. We collected demographic data and patient history (ASA score, age, sex, BMI). We also specified the type of ureteroscopy, and characteristics of stones (density, location, size). We noted operative time and the short-term complications.

Outpatient surgery criteria

All patients met the criteria for outpatient surgery under the SFAR (French Anesthesiology and Reanimation Society) and AFU (French Urology Association) [2] recommendations:

- Patient consent
- Must be escorted home by a third party and should not be alone the first night following surgery
- Must be able to understand and respect the postoperative surveillance guidelines
- Must not have psychiatric problems preventing collaboration with the Ambulatory Surgery Unit
- Must live in acceptable conditions with access to a phone

Patients were initially evaluated by anesthesiologists who validated the procedure feasibility as an outpatient modality. In the same time, 220 ureteroscopies (rigid and flexible) were performed in a conventional hospitalization setting because patients did not meet the criteria for outpatient surgery (see above).

Surgical technique

For patients with no previous double pigtail stent, surgery was scheduled to attempt a ureteroscopy. If the non-prepared ureter did not allow performing ureteroscopy, a double pigtail stent was placed and the ureteroscopy was scheduled two weeks later. Before surgery, all patients had a sterile urine culture. During the procedure, performed under general anesthesia, all patients received intravenous antibioprophylaxy with 2nd or 3rd generation cephalosporins. Ureteroscopy used an Olympus flexible ureterscope P5 8.4 French (Fr) and an Olympus 7.8 semi-rigid ureteroscope and were performed using a standard safety wire. The majority of stones were treated with a Holmium:YAG laser (Stonelight; AMS) or removed intact with an endoscopic basket. A double pigtail stent was placed as indicated by the operator following a long procedure, in case of repeated endo ureteral maneuvers or in placing the access sheath. After the procedure the patient was discharged after a decision taken in common by the surgeon and the anesthesiologist, at least 4 to 6 h after the ureteroscopy. Postoperative analgesia was ensured by intravenous paracetamol (1 g/6 h) completed by intravenous tramadol 100 mg/8 h) if necessary. This treatment was continued per os after discharge. Criteria to consider hospitalization after surgery (except anaesthetic issues) were an acute urine retention, pain with need for continued intravenous treatment or fever. The double pigtail stent was removed in the outpatient clinic.

Legislation and statistics

Data collection followed French legislation concerning prospective interventional studies to evaluate routine care (Article Art. L1121-1-2 of French Public Health Code (Code de santé publique français)). Institutional review board approval was obtained to prospectively collect data on patients who underwent Ureteroscopy. The study did not require submitting to a Consultative Committee for Persons' Protection in Biomedical Research (CCPPRB). Patients were informed verbally and received an information document edited by the French Urology Association (http://urofrance.org/nc/lurologie-grandpublic/fiches-patient/resultats-de-la-recherche/html/ureteroscopie.html). Categorical variables were analyzed using the chi-square test and Fisher's exact test when applicable. Continuous variables were analyzed parametrically using Student's t-test and non-parametrically using the Kruskal–Wallis test or the Mann and Whitney test. For univariate analysis, $p < 0.05$ defined statistical significance.

Results

In total, 100 procedures in 87 patients were included. The patients all meet the criteria for outpatient surgery; their characteristics are summarized in Table 1. The

Table 1 Patients characteristics by treatment groups

		Rigid ureteroscopy N = 31	Flexible ureteroscopy N = 44	Rigid + flexible ureteroscopy N = 25	p
Multiple procedures		1	9	3	0.05
Gender	F	8 (26.7 %)	17 (44.7 %)	9 (40.9 %)	0.07
	M	22 (73.3 %)	18 (55.3 %)	13 (59.1 %)	
Median age at TT (years old)		54.2 (35.8–66.2) (25.3–82.4)	43.4 (25.1–60) (21–76.4)	54.7 (39–61) (26.8–76.4)	1
ASA 1		22	30	10	
ASA 2		8	5	12	
Median BMI (kg/m^2) (IQR) (Min-max)		25.4 (24–28.3) (17.3–37.8)	26 (24.3–29.3) (18.9–38.1)	26.8 (23.9–28) (21–39.9)	0.014
History of urinary stones treatment (same side)	ESWL	1	4	1	
	URS	2	4	0	
	PCNL	0	3	0	
Preoperative JJ stent		24 (77.4 %)	35 (79.5 %)	23 (92 %)	0.2
Median time between diagnosis and TT (days) (IQR) (min-max)		58 (30–92.5) (7–146)	63 (33–80.5) (14–127)	57.4 (41–80) (14–213)	0.9
Stones size (mm) (IQR) (min-max)		7 (6–10) (4–30)	12.5 (10–17.5) (6–30)	8 (6.5–14) (4–34)	0.0008
Median stones density (UH) (IQR) (min-max)		1000 (900–1200) (550–1330)	920 (800–1000) (500–1580)	895 (525–1150) (433–1450)	0.13
Median operative time (min) (IQR) (min-max)		41.5 (31–59.5) (10–90)	60 (52.5–79) (20–150)	60 (46.2–66.7) (31–90)	<0.0001
Postoperative double pigtail stent		19 (61.3 %)	33 (75 %)	14 (56 %)	0.2
Stone free		27/30 (90 %)	25/35 (71.4 %)	21/22 (95.4 %)	0.03
Postoperative complications	Clavien 2	0	2 APN 1 APr	0	0.3
	Clavien 3	2 Renal colics	1 Urinoma	0	

majority of patients were male with 53 men (sex ratio M/F 1.13), with a median age of 56 years old (Interquartile range (IQR) 39–64.5; min 23.4-max 82.5). Patients were exclusively ASA 1 ($n = 62$; 71.3 %) and ASA 2 ($n = 25$; 28.7 %).

Descriptive analysis of operating characteristics
The median time between the date of diagnosis and ureteroscopy was 82.5 days (IQR 57.2–119.3; min 13-max 739). 44 % of ureteroscopies were FURS, 31 % were RURS and 25 % associated rigid and flexible ureteroscopy if there were several locations or the original ureteral stone was flushed in the kidney (22 patients). One failure of FURS (procedure stopped after 30 min) was secondary to ureteral wound probably during the ascension of the access sheath. The median operating time was 60 min (IQR 45–75; min 20- max 150). A majority of patients had a double pigtail stent preoperatively placed during an acute episode of renal colic ($n = 52$) or obstructive pyelonephritis ($n = 14$) or simply to prepare the endoscopic procedure ($n = 22$). Twelve procedures could be performed without a previous double pigtail stent. The median time between double pigtail stent placement and ureteroscopy was 63.5 days (IQR 35–92; min 7- max 213). Postoperatively a double pigtail stent was left in place after 66 procedures (66 %).

Urinary stone characteristics
82.9 % of patients were carrying a single stone and 17.1 % ($n = 14$) two or more. One hundred fourteen stones were treated (Fig. 1). The distribution and mean size of urinary stones are presented in Table 2. The mean stone density evaluated on preoperative CT scans was 964.9 ± 286.7 HU. The median stone load was 8 mm (IQR 6,3–13; min 2- max 30). Kidney urinary stones under 6 mm in size were processed at the same time as the main stone.

Postoperative complications
Postoperative complications were first of all infectious (Clavien stage 2): acute prostatitis at day 13, 2 pyelonephritis 48 h after surgery. Three complications were Clavien stage 3b: 2 renal colic requiring ureteral stenting 48 h after ambulatory discharge, and a symptomatic perirenal urinoma 48 h after surgery. Complications rate was 6 %.

There was one intraoperative complication (1 %): an ureteral lesion with contrast leakage requiring ureteral stent and the cessation of the procedure after 30 min.

The conventional hospitalization conversion rate was 2 % (2/100) and included the patient with an intraoperative ureteral wound and a patient with poorly controlled postoperative pain. Gvien the low rate of complications it was not possible to identify patients or procedures at risk of complications.

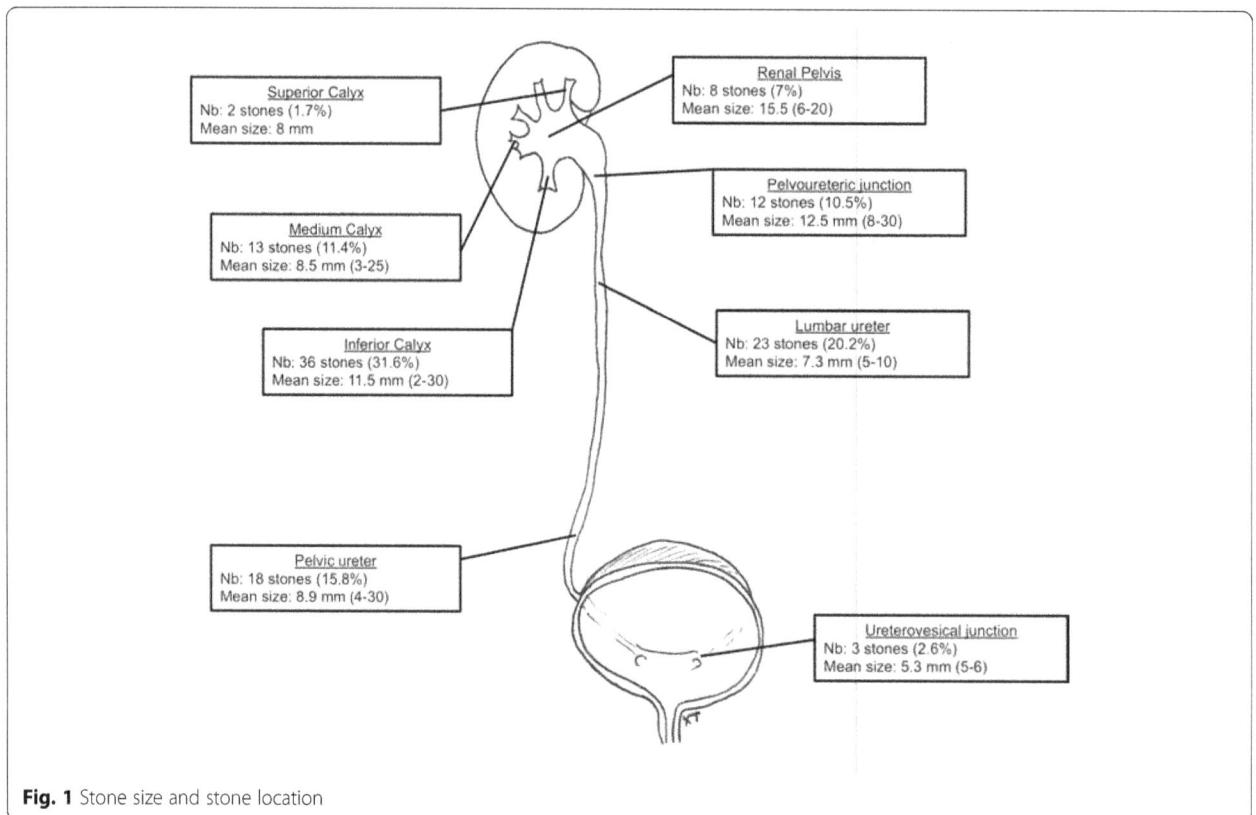

Fig. 1 Stone size and stone location

Table 2 Patients characteristics by stone localization

		Distal ureter stones N = 16	Proximal ureter stones N = 22	Renal stones N = 62	p
Multiple procedures		0	2	11	
Rigid ureteroscopy		14	12	3	
Flexible ureteroscopy		0	2	43	
Both		2	8	16	
Gender	Female	6	8	24	
	Male	10	12	27	
Median age at TT (years old) (IQR) (Min-max)		54 (35–54) (25–82)	52 (23–67) (23–80)	57 (25–65) (25–76)	0.8
ASA 1		14	18	34	
ASA 2		2	2	17	
Median BMI (kg/T^2) (IQR) (Min-Max)		25 (24–28) (21–32)	27 (25–29) (17–40)	26 (24–28) (19–38)	0.47
History of urinary stones treatment (same side)	ESWL	0	0	6	0.035
	URS	1	0	5	
	PCNL	0	0	3	
Preoperative JJ stent		14 (87.5 %)	18 (81.8 %)	49 (79 %)	0.74
Median time between diagnosis and TT (days) (IQR) (Min-max)		86 (50–109) (13–289)	67 (38–93) (21–151)	93 (65–156) (25–739)	0.053
Median Stone size (mm) (IQR) (Min-max)		7 (5.3–10) (4–30)	7 (6.3–8) (4–10)	10 (6.6–13) (2–30)	0.014
Median stone density (UH) (IQR) (Min-max)		1003 (930–1125) (550–1310)	1000 (660–1200) (433–1330)	943 (618–1000) 500–1580)	0.24
Median operative time (min) (IQR) (Min-max)		40 (30–45) (20–60)	45 (35–60) (10–90)	60 (50–75) (20–150)	<0.0001
Postoperative double pigtail stent		8 (50 %)	15 (68.2 %)	43 (69.35 %)	0.33
Stone free after multiple procedures		15/16 (93.7 %)	19/20 (95 %)	38/51 (74.5 %)	0.053
Postoperative complications	Clavien 2		1 AProst	2 APN	
			1 Renal colic	1 Renal colic	
	Clavien 3			1 Urinoma	

Statistical analysis and follow up

The mean operative time of patients who had postoperative complications or who were converted to conventional hospitalization was not different from the mean operative time of other patients (64,6 vs. 57,2 min; $p = 0.4$). In the same way, ureteroscopy type (rigid, flexible or both) was not associated to postoperative complications ($p = 0.3$). Median follow up was 3.5 months (IQR 2.1-5.5; min 0.7-max 9.4). Seventy-two patients were assessed post operatively for residual fragments by CT-scan and 15 by US. On the one hand, studying the patient groups "stone Free" and the patient group "not stone free," we found no significant difference in the number of urinary stones before surgery ($p = 0.37$) nor in terms of their density ($p = 0.85$). On another hand, the impact of stone size on the stone-free status and the need for one or more sessions was highly significant ($p < 0.0001$). In addition, there was a significant correlation between operative time and stone size ($p < 0.0001$; $r = 0.59$), but not between the operating time and stone density ($p = 0.8$). Bigger urinary stones were treated by FURS ($p = 0.0008$) on patients with longer histories of urinary stone treatment ($p = 0.014$). Mean operative time was higher for FURS ($p < 0.0001$). At the end of 34 procedures, double pigtail stent was not required. Median time of ureteral catheter removal after ureteroscopy was 22 days (IQR 17.5-34.5; min 8- max 119).

Discussion

In Urology, several procedures can be done in outpatient surgery: female urethral sling, ACT balloons, male genital organ surgery, and prostate laser surgery. Radical prostatectomies and nephrectomies are currently under investigation [6, 7] as well as Percutaneous Nephrolithotomy [8, 9] with case reports and small series. Ambulatory surgery is encouraged in all countries by different national health systems with a view to its economic advantages [2]. An american study evaluated that ambulatory surgery could generate savings of 363 to $1000 US dollars per outpatient case [10]. Rigid or semi-rigid ureteroscopy are routinely performed in many countries especially in the US. Indeed in 1994, Wills asked whether ureteroscopy could be performed as an outpatient surgery [11]. Most of the studies of ureteroscopy describe procedures during conventional inpatient hospitalization or a day-case procedure with an overnight stay. In a strictly defined outpatient setting, patient admission and discharge should occur on the same day. The first study describing results of ambulatory rigid ureteroscopy with laser stone fragmentation was published in 1998 by Yip [12]. The complication rate in 69 patients was 10 % with 6 % of unplanned readmission. This study demonstrated that rigid ureteroscopy for ureteric stones can be performed in an outpatient surgery department, with an acceptable rate of unplanned readmissions and an acceptable rate

of complications. Several other studies followed confirming these results [13, 14]. Others publications studied factors influencing JJ stent placement after outpatient procedures [15], or preoperative predictors of postoperative events [16]. Ureteroscopy had to be compared to other outpatient procedures to treat upper urinary tract stones, namely extracorporeal shockwave lithotripsy [17, 18]. Jeong reported that shockwave lithotripsy was more painful with a lower rate of stone free patients.

Ureteroscopy is not dependent on stone radiolucent characteristic: any kind of urinary stone can be treated. FURS is a widely used procedure, but documentation on the safety and efficacy of this treatment modality in an outpatient setting is scarce. There were only two studies in the literature analyzing results of FURS in a true outpatient setting, but these studies were retrospective reviews. Bromwich [5] reported a study with the same design than ours. 64 rigid and flexible ureteroscopies were performed in outpatient surgery. 45 patients were treated for urinary stones including 13 FURS. Rate of immediate admission was 6.25 % ($n = 4$) mostly following postoperative uncontrolled pain. Rate of unplanned readmission after discharge was 4.7 % ($n = 3$) with one urinary retention, one clot retention and one for social reasons. Tan [19] studied the rate of immediate unplanned hospital admission and factors associated with admission for outpatient ureteroscopy for stone disease. For 1798 consecutive outpatient ureteroscopic procedures for urolithiasis, there were 70 immediate unplanned admissions (3.9 %). The authors found after multivariate analysis that the significant factors associated with unplanned admission were: previous admission related to stones, history of psychiatric illness and bilateral procedure. Unfortunately, the number of FURS included in this study was not specified. In the latest study of outpatient ureteroscopy for kidney stones, 82 % of the patients were considered stone free after one procedure and an overall stone-free rate of 85 % was found. Several studies have found stone-free rate higher than 90 % after one procedure [5, 19, 20]. However, most of these studies included small study populations and the outpatient setting was unclear, which makes comparison of the findings difficult. Moreover there is, no standardized definition of "stone-free rate" in the literature, and this fact makes comparisons across studies difficult [21]. At the time of surgery, 51.7 % of the patients had renal stones, which fact could explain variability in operative time (20 to 150 min). This is well known, as many steps in this procedure, such as ascension of the access sheath, laser stone vaporization and basket removal of stone fragments can take varying times and are difficult to predict. This high variability in operating times shows that ureteroscopic stone removal is a challenging procedure with a tight schedule in an outpatient surgery department. Accurately estimating operating times is essential in an outpatient surgery department. Recently, Lasselin [22] demonstrated that rate of ureteroscope damage is associated with operative time and cumulative duration of intervention. Its therefore important to limit ureteroscopy operating time in outpatient surgery in order to limit ureteroscope damage and to ensure good patient outcomes. With a low rate of surgical and anesthesiology complications, these procedures can be repeated to achieve upper urinary tract stone treatment whatever the initial stone load. The remaining question is the rate of ureteral stricture which is a medium and long follow up complication after ureteroscopy, occurs in 3–6 % of the surgeries and could be treated conservatively with a JJ stent according to Preminger [23]. The major strength of the present study is the availability of detailed medical records for each patient, and the prospective design that provided very comprehensive data. There are some limitations to this study. Only complications leading to contact with the hospital were registered and patients could have experienced other complications at home. Another limitation is the lack of a standardized definition of stone-free status.

Conclusion

Rigid as well as flexible ureteroscopy is a safe and efficient procedure that can easily be carried out in an outpatient department to treat upper urinary tract stones. It can reduce the need for admissions and thus cut healthcare costs. Most kidney urinary stones can be treated by flexible ureteroscopy in outpatient surgery with a low rate of complications and no difference from rigid ureteroscopy. Multiple locations and high stone load were associated with multiple procedure with no increase in morbidity rate. If ESWL is not available, FURS is a good treatment in an outpatient setting whatever the stone size and location.

Ethics approval and consent to participate

Study approved by Caen University Hospital ethic committee (no reference number provided).

Patients were informed verbally and received an information document edited by the French Urology Association.

Abbreviations

FURS: flexible ureteroscopy; ESWL: extracorporeal shock wave lithotripsy; RURS: rigid ureteroscopy.

Competing interests

The authors declare that they have no competing interests.

Authors' contributions

AO: wrote the paper. AD: wrote the paper. SLG: data prospective collection, bibliographic research. CC: data prospective collection; statistical analysis. XT: study design, statistical analysis, correct the paper. All authors read and approved the final version of the manuscript.

Acknowledgments

Dr Sylvie Collon and Mr Channing Bates for English editing.

Funding

None.

References

1. Chabannes É, Bensalah K, Carpentier X, Bringer J-P, Conort P, Denis É, et al. Management of adult's renal and ureteral stones. Update of the Lithiasis Committee of the French Association of Urology (CLAFU). General considerations. Prog Urol. 2013;23:1389–99.
2. Chirurgie ambulatoire en Urologie Argumentaire Recommandations AFU/SFAR/AFCA/ANAP, n.d. http://urofrance.org/nc/science-et-recherche/base-bibliographique/article/html/chirurgie-ambulatoire-enurologie-argumentaire.html.
3. Hyams ES, Shah O. Percutaneous nephrostolithotomy versus flexible ureteroscopy/holmium laser lithotripsy: cost and outcome analysis. J Urol. 2009;182:1012–7.
4. Geavlete P, Georgescu D, Niță G, Mirciulescu V, Cauni V. Complications of 2735 retrograde semirigid ureteroscopy procedures: a single-center experience. J Endourol. 2006;20:179–85.
5. Bromwich EJ, Lockyer R, Keoghane SR. Day-case rigid and flexible ureteroscopy. Ann R Coll Surg Engl. 2007;89:526–8.
6. Baldini A, Golfier F, Mouloud K, Bruge Ansel M-H, Navarro R, Ruffion A, et al. Day case laparoscopic nephrectomy with vaginal extraction: initial experience. Urology. 2014;84:1525–8.
7. Martin AD, Nunez RN, Andrews JR, Martin GL, Andrews PE, Castle EP. Outpatient prostatectomy: too much too soon or just what the patient ordered. Urology. 2010;75:421–4.
8. Kokorovic A, Wilson JWL, Beiko D. Outpatient bilateral supracostal tubeless percutaneous nephrolithotomy for staghorn calculi. Can Urol Assoc J. 2014; 8:E273–5.
9. Shahrour W, Andonian S. Ambulatory percutaneous nephrolithotomy: initial series. Urology. 2010;76:1288–92.
10. Munnich EL, Parente ST. Procedures take less time at ambulatory surgery centers, keeping costs down and ability to meet demand up. Health Aff. 2014;33:764–9.
11. Wills TE, Burns JR. Ureteroscopy: an outpatient procedure? J Urol. 1994;151:1185–7.
12. Yip KH, Lee CW, Tam PC. Holmium laser lithotripsy for ureteral calculi: an outpatient procedure. J Endourol. 1998;12:241–6.
13. Taylor AL, Oakley N, Das S, Parys BT. Day-case ureteroscopy: an observational study. BJU Int. 2002;89:181–5.
14. Chen JJC, Yip SKH, Wong MYC, Cheng CWS. Ureteroscopy as an out-patient procedure: the Singapore General Hospital Urology Centre experience. Hong Kong Med J. 2003;9:175–8.
15. Cheung MC, Yip SK, Lee FC, Tam PC. Outpatient ureteroscopic lithotripsy: selective internal stenting and factors enhancing success. J Endourol. 2000;14:559–64.
16. Cheung MC, Lee F, Leung YL, Wong BB, Chu SM, Tam PC. Outpatient ureteroscopy: predictive factors for postoperative events. Urology. 2001;58:914–8.
17. Jeong BC, Park HK, Kwak C, Oh S-J, Kim HH. How painful are shockwave lithotripsy and endoscopic procedures performed at outpatient urology clinics? Urol Res. 2005;33:291–6.
18. Ghalayini IF, Al-Ghazo MA, Khader YS. Extracorporeal shockwave lithotripsy versus ureteroscopy for distal ureteric calculi: efficacy and patient satisfaction. Int Braz J Urol. 2006;32:656–64. discussion 664–7.
19. Tan H-J, Strope SA, He C, Roberts WW, Faerber GJ, Wolf JS. Immediate unplanned hospital admission after outpatient ureteroscopy for stone disease. J Urol. 2011;185:2181–5.
20. Chan KY, Zulkifli MZ, Nazri MJ, Rashid MO. A review of day care ureteroscopy of a teaching hospital in Malaysia. Med J Malaysia. 2005;60:5–9.
21. Deters LA, Jumper CM, Steinberg PL, Pais VM. Evaluating the definition of "stone free status" in contemporary urologic literature. Clin Nephrol. 2011;76:354–7.
22. Lasselin J, Viart L, Lasselin-Boyard P, Raynal G, Saint F. Flexible ureteroscope damages. Evaluation of university hospital service equipment. Prog Urol. 2015;25:265–73.
23. Preminger GM, Tiselius H-G, Assimos DG, Alken P, Buck AC, Gallucci M, et al. 2007 Guideline for the management of ureteral calculi. Eur Urol. 2007;52: 1610–31.

15

A Randomized Study of Minimally Invasive Percutaneous Nephrolithotomy (MPCNL) with the aid of a patented suctioning sheath in the treatment of renal calculus complicated by pyonephrosis by one surgery

Jianrong Huang[1†], Leming Song[1*†], Donghua Xie[1,2*†], Monong Li[3†], Xiaolin Deng[1†], Min Hu[1], Zuofeng Peng[1], Tairong Liu[1], Chuance Du[1], Lei Yao[1], Shengfeng Liu[1], Shulin Guo[1] and Jiuqing Zhong[1]

Abstract

Background: Calculus pyonephrosis is difficult to manage. The aim of this study is to explore the value of a patented suctioning sheath assisted minimally invasive percutaneous nephrolithotomy (MPCNL) in the treatment of calculus pyonephrosis.

Methods: One hundred and eighty two patients with calculus pyonephrosis were randomizely divided into observation group ($n = 91$) and control group ($n = 91$). The control group was treated with MPCNL traditionally using peel-away sheath while the observation group was treated with MPCNL using the patented suctioning sheath.

Results: All the patients in the observation group underwent one stage surgical treatment, 14 patients in the control group underwent first-stage surgery with the rest of the group underwent one stage surgery. The complication rate was 12.1% in the observation group, significantly lower than the rate in the control group which was 51.6%; One surgery stone clearance in the observation group was 96.7% while it was 73.6% in the control group; operative time in the observation group was (54.5 ± 14.5) min, compared to (70.2 ± 11.7) min in the control group; the bleeding amount in the observation group was (126.4 ± 47.2) ml, compared to (321.6 ± 82.5) ml in the control group; the hospitalization duration for the observation group was (6.4 ± 2.3) days, compared to (10.6 ± 3.7) days in the control group. Comparison of the above indicators, the observation group was better than the control group with significant difference ($p < 0.001$ each).

Conclusions: Minimally invasive percutaneous nephrolithotomy with the aid of the patented suctioning sheath in the treatment of calculus pyonephrosis in one surgery is economic, practical, and warrants clinical promotion.

Keywords: Calculus pyonephrosis, Suctioning lithotripsy and stone clearance sheath, MPCNL

* Correspondence: xdhmd666@hotmail.com; xiedh07@gmail.com
†Equal contributors
[1]Department of Urology, The Affiliated Ganzhou Hospital of Nanchang University, 17 Hongqi Avenue, Ganzhou, Jiangxi 341000, China
Full list of author information is available at the end of the article

Background

Currently MPCNL has become one of the most important means in the treatment of upper urinary calculi. However, inappropriate infusion or poor drainage both can lead to significantly increased renal pelvic pressure, resulting in renal damage at various degrees, liquid reflux or extravasation, infection spread, urosepsis, or infectious shock. Patients undergo surgeries for complicated stones with pyonephrosis are more liable to worsening infection and urosepsis [1]. We designed a patented system with suctioning ability to facilitate minimally invasive PCNL (MPCNL). This patented system was found to be safe and highly efficient in managing renal stones in the previous study [2–4]. However, we did not know the success and complication rates of our MPCNLs in treating renal calculus complicated by pyonephrosis by one surgery. In this study, we performed one-stage MPCNLs using a self-designed and patented suctioning lithotripsy sheath [4] (thereafter referred to as the patent sheath, see Fig. 1) in treating renal and upper ureteral calculi complicated by pyonephrosis in 91 cases to clear stone by one surgery, avoided two stage surgeries including first-stage percutaneous nephrostomy and second-stage stone lithotripsy. We thus reported the outcome as below.

Methods

Patients

From March 2011 to April 2013 one hundred eighty two patients with calculus pyonephrosis were admitted and treated at Ganzhou Hospital of Nanchang University, China. Among them 110 were males while 72 were females. The age ranged from 21 to 82 years old with a mean age at 44.1 ± 3.7 years old. There were 98 cases with left renal calculus while 84 cases with right renal calculus. Calculus dimension ranged from 8.8 to 22.5 cm^2 with a mean dimension at 15.1 ± 6.5 cm^2. All patients had costovertebral angle (CVA) tenderness by physical exam. Urinalysis revealed white blood cell (WBC) ++ ~ +++. Seventy four patients were found to have Temperature ≥ 37.8 °C. The stone diseases were diagnosed by B ultrasonography, KUB (Kidneys, ureters, and bladder x-ray), or intravenous urography (IVU). Computed tomography (CT) scan was performed for each patient to confirm. Patients with systemic coagulopathy

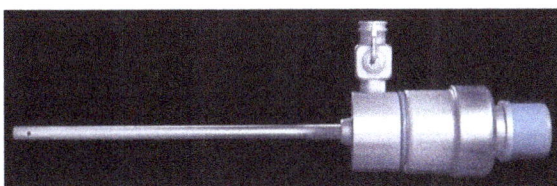

Fig. 1 Patented suctioning lithotripsy sheath

were ruled out from the study. These enrolled patients were randomized into either control group($n = 91$) or observation group($n = 91$) in a ratio of 1:1 according to the random number table. As shown in Table 1, comparisons of the two groups on sex, age, stone location, and course of disease revealed no significant difference ($P > 0.05$ each).

Surgical procedure

Surgery was performed under general anesthesia for all 182 patients, all the surgeries were performed by one surgeon. Patients in the observation group underwent patented sheath assisted MPCNL. Patients in the control group were treated using traditional MPCNL without the assistance of the patented sheath but peel-away sheath. Patients in both groups were administered antibiotic pre and post surgery. The patient was first placed

Table 1 General clinical data comparison(n = 91 each, $\bar{x}$ ±s)

Variable	Observation group	Control group	P value
Age (year)	43.5 ± 2.9	44.1 ± 3.2	>0.05
Sex			
Male: Female	53:38	51:40	>0.05
BMI(kg/cm2)	21.6 ± 5.7	22.5 ± 1.1	>0.05
Stone size(mm)	16.7 ± 5.8	15.1 ± 6.3	>0.05
Stone location			>0.05
Renal pelvis and upper segment of ureter	27 (29.7%)	29 (31.9%)	
Upper renal calyx	25 (27.5%)	21 (23.1%)	
Mid renal calyx	9 (9.9%)	7 (7.7%)	
Lower renal calyx	30 (33.0%)	34 (37.4%)	
Renal insufficiency (n,%)	8 (8.8%)	11 (12.1%)	>0.05
H/o ESWL (n,%)	15 (14.3%)	17 (12.8%)	>0.05
H/o surgery to remove stone (n,%)	13 (14.3%)	14 (15.4%)	>0.05
Comorbidities			>0.05
Hypertension	7 (7.7%)	6 (6.6%)	
Diabetes mellitus	4 (4.4%)	6 (6.6%)	
Heart disease	5 (5.5%)	3 (3.3%)	
Stone composition			>0.05
Calcium oxalate	44 (48.4%)	43 (47.3%)	
Calcium phosphate	11 (12.1%)	15 (16.5%)	
Cystine	2 (2.2%)	1 (1.1%)	
Struvite	19 (20.9%)	17 (18.7%)	
Uric acid	7 (7.7%)	5 (5.5%)	
Mixed	8 (8.8%)	10 (11.0%)	
Hydronephrosis			>0.05
Mild	13 (14.3%)	17 (18.7%)	
Moderate	47 (51.6%)	49 (53.8%)	
Severe	31 (34.1%)	25 (27.5%)	

in a lithotomy position. A 5 F ureteral catheter was then inserted retrogradely into the renal pelvis through cystoscopy or ureteroscopy, and continuous infusion of saline was used to produce artificial hydronephrosis. After this, a Foley catheter was inserted; the patient was then changed to the prone position. Ultrasonography-guided percutaneous punctures were made with an 18-gauge coaxial needle into the targeted calyx. The puncture point was in the 11th intercostal space or the 12 th subcostal margin, between the posterior axillary line and scapula line. The puncture was judged successful if there was urine overflow or if it touched a stone. Zebra guidewire was inserted and fixed. The puncture needle was then taken out. After a 0.5–0.7 cm skin incision, the dilation of the percutaneous tract was performed serially over the guidewire with a fascial dilator from 8 F to 16 F. A 16 F patented sheath was then placed at the percutaneous access port and was connected to a vacuum aspiration machine. The pressure was maintained at 0.01–0.02 MPa. Subsequently, a small diameter nephroscope was inserted through the sheath. Initially, pus or purulent bolts were sucked out using the vacuum suctioning device (See Fig. 2). A holmium laser was then used to break the stones, and a vacuum suctioning device was used to clear gravel through the patented sheath until complete clearance. We then inspected renal pelvis and each renal calyx carefully. After finding that all stones were cleared, we indwelled a 6 F ureteral stent and a 16 F nephrostomy tube which will be removed 4–5 days after surgery. Occurrence of renal pelvic perforation was investigated at the end of the procedure via nephrostogram.

For any patient in the two groups with the following intraoperative occurrences, the surgery was converted to a simple nephrostomy: (1) body temperature lower than 36 °C or higher than 38 °C; (2) heart rate higher than 90 beats per minute; (3) respiratory rate greater than 20 breaths per minute or PaCO2 less than 32 mmHg [5]; (4) excessive bleeding;(5) suctioning channel was blocked due to thick pus.

Observation index

Perioperatively, vital signs were closely monitored. Also, the complete blood count, serum electrolytes, BUN/creatinine, and calcitonin were checked. Patients were evaluated on postoperative day 30 by KUB assess stone-free status. For patients with radiolucent or residual stones, CT scan was performed. Successful stone clearance was defined as no residual stone or residual stone size < 4 mm. Patients in the two groups were compared for operation time, bleeding amount, stone clearance rate, complication rate, and average days of hospitalization.

Statistical analysis

We used Excel for data input. SPSSll.5 statistical software package was used for data analysis. The measurement data were represented as mean ± standard deviation ($\bar{x}$ ±s) and analyzed using t test. Count data was analyzed using χ^2 test. $P < 0.05$, with statistically significant difference.

Results

All patients in the observation group were treated with patented sheath assisted MPCNL successfully by one surgery without major complication including surrounding organ injury, pleural effusion, or major bleeding. There were 75 cases stones were cleared through one percutaneous tract, 15 cases stones was cleared through two percutaneous tracts, and two cases stones were cleared through three percutaneous tracts. There were ten cases with temperature ≥ 38.5 °C on postoperative day 2. There was one case in this group with complication of renal pelvic perforation. For the patients in the control group, 14 cases underwent first-stage percutaneous nephrostomy due to the difficulty in doing lithotripsy in the first surgery, while the rest of this group underwent one stage MPCNL. There were 15 cases with bleeding ≥ 800 ml and were transfused. There were 25 cases with temperature ≥ 38.5 °C on postoperative day 2. There were seven cases in this group with complication of renal pelvic perforation. In the observation group each index is better than the control group with significant difference ($P < 0.001$ each, see Table 2). Body temperatures returned to normal for those patients with

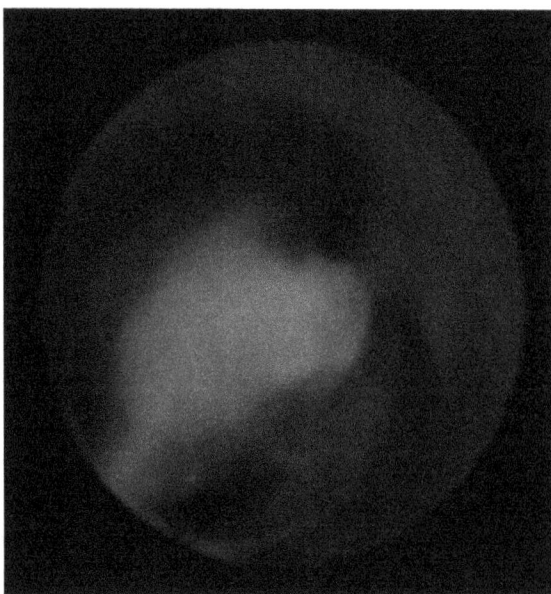

Fig. 2 Endoscopic view of renal calculus complicated by pyonephrosis

Table 2 Operative outcome comparison between two groups($\bar{x}$ ±s)

Variables	Observation group	Control group	P value
Operation time (min)	54.5 ± 14.5	70.2 ± 11.7	<0.001
Bleeding amount (ml)	126.4 ± 47.2	321.6 ± 82.5	<0.001
Stone-free rates	96.7% (88)	73.6% (67)	<0.001
Incidence of complication			
Fever ≥ 38.5 °C	10	25	<0.001
Bleeding amount ≥ 800 ml	0	15	<0.001
Renal pelvic perforation	1	7	<0.001
Days for hospitalization	6.4 ± 2.3	10.6 ± 3.7	<0.001

postoperative fever after strengthening anti-infection treatment without the occurrence of sepsis or pyemia. After a follow up of 3 months, serum creatinine (Scr) and blood urea nitrogen (BUN) in 74 cases that had elevated preoperative Scr and BUN preoperatively were reduced to varying degrees (See Table 2 and Fig. 3).

Discussion

Upper ureter or renal stones often were treated with MPCNL and most patients can achieve the purpose of cure. Due to the pressure limit of renal parenchymal reflux is 30 mmHg [6], when the MPCNL is performed under high pressure perfusion it is easy to cause the intrapelvic pressure over 30 mmHg, and the operation manipulation, the integrity of the pelvic wall epithelium could be injured and thereafter leads to direct exposure of venous and lymphatic system followed by renal parenchyma reflux [7]; When the stones and infection occur at the same time, tissue edema and congestion are more likely to cause pelvic fluid absorption. A large amount of short-term liquid absorption can cause the perfusion fluid syndrome, and when the bacteria and its toxin reflux into the blood, complications like bacteremia,

sepsis, or postoperative fever occur [8]. MPCNL surgery complication is related to the amount of liquid absorption. It is a positive correlation between the integrity of the epithelial cells, renal pelvic pressure, and the operation time [6, 9]. Performing MPCNL through irrigation can cause stones shift. When the collection system is connected to the renal abscess pus, due to the blurring of vision, it is not easy to find the pelvic outlet so the surgeon is often forced to abandon stone lithotripsy in which circumstance usually a percutaneous nephrostomy is performed as a first-stage surgery. In the current study, incidence rate of surgical complications in the control group was 51.6%% with 14 cases needing two staged operation. Therefore, how to improve success rate of surgery and reduce postoperative complications for calculus pyonephrosis is always a challenge in the field of Urology [10].

According to a previous report, when the intra-pelvic pressure is below 20 mmHg, it is feasible to use the EMS LithoClast master for one-phase PCNL of the relatively symptomatically stable patients with calculous pyonephrosis. Nevertheless, this surgical procedure has always carried high risks and its advantages and disadvantages should be validated by further studies of larger sample sizes [11, 12]. Patented sheath connected during surgery remains 0.01–0.02 MPa negative pressure suction to keep renal pelvis in a negative pressure state, so that the discharge of perfusion fluid and pus went smoothly, avoided lavage, bacteria, toxins reflux and spread to surrounding tissues, reduced fever infection complications after surgery. In the current study, only 10 patients in the observation group were found to have temperature ≥ 38.5 °C, significantly lower than those in the control group; Negative pressure adsorption can remove the effect of blood clots and floc, the vision can be more clear. With negative pressure "adsorption" effect on the gravel, small stones and pus hidden in the calyces can be automatically removed by suction. Due to a big

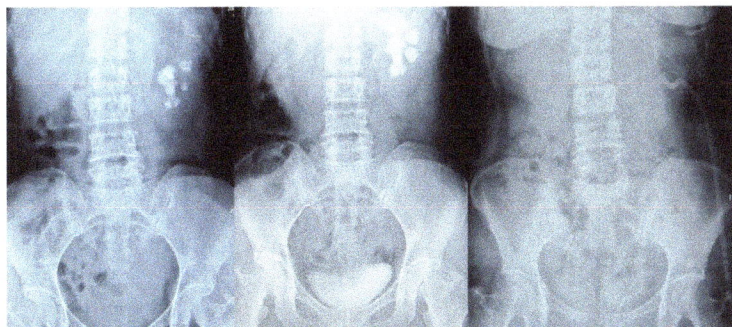

Fig. 3 Left: Preoperative KUB for a patient with staghorn renal calculus complicated by pyonephrosis; Middle: Preoperative IVU for a patient with staghorn renal calculus complicated by pyonephrosis; Right: Post-MPCNL KUB for a patient with staghorn renal calculus complicated by pyonephrosis, with the aid of the patented suctioning sheath

discharge cavity of the sheath which is not easy to be blocked, there is no need of lithotomy forceps or stone basket, without the need for repeated importing a ureteroscope to flush, either. We are thus able to improve the efficacy of lithotripsy and stone clearance, shorten operation time, and reduce the operation complications such as bleeding [3]. In this study, all patients in the observation group were successfully treated with the MPCNL by one surgery with a stone clearance rate of 96.7%. There were no adjacent organ injury and major bleeding, compared with the control group, with significant difference. With improved success rate of surgery and reduced rate of complication, the hospitalization time was shortened and the cost of hospitalization was reduced. Of course, surgeons may have been more aggressive using the patented sheath and less aggressive with the peel-away sheath due to the aims of this study, therefore getting higher stone-free rates in patients in the observation arm. Other limitation of this study is that we did not measure intrarenal pelvic pressure for every patient during the surgery, even though we have had previous research data revealing that the patented sheath could reduce intrarenal pressure.

Conclusion

In summary, through analysis and comparison the observation group was better than the control group reflected by multiple clinical indexes. Managing calculus pyonephrosis using patented sheath assisted MPCNL is safe, economic with fewer complications.

Abbreviations

BUN: Blood urea nitrogen; CT: Computed tomography; CVA: Costovertebral angle; IVU: Intravenous urography; KUB: Kidneys, ureters, and bladder x-ray; MPa: Megapascal; MPCNL: Minimally invasive percutaneous nephrolithotomy; PaCO2: Partial pressure of carbon dioxide in arterial blood; PCNL: Percutaneous nephrolithotomy; Scr: Serum creatinine (Scr); WBC: White blood cell

Acknowledgements

Not applicable.

Funding

Major Scientific Fund from Science and Technology Department of Jiangxi Province to L.M.S.

Authors' contributions

DX, ML, and XD were involved in analysis and interpretation of data, and drafting the report; JH, LS, DX, MH, ZP, TL, CD, LY, SL, SG and JZ were involved in data acquisition; LS, JH, DX, and ML were involved in conception and design; All authors read and approved the final manuscript.

Competing interests

Dr. Leming Song is the owner of the patent.

Ethics approval and consent to participate

The study was performed with the approval of ethics committee at the Affiliated Ganzhou City People's Hospital of Nanchang University, China, in compliance with the Helsinki Declaration. Written informed consent was obtained from every patient for participation in this study prior to undergoing treatment.

Statement

We have adhered to CONSORT methodology for this study.

Author details

[1]Department of Urology, The Affiliated Ganzhou Hospital of Nanchang University, 17 Hongqi Avenue, Ganzhou, Jiangxi 341000, China. [2]Department of Urology, Detroit Medical Center, Detroit, MI 48201, USA. [3]Department of Urology, The affiliated Qingdao Municipal Hospital of Medical College of Qingdao University, Qingdao, Shandong 266021, China.

References

1. Zeng G, Mai Z, Zhao Z, Li X, Zhong W, Yuan J, Wu K, Wu W. Treatment of upper urinary calculi with Chinese minimally invasive percutaneous nephrolithotomy: a single-center experience with 12,482 consecutive patients over 20 years. Urolithiasis. 2013;41(3):225–9.
2. Deng X, Song L, Xie D, Huang J, Zhu L, Wang X, Fan D, Peng Z, Hu M, Yang Z et al. Predicting Outcomes after Minimally Percutaneous Nephrolithotomy with the Aid of a Patented System by Using the Guy's Stone Score. Urol Int. 2016;97:67–71.
3. Yang Z, Song L, Xie D, Hu M, Peng Z, Liu T, Du C, Zhong J, Qing W, Guo S. Comparative study of outcome in treating upper ureteral impacted stones using minimally invasive percutaneous nephrolithotomy with Aid of patented system or transurethral ureteroscopy. Urology. 2012;80(6):1192–7.
4. Song L, Chen Z, Liu T, Zhong J, Qin W, Guo S, Peng Z, Hu M, Du C, Zhu L. The application of a patented system to minimally invasive percutaneous nephrolithotomy. J Endourol. 2011;25(8):1281–6.
5. Erdil T, Bostanci Y, Ozden E, Atac F, Yakupoglu YK, Yilmaz AF, Sarikaya S. Risk factors for systemic inflammatory response syndrome following percutaneous nephrolithotomy. Urolithiasis. 2013;41(5):395–401.
6. Guohua Z, Wen Z, Xun L, Wenzhong C, Yongzhong H, Zhaohui H, Ming L, Kaijun W. The influence of minimally invasive percutaneous nephrolithotomy on renal pelvic pressure in vivo. Surg Laparosc Endosc Percutan Tech. 2007; 17(4):307–10.
7. Hinman F, Redewill FH. Pyelovenous back flow. J Am Med Assoc. 1926; 87(16):1287–93.
8. De La Rosette J, Denstedt J, Geavlete P, Keeley F, Matsuda T, Pearle M, Preminger G, Traxer O. The clinical research office of the endourological society ureteroscopy global study: indications, complications, and outcomes in 11,885 patients. J Endourol. 2014;28(2):131–9.
9. Zhong W, Zeng G, Wu K, Li X, Chen W, Yang H. Does a smaller tract in percutaneous nephrolithotomy contribute to high renal pelvic pressure and postoperative fever? J Endourol. 2008;22(9):2147–52.
10. Chen L, Li J, Huang X, Wang X. Analysis for risk factors of systemic inflammatory response syndrome after one-phase treatment for apyrexic calculous pyonephrosis by percutaneous nephrolithotomy. Beijing da xue xue bao Yi xue ban = J Peking Univ Health Sci. 2014;46(4):566–9.
11. Zhou DQ, Wang J, Li WG, Pang X, Liu SW, Yu XX, Jiang B. Treatment of calculous pyonephrosis with percutaneous nephrolithotomy via the standard access. Nan fang yi ke da xue xue bao = J South Med Univ. 2009;29(7):1417–9.
12. Wang J, Zhou DQ, He M, Li WG, Pang X, Yu XX, Jiang B. One-phase treatment for calculous pyonephrosis by percutaneous nephrolithotomy assisted by EMS LithoClast master. Chin Med J. 2013;126(8):1584–6.

16

Minimally invasive surgical treatment on delayed uretero-vaginal fistula

Xinying Li, Ping Wang, Yili Liu and Chunlai Liu[*] (ORCID)

Abstract

Objective: To evaluate the procedure of endoscopic surgery for ureterovaginal fistula (UVF) and its clinical efficacy.

Materials and methods: A retrospective analysis of 46 patients needing treatment for UVF with endourology technology was conducted (all patients had unilateral ureteric injury, 27 left and 19 right). Transurethral retrograde ureteric stenting or realignment retrograde/antegrade approach stenting was used to treat the fistula, and the relation between treatment and prognosis was analyzed.

Results: One case failed, the patient undergoing percutaneous nephrostomy instead. Success was achieved in 45 cases, and urinary leakage was stopped 48 h after surgery. Of the 45 patients operated on, 16 had their double-J stents removed after 3–6 months, and 29 needed replacement every 6–12 months. In a postoperative follow-up of 6–36 months, 10 patients had recurrent stenosis needing ureteroscopic endoureterotomy or reexpansion with a balloon. No other complications occurred.

Conclusions: Endoscopic surgery is an effective technology in the treatment of UVF, with the advantages of being effective, reliable, less invasive, and readily accepted by patients.

Keywords: Ureter injury, Minimally invasive surgical, Endoscopy, Percutaneous nephroscopy, Ureterovaginal fistula

Introduction

A ureterovaginal fistula (UVF) is an abnormal channel between the ureter and vagina, which is a severely disabling complication resulting in incontinence, infection, and discomfort; it is often diagnosed postoperatively [1]. The incidence of UVF has been increasing due to the growing use of the laparoscopic surgical technique [2]. Traditionally, a laparotomy or laparoscopic surgery has been used to repair the delayed UVF [3, 4]; however, the serious local inflammatory response has slowed surgical repair. In recent years, minimally invasive treatment has been widely used for this disease. We have retrospectively analyzed 46 patients who were treated with minimally invasive treatment of UVF at our hospital from 2006 to 2016. In this review, we discuss the treatments to repair UVF, the required techniques, and postoperative recommendations.

* Correspondence: lixinying99@foxmail.com
Department of Urology, The Fourth Hospital of China Medical University, 4 Chongshan Road, Shenyang 110032, China

Patients and methods

The mean age of selected patients suffering from ureterovaginal fistula was 42.5 years (range, 34–53). They all had unilateral ureteric injury (27 left and 19 right). All patients who were followed had delayed UVF after laparoscopic total hysterectomy (56.5%), laparoscopic radical resection of cervical cancer (34.8%), and laparotomy cervical cancer resection procedures (8.6%). The injuries were diagnosed in a median 3.7 days (range, 24 h to 42 days) after the primary procedure, when they were typically discovered having a urine leak from the vagina. The lesion-side ureters of these patients were opened; in the retroperitoneum, extravasation of contrast medium from the computed tomography urogram (CTU) of the distal ureter was revealed. The CTU revealed 35 patients with delayed kidney development lateral to the injuries. In the other 11 patients, renal imaging was normal. Ultrasound showed all of them to have hydronephrosis—19 mild and 27 moderate. A routine chemistry examination of the vaginal leakage revealed that urea and creatinine levels were close to normal urine. Flexible cystoscopy showed that the bladder mucosa was normal and that there was no blue-tinged urine extravasation in the vagina after injecting indigo carmine or methylene blue in the bladder to help rule out vesicovaginal fistula.

Treatment
Ureteroscopy
Under continuous epidural or general anesthesia, all 46 patients were placed in the flank-reclining, split-leg position for simultaneous antegrade and retrograde ureteroscopy. We inserted an F16 ureteroscope in the bladder through the urethra. First, we made a ureteroscopic observation to again rule out vesicovaginal fistula. Then, a Zebra urological guide wire, carrying a ureteral scope, was inserted in the injured side of the ureter as far as the injury site. A Holmium laser was used when the cavity was too narrow or the surgery suture was met. Forty-six patients having a definitive diagnosis of delayed UVF were classified according to the lesion's description, as follows:

Class 1: The ureteric injuries were only fistulas, the ureteral mucosa was continuous, and the Zebra urological guide wire could be uplinked into the renal pelvis along the ureteral mucosa (34 cases).
Class 2: More than half the diameter of the ureter was lacerated, a segment of the ureteral wall was a coloboma or collapsed, and the Zebra guide wire would not pass through the injury (9 cases).
Class 3: The ureters were completely avulsed and the lacerated ends were filled in by the adjacent tissue (2 cases).
Class 4: The injured ureter was completely atretic (1 case).

Ureteric stent placement
For Classes 1, two or three double-J (D-J) stents were indwelled over the injury through the Zebra guide wire, which uplinked into the renal pelvis along the ureter's mucous membrane. The stents were confirmed to be in their appropriate positions during the operation with ultrasonography.

Endoscopic realignment for treatment [5]
The ureters of Class 2 were injured so seriously that the guide wire could hardly pass through the damaged region to reach the pelvis by retrograde ureteroscopy. Percutaneous nephroscopy had to be used to admit a flexible ureteroscope into the injury and insert the guide wire into the retroperitoneal space. A rigid ureteroscope was inserted retrogradely through the distal ureter to the injury. Then, a double ureteroscopic joint exploration and realignment was accomplished.

The guide wire was detected by the rigid ureteroscope, which was seized by the tip with an endoscopic grasping forceps and pulled out from urethra (using the foreign-body clamp in the ureteroscope to clip the guide wire outside the body through the diseased side of the distal ureter, bladder,

and urethra), placing three D-J stents along the guide wire and over the fistula.

Treatment of ureteral occlusion
The ureters of Classes 3 and 4 were in complete occlusion, with the ureteroscope and guide wire unable to open the occluded portion. Therefore, a "cut-to-the-light" technique was employed [6], with the ureteral segments being aligned via ultrasonographic and endoscopic control. The room light was dimmed and the rigid ureteroscope's light was turned off. Using the light source of the flexible ureteroscope that was inserted through the nephrostomy as a guide, we used the Holmium laser to restore ureteral continuity. A guide wire was indwelled across the area and uplinked to the renal pelvis, then three D-J stents were placed along the guide wire.

Treatment of secondary ureteric stricture
Ten patients had recurrent stenosis, which needed ureteroscopic endoureterotomy. First, we made an adequate longitudinal endoluminal incision of the strictured segment of the ureter and vaporized the scars until the periureteral fat was seen. Then, we indwelled three D-J stents for at least 6 weeks. We repeated the internal urethrectomy and replaced the stents after 6–12 months if the narrowing reappeared.

Results
Results of the surgical treatment are shown in Table 1 and Table 2. Urine leakage decreased significantly and no obvious leakage became evident within 48 h postoperatively.

For Class 1, of the 34 patients who successfully underwent retrograde ureteric stenting,16 had their stents removed after 3–6 months. The other 18 needed to have stent replacement or have their endoureterotomy re-expanded every 6–12 months. The mean operating time was 35 min (range, 25–60 min), and the mean hospital stay was 3.8 days (range, 3–5 days).

Eleven Class 2, 3, and 4 patients underwent realignment of rigid and flexible ureteroscopy for stenting, needing replacement of their D-J stents or reexpanded with incision every 6 months. The antegrade flexible ureteroscopy ensured that the stents formed in the correct position and that the nephrostomy drainage was placed. The nephrostomy tube was left in place for 1–2 weeks to decrease intravesicular pressure and minimize reflux through stents. The other Class 2 patient, whose injury was healed by scar tissue, was diagnosed 42 days after the initial operation. After the ureteroscope was withdrawn, the scar's "pseudo" tunnel narrowed again, requiring a repeat nephrostomy.She had to change the nephrostomy tube every month. The mean operating time was 80 ± 2 min (range, 60–110 min), and the mean hospital stay was 8.2 days (range, 6–10 days). To avoid

Table 1 Results list

	Age-bracket(y)	Side	Extent of injury	Initial operation	Time of recognition(days)	Operative time(min)	Hospital time(days)	Subsequent procedure
1	40–45	R	Class 1	a	8	30	3	III
2	35–40	L	Class 1	b	3	40	3	I
3	40–45	L	Class 1	b	6	40	3	I
4	40–45	L	Class 1	a	5	35	5	III
5	35–40	R	Class 1	b	2	30	3	I
6	45–50	R	Class 1	a	3	30	5	III
7	40–45	R	Class 1	c	4	35	4	III
8	40–45	L	Class 1	b	7	30	4	I&II
9	40–45	L	Class 1	b	2	30	3	III
10	45–50	R	Class 1	a	1	25	3	I
11	40–45	L	Class 1	a	2	25	4	I
12	25–35	L	Class 1	a	5	25	4	I&II
13	35–40	R	Class 1	a	2	35	4	III
14	40–45	L	Class 1	a	3	30	4	I
15	50–55	L	Class 1	a	2	40	5	I&II
16	40–45	L	Class 1	a	2	40	4	I
17	45–50	R	Class 1	b	1	60	3	I
18	35–40	L	Class 1	a	2	50	5	III
19	40–45	L	Class 1	b	8	50	3	III
20	35–40	L	Class 1	a	1	40	3	III
21	40–45	R	Class 1	a	5	40	4	I
22	25–35	R	Class 1	b	6	30	4	I&II
23	50–55	R	Class 1	a	2	30	3	III
24	50–55	R	Class 1	a	4	25	4	III
25	40–45	L	Class 1	b	5	30	4	I
26	45–50	L	Class 1	a	10	40	4	III
27	50–55	R	Class 1	b	4	40	4	I
28	40–45	L	Class 1	b	6	35	3	III
29	40–45	L	Class 1	b	1	30	5	III
30	40–45	R	Class 1	a	3	40	5	III
31	25–35	L	Class 1	a	3	35	4	I
32	35–40	L	Class 1	a	3	40	3	I
33	35–40	R	Class 1	b	1	40	3	III
34	45–50	R	Class 1	a	5	45	4	I
35	25–35	L	Class 2	a	6	80	9	I&II
36	35–40	L	Class 2	c	3	75	10	I&II
37	45–50	L	Class 2	a	3	70	7	I
38	45–50	R	Class 2	c	42	70	8	IV
39	45–50	L	Class 2	a	2	65	7	I
40	45–50	R	Class 2	c	4	60	10	I&II
41	45–50	R	Class 2	b	4	60	7	I
42	40–45	L	Class 2	a	3	90	7	I
43	40–45	L	Class 2	b	8	75	9	I&II

Table 1 Results list *(Continued)*

	Age-bracket(y)	Side	Extent of injury	Initial operation	Time of recognition(days)	Operative time(min)	Hospital time(days)	Subsequent procedure
44	45–50	L	Class 3	b	1	90	6	I
45	50–55	R	Class 3	a	1	90	8	I&II
46	40–45	L	Class 4	a	4	110	10	I&II

Abbreviation: *a* Laparoscopic total hysterectomy, *b* Laparoscopic radical resection of cervical cancer, *c* Laparotomic cervical cancer resection procedures, *I* Replace D-J stents every 6–12 months, *II* Ureteroscopic endoureterotomy or re-expand with balloon every 6–12 months; *III* Removed the double-j stents after 3–6 months, *IV* Exchange nephrostomy tube every month

sepsis and infection during hospitalization, the antibiotics should be used for 3 days routinely.

The catheter was indwelled in all 46 patients at the end of the operation and removed 2 weeks later. The overall catheterization success rate was 97.8%. There were no major complications, and blood loss was minimal. In the 6-month-to-3-year follow-ups (average, 18.6 months), ultrasound and intravenous pyelograms showed the ureter to be unobstructed, with the pelviureteric hydrocele significantly reduced or eradicated.

Discussion

Almost all UVFs are linked to an iatrogenic lesion, which usually follows pelvic and gynecological surgery [7, 8]. It occurs as one of the rare and serious surgical complications [9]. The incidence of UVF can be attributed to the surgical technique [10] and its technical difficulty [11], although the risk factors for the underlying pathology of individual patients are not identical. Based on the surgical history, clinical symptoms, and auxiliary examination, diagnosis of UVF is not complicated [12].

For economic reasons, many surgeons dislike taking a patient who has undergone previous ureteral surgery, so UVF patients are often difficult to diagnose intraoperatively [13], with a median time to diagnosis of 3–30 days post injury. The basic tenet in treating a UVF is to restore the continuity of the urinary tract, protect kidney function, reduce localized stenosis, and avoid urinary fistula formation [14].

Due to secondary renal damage resulting from ureter-repair surgery or reconstruction, preoperative excretory urography or other auxiliary methods are needed to determine contralateral renal function, which is of great value in

Table 2 Statistical of Results

	Successful operation		Failure operation	Total
	Removed D-J stents post operation	Replace D-J stents regularly		
Class 1	16	18	0	34
Class 2	0	8	1	9
Class 3	0	2	0	2
Class 4	0	1	0	1
Total	16	29	1	46
	45			

deciding how to deal with the damaged ureter. Urologists should adopt a comprehensive protocol according to the type, position, and degree of injuries.

Although the success rate, operative complications, and long-term outcome of traditional early surgical treatment for UVF are similar to delayed operation [15, 16], we suggest that UVF repair surgery or ureteric reimplantation be completed in the early stages [17, 18], which might avoid renal damage and reduce patient's pain and financial burden. Generally, first-stage repair surgery should be available intraoperatively or within 24 h after ureteral injury. But for the delayed diagnosis cases and severe shockers with complicated injuries, repair surgery should be put off for 3–6 months after urine transfer [19].

In recent years, retrograde ureteric stenting has been recommended for the first stage of UVF, which reduces urine leakage in internal drainage and in inflammatory lesions [20]. UVF can typically be treated successfully by ureteric stenting as long as the ureter wall is continuous.

Generally speaking, there is no need to disconnect the ureter during transurethral ureteroscopy and retrograde stenting, UVF can typically be treated successfully by placing a D-J stent [21],which can replace the patient's mental and physical trauma with easy acceptance, short hospitalization time, and fast recovery. Even if the UVF fails to heal, it can be used in first-stage treatment in full drainage to protect renal function and lay a good foundation for stage II surgery.

For some severe ureteric injuries, retrograde stenting is sometimes unsuccessful. Combining our practice with the literature review, we believe that the realignment retrograde/antegrade stenting approach is feasible by inserting the guide wire into the injury from the percutaneous nephroscope channel [22] and using the ureteroscope to grasp the guide wire out from the urethra, then pass the D-J stent along the guide wire and over the injury.

In a minority of situations, in which a patient presents with a severe ureteral injury—completely lacerated or atretic—such that a guide wire cannot be passed in either in a retrograde or antegrade fashion, endoscopic realignment for treatment and "cut-to-the-light" technique should be employed [6].

Compared with retrograde stenting, the extravasation of urine and washing fluid can be smoothly accomplished provided there is sufficient time and operating space for surgery. It would made stenting easier, more readily available, safer, and less invasive.

Therefore, it is appropriate for patients with a history of open pelvic and radical gynecologic surgery, multiple casualties, and those with severe fever, local inflammatory reaction, or severe shock.

Additional advantages of this method are as follows:

1. It is easy to find both ends of ureteral injury and approach its focus along the nephrostomy channel by means of double ureteroscopic realignment, which increases the success rate of prograde or retrograde ureteric stenting, avoiding additional surgery, or ureteric reimplantation or placement of a percutaneous nephrolithotomy (PCN) tube.
2. It ensures that the guide wire reaches the injury using direct vision and avoids exacerbating the ureter injury during adjustment of the guide wire's position and direction during the procedure.
3. It is particularly appropriate for patients with failing retrograde ureteric stenting; patients who suffer from a severed ureter, severe injury, or ureter distortion; those who cannot tolerate long-term indwelling of a urinary catheter; and those with an advanced tumor.
4. The flank-reclining, split-leg position provides sufficient operating space to perform a PCN and retrograde ureteroscopy simultaneously.

Although the endoscopic realignment was successfully used, some obvious disadvantages of the method are as follows: In some cases with normal or mild hydronephrosis, it is difficult to gain access to a nondilated renal collecting system because of urine leakage. The ureter is easy to collapse and block after pulling out the ureteral stent in patients who have long suffered from defects of ureteric avulsion or transection (usually > 2 cm), serious stricture formation, repeated surgeries, or serious fibrosis of the ureteral surroundings. In addition, this procedure should be performed before the flexible ureteroscopy's light no longer penetrates the tissue between the ureteroscopes. However, more studies with longer, consecutive follow-ups and mass cases are necessary to predict prognosis in the future.

Conclusions
UVF is an uncommon iatrogenic complication of gynecologic surgery and difficult to diagnosis early. The incidence is more common in patients who have had radical hysterectomy. Minimally invasive methods using the D-J stent are safe and effective techniques for managing delayed UVF. We strongly recommend minimally invasive

treatment of fistulae assisted with the ureteroscope to raise the cure rate, reduce the period of pain, and improve the survival rate.

Abbreviations
D-J: Double J; PCN: Percutaneous nephroscopy; UVF: Uretero-vaginal fistula

Acknowledgements
We thank all participants. We are grateful to the research study coordinators and members of the Department of The Fourth Affiliated Hospital of China Medical Universitywho contributed to this study: Chundong Zhang,MD,Junzhe Jin,PHD,Xiling Zhang,PHD. We also thank Salvatore Micali, M.D. for careful reading and editing of this manuscript.

Funding
Not applicable.

Authors' contributions
Participate in the conception and initial design: CL. Participate in the acquisition: CL, PW, YL, XL. Participate in the analysis and interpretation: CL, PW, YL, XL. Participate in the drafting and/or revision of the manuscript: CL, PW, YL,XL. All authors read and approved the final manuscript.

Competing interests
The authors declare that they have no competing interests.

References
1. Comiter CV, Vasavada SP, Raz S. Ureterovaginal Fistula. London: Springer; 2003.
2. Parpala-Spårman T, Paananen I, Santala M, Ohtonen P, Hellström P. Increasing numbers of ureteric injuries after the introduction of laparoscopic surgery. Scand J Urol. 2008;42:422.
3. Modi P, Goel R, Dodiya S. Laparoscopic ureteroneocystostomy for distal ureteral injuries. Urology. 2005;66:751–3.
4. El-Lamie IK. Urogenital fistulae: changing trends and personal experience of 46 cases. Int Urogynecol J. 2008;19:267–72.
5. Liu C, Zhang X, Xue D, Liu Y, Wang P. Endoscopic realignment in the management of complete transected ureter. Int Urol Nephrol. 2014;46:335–40.
6. Goda K, Kawabata G, Yasufuku T, Hara I, Fujisawa M, Kamidono S, Okada H. Cut-to-the-light technique and potassium titanyl phosphate laser ureterotomy for complete ureteral obstruction. Int J Urol. 2004;11:427.
7. Akman RY, Sargin S, Özdemir G, Yazicioğlu A, Çetin S. Vesicovaginal and Ureterovaginal Fistulas: A Review of 39 Cases. Int Urol Nephrol. 1999;31:321.
8. Alotaibi KM. Ureterovaginal fistulas: the role of endoscopy and a percutaneous approach. Urology Annals. 2012;4:102–5.
9. Oh BR, Kwon DD, Park KS, Ryu SB, Park YI, Jr PJ. Late presentation of ureteral injury after laparoscopic surgery. Obstet Gynecol. 2000;95:337–9.
10. Lim MC, Lee BY, Lee DO, Joung JY, Kang S, Seo SS, Chung J, Park SY. Lower urinary tract injuries diagnosed after hysterectomy: seven-year experience at a cancer hospital. J Obstet Gynaecol Res. 2010;36:318–25.
11. Brandes S, Coburn M, Armenakas N, McAninch J. Diagnosis and management of ureteric injury: an evidence-based analysis. BJU Int. 2004;94:277–89.
12. Boateng AA, Eltahawy EA, Mahdy A. Vaginal repair of ureterovaginal fistula may be suitable for selected cases. Int Urogynecol J. 2013;24:921–4.
13. El OM, Jlif H, Boujnah B, Ayed M, Zmerli S. Uretero-vaginal fistula. Apropos of 30 cases. J De Gynécologie Obstétrique Et Biologie De La Reprod. 1989; 18:891–4.
14. Wagner JR, Paul Russo MD. Urologic complications of major pelvic surgery. Semin Surg Oncol. 2000;18:216–28.
15. Abraham GP, Das K, Ramaswami K, George DP, Abraham JJ, Thachil T. Laparoscopic reconstruction of iatrogenic-induced lower ureteric strictures: does timing of repair influence the outcome? Indian J Urol Iju Journal of the Urological Society of India. 2011;27:465.

16. Mahendran HA, Praveen S, Ho C, Goh EH, Tan GH, Zuklifli MZ. Iatrogenic ureter injuries: eleven years experience in a tertiary hospital. Med J Malaysia. 2012;67:169–72.

17. Singh V, Jhanwar A, Sinha RJ. Transperitoneal laparoscopic ureteric reimplantation for lower ureteric strictures and ureterovaginal fistulas: a study from North India. Afr J Urol. 2017;23:43–7.

18. Wong WY, Tsu JH, Ng AT, Wong EM, Ho KL, Yiu MK. Iatrogenic ureteral injuries: a 20-year retrospective review in a university teaching hospital; 2014. p. 11.

19. Kim SK, Lee YR, Min SK, Choi JS. Transrenal ureteral occlusion with the use of microcoils in five patients with ureterovaginal fistulas. Abdom Radiol. 2008;33:615–20.

20. Pocock RD, Stower MJ, Ferro MA, Smith PJB, Gingell JC. Double J stents: a review of 100 patients. Br J Urol. 1986;58:629–33.

21. Yates DR, Mehta SSSpencer PA, Parys BT. Combined antegrade and retrograde endoscopic retroperitoneal bypass of ureteric strictures: a modification of the 'rendezvous' procedure. BJU Int. 2010;105:992.

22. Trouillon R, Kang DK, Park H, Chang SI, O'Hare D. Percutaneous minimally invasive management of iatrogenic ureteral injuries. J Endourol. 2010;24:1921–7.

17

A modified neo-vagina procedure in a low resource urogynecological unit: a case report of a 21 year old with Mayer-Rokitansky-Küster-Hauser (mrkh) Syndrome operated at Mbarara referral hospital, Southwestern Uganda

Musa Kayondo[1,2*], Joseph Njagi[1,2], Peter Kivuniike Mukasa[3] and Tom Margolis[4,5]

Abstract

Background: Although vaginal agenesis as may occur in Mayer-Rokitansky-Küster-Hauser (MRKH) syndrome is a rare condition, it is associated with not only anatomical problems but also serious psychological and social problems like painful sexual intercourse, primary amenorrhea and infertility. Surgery, which is aimed at reconstruction of a vagina of adequate length and width to serve the function, is the main method of treatment. Many methods for vaginal reconstruction have been described but each has its complications and limitations. The most commonly preferred procedure for treating this condition is the McIndoe vaginoplasty which involves dissection into the recto-vesical space, inserting two split thickness skin grafts folded over a mold in this newly created space and regular dilatation of the neovagina postoperatively to avoid stenosis. However surgeons with this expertise in this part of the world are rare to find and where they are available, the special molds on which to fold the skin grafts into the neovaginal space are not readily available.

Case presentation: A 21-year-old female with vaginal agenesis was operated on using a modification of the McIndoe procedure using a cylinder of a 60cm^3 syringe as a vaginal mold/form and kept in place. We left a Foley in place for 10 days and we did a dye test after removing the syringe to ensure that there was no leakage resulting from fistula formation.

Conclusion: The operation was successful and on subsequent monthly reviews of the patient, she has a patent functional vagina of about 9 cm in length at 8 months after the operation with resumption of sexual intercourse.

Keywords: Vaginal agenesis, Mayer-Rokitansky-Küster-Hauser syndrome, Skin grafts, Neovagina, Vaginal molds, Case reports

* Correspondence: kayondo100@yahoo.com
[1]Faculty of Medicine, Mbarara University of Science and Technology, P.O. BOX 1410 Mbarara, Uganda
[2]Department of Obstetrics and Gynecology, Mbarara Regional Referral Hospital, P.O. BOX 40 Mbarara, Uganda
Full list of author information is available at the end of the article

Background

The vagina is an important organ in females not only forming a part of the birth canal but also serving as the main organ for sexual intercourse. Congenital absence of the vagina which usually occurs in Mayer-Rokitansky-Küster-Hauser syndrome, Androgen insensitivity syndrome and other embryological disorders usually presents with social problems ranging from failure to have sexual penetration, painful coitus and sometimes broken marriages which if not taken care of often lead to serious psychological problems like depression and rejection [1]. Such women require construction of a new vagina (neo-vaginal procedure) so that they can at least have sexual pleasure [1–3]. In most centers these women are turned away due to lack of surgeons with expertise to handle this problem. Even in places where the expertise is available, resources required for this complex procedure are not available. Known conventional neo-vaginal surgical procedures include McIndoe vaginoplasty, rectosigmoid vaginoplasty and the modified vacchietti [1, 3, 4]. The most widely used among these methods is the classical McIndoe which involves dissection and creation of a neo-vagina in the rectovesical space and insertion of 2 skin grafts from the inguinal regions folded over a vaginal mold (form) into this space. Split-thickness skin grafts have over the time been used in this operation. The skin is harvested from a region of the body, which is hair free notably from the inguinal region, buttocks and inner thighs. The skin is harvested using an air powered or electrical dermatome. The harvested skin is folded over a foam mold and inserted in the newly dissected recto-vesical space. Closure of the donor site is done with a vicryl 2/0 suture inserted subcutaneously to ensure hemostasis and cosmesis. The vaginal mold prevents restenosis of the neovagina and is kept in for a period of at least 10 days [2–5]. These procedures are relatively complex and inappropriate in a low resource setting like our hospital because the vaginal molds to prevent restenosis of the neovagina are not readily available and neither are the electric or air powered dermatomes for harvesting skin.

Another procedure that has been described for treatment of MRKH syndrome is the Vacchietti procedure. This procedure utilizes a laparoscope to produce a neo-vagina whose dimensions are comparable to those of a normal vagina. In this procedure, a small sphere that is made of plastic ("olive") is fixed on the vaginal dimple; the strings on the olive are passed through the mucosa of the vagina into the peritoneal cavity and through the navel. The strings are attached on to a traction device, which is then adjusted daily such that the "olive" is pulled inwards. This serial pull stretches the vagina by approximately 1 cm per day hence forming a vagina, which is approximately 7 cm wide, and 7 cm in depth. With regards to restoration of vaginal anatomy and function in patients with MRKH syndrome, the laparoscopic Vacchietti technique has better success rates when compared to other treatments [6–8]. Laparoscopy is not available in this part of the world hence this procedure is not possible at our hospital.

Therefore in this case we designed a relatively easier procedure (modified McIndoe) where we harvested 2 full thickness skin flaps from the inguinal region using a scalpel instead of an electric dermatome which was folded on to a cylinder of a 60cm^3 syringe to act as the vaginal mold to prevent restenosis of the reconstructed vagina in a 21-year-old woman with vaginal agenesis due to Rokitansky's syndrome. A surgeon, with skill in vaginal surgery can easily do this procedure.

Case presentation

A 21-year-old woman was admitted to the gynecology ward of Mbarara Regional Referral Hospital (MRRH) with primary amenorrhea, failure to conceive and painful coitus. All these had affected her marriage of three years to a point of divorce. On evaluation she was found to have a normal female genotype with well-developed secondary sexual characteristics. Pelvic examination revealed a vaginal dimple with no palpable uterus (Fig. 1). An abdominal ultrasound scan revealed presence of both ovaries with a streak like or rudimentary uterus. The rest of the pelvic organs were normal. A preoperative diagnosis of vaginal agenesis due to MRKH syndrome was made. A decision to do surgery of creating a new vagina by using a modification of the McIndoe procedure was decided. Counseling of the patient about the surgical procedure with emphasis on the expectations was done. We explained to the patient that the procedure would improve her sexual life but would have no effect on her ability to conceive which she accepted and consented to the operation. Bowel preparation using soap enema plus overnight fasting was done prior to the operation. After induction of anesthesia, the patient was put in lithotomy position. The vulva was cleaned with antiseptic solution then draped. A urethral catheter of size 16 was inserted into the bladder. A transverse incision was made on the vaginal dimple to open into the rectovesical space. Bunt dissection was continued until a length of about 9 cm and 3 cm in width was achieved. A methylene blue dye was introduced into the bladder to make sure that there was no accidental bladder injury and a finger was also introduced into the rectum to ensure that there was no rectal injury.

Two full thickness hair free folds of skin measuring 12 by 6 cm in length and width were harvested from each lateral side of the abdominal wall starting from the anterior superior iliac spines. We used the lateral side instead of the skin over the inguinal ligament as done in

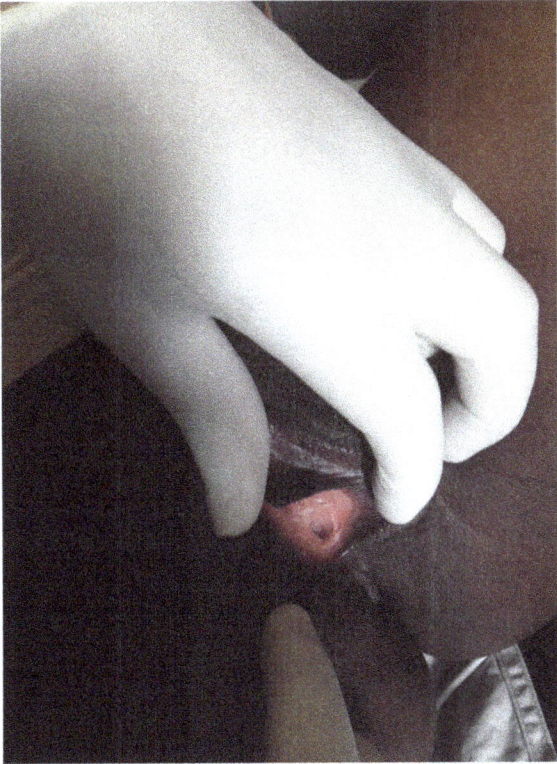

Fig. 1 Showing the Vaginal dimple of the 21 year old patient with vaginal agenesis before surgery

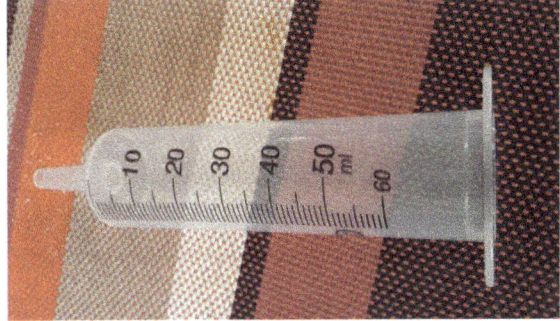

Fig. 2 The cylinder of a 60cm³ syringe, which was used as a mold instead of the conventional vaginal form on which the skin grafts were folded to prevent stenosis of the neovagina

the McIndoe method because our patient was too skinny for us to get adequate length and width of skin in this area. The folds were prepared by first immersing them in normal saline then the subcutaneous fat from each of the folds was removed using a sharp scissor. The assistant closed the sites from which the grafts were harvested using nylon 2/0 sutures interrupted vertical matrix as the lead surgeon prepared the grafts.

Unlike in the McIndoe method were the skin flaps are folded on a vaginal mold/form, here we used the cylinder of a 60 ml bladder syringe to act as a stent for the grafts in place of the vaginal form due to lack of the foam rubber to make a vaginal form (Fig. 2). The tip of the syringe was cut off before it was inserted. The skin grafts were folded on the cylinder of the syringe with the epidermal sides lying on the cylinder using interrupted vicryl 3/0 sutures. The excess lengths of the grafts were trimmed off.

The graft with its cylinder was then carefully inserted into the newly created rectovesical space after achieving hemostasis. In order to secure the graft in place, the cylinder of the syringe was fixed to the labia majora on either side using a nylon 2/0 suture unlike in the McIndoe method where the labia are sutured in the midline. The cylinder stent was maintained for 10 days to keep the neovagina patent. The urethral catheter was also kept in for the same duration to ease the patient's voiding and to also

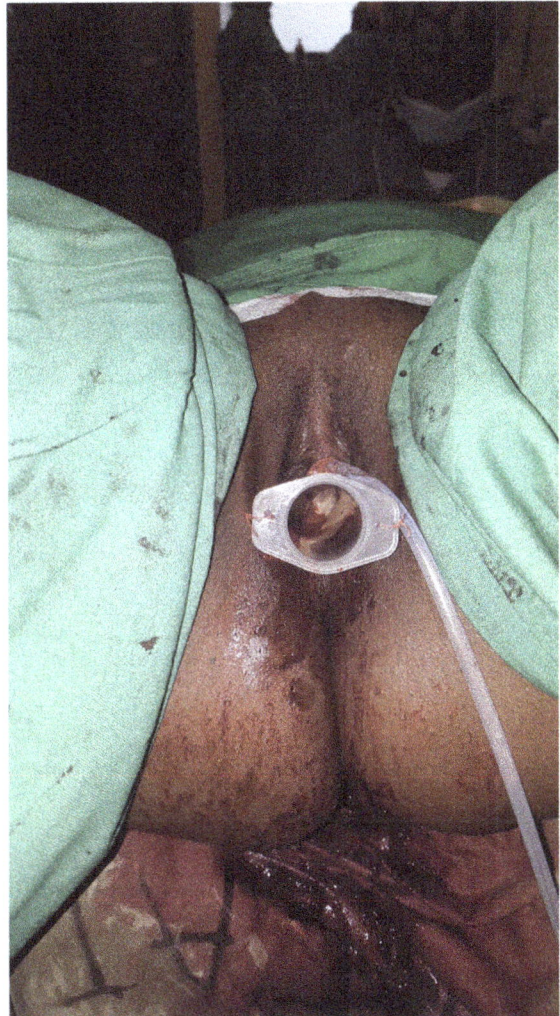

Fig. 3 Showing the cylinder of the syringe inserted into the neovagina and fixed on to the labia majora by a stitch on either side for 10 days to prevent restenosis

rest the bladder and urethra to guard against pressure necrosis that could be caused by the prolonged pressure on the urethra by the cylinder hence causing a fistula. A low residue diet was prescribed for the patient to prevent constipation and hard stools. She was also put on oral antibiotics and analgesia to prevent post surgical infection and pain for about 5 days. We used antibiotics, which were readily available in the hospital (Ceftriaxone and metronidazole). The labial stitches anchoring the cylinder stent were removed on the 10th postoperative day on the ward. She was examined and there was no any postoperative complication like infection, graft rejection or bleeding (Fig. 3). A methylene blue test was done before the Foley catheter was removed to ensure that there was no fistula formed as a result of pressure necrosis by the cylinder on the urethra. After removal of the cylinder stent she was taught self-serial dilatation using a condom rolled on to a candle to prevent stricture of the neovagina. She was advised to do this self-dilatation for at least 3 months.

She was discharged with a patent neovagina and the skin donor sites had healed after removal of the skin sutures. She has been followed up every 2 months for the last 8 months after operation and on examination the neovagina is patent (Figs. 4, 5 and 6) and she has

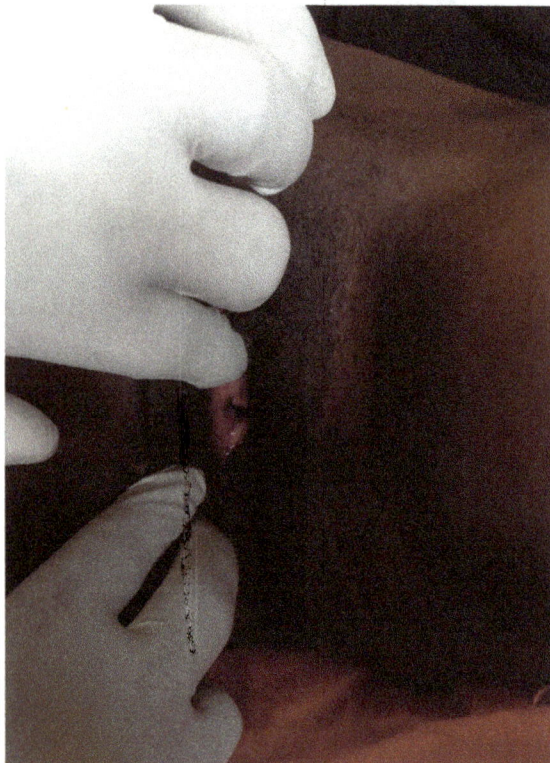
Fig. 4 Opening to the newly reconstructed vagina on the 11th post operative day after removal of the cylinder that acted like the vaginal stent/mold

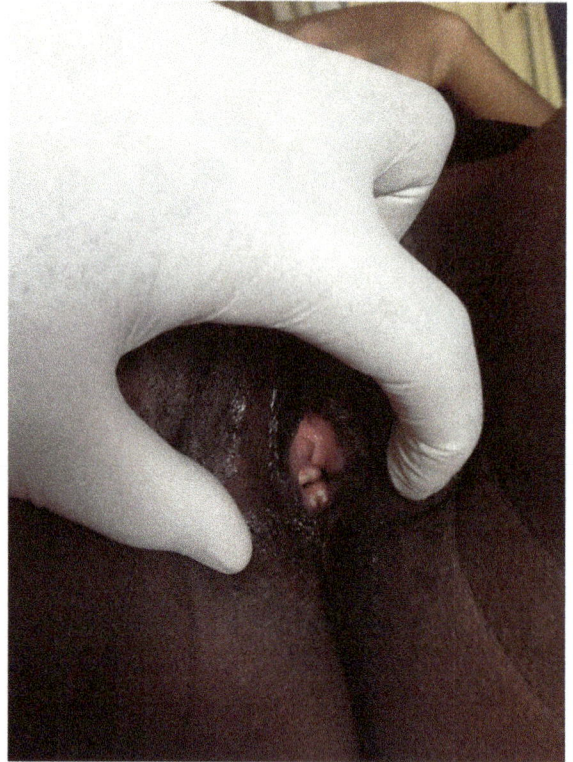
Fig. 5 Appearance of the Neovagina at 3 months post operative

resumed sexual intercourse, which has really improved her marital life.

Discussion

Although vaginal dysgenesis seems to be a rare condition with reported incidences ranging from 1 in 4000 to 1 in 10,000 females, it is associated with adverse psychological and social effects in women [1]. Therefore the surgery to rectify this problem not only does it restore the anatomy but it also improves the psychological and social state of these girls and women like enabling them to enjoy penetrative sex thus preventing divorce [1, 3, 9].

In low resource countries like Uganda such women find it hard to get any medical help because there are a few or no surgeons with the expertise to handle these conditions. Even where expertise is available, the equipment and supplies like vaginal molds (forms) are not easy to come by.

In this case of the 21 year old with vaginal dysgenesis we started off the procedure same way as in the conventional McIndoe method. The difference of our procedure from the classical McIndoe is that we used full thickness skin flaps instead of the split skin grafts. The full thickness grafts are easier to harvest than the split thickness ones when an electrical dermatome is not readily available like in our case. The full thickness grafts have also been found to take a longer time to shrink during the

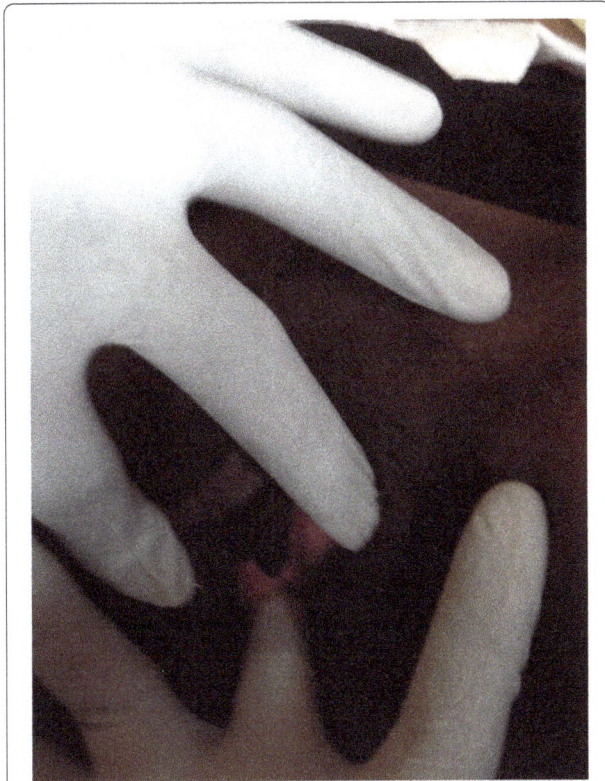

Fig. 6 The neovagina still patent at 3 months post operation and able to admit at least one finger

postoperative period when compared to the split thickness grafts. This therefore shortens the time required in utilization of the vaginal foam [3–5]. Therefore in our case we kept the stent in situ for only 10 days because we used the full thickness skin grafts yet it would have stayed in longer if we had used the split thickness skin grafts which is usually uncomfortable to the patient.

In contrast to the McIndoe, we introduced methylene blue dye in the bladder to make sure that there was no bladder perforation during dissection of the rectovesical space. We also harvested skin folds from the hairless skin area above the anterior superior iliac spine in contrast to the McIndoe method, which uses the skin over the inguinal region. This was because our patient was very skinny that we couldn't get enough skin over the inguinal region. It proved to be enough skin and a good area for harvesting skin in these circumstances.

The McIndoe method uses a specifically designed vaginal mold from foam rubber to prevent restenosis of the reconstructed vagina [2, 4, 5]. Since we couldn't get the special vaginal mold, we improvised by using a cylinder of a 60cm^3 syringe. This is the one that acted as a mold for the skin grafts inserted into the neovagina. These syringes are very easy to come by in our hospital; they cause minimal discomfort to the patient and can easily

be removed after 10 days without distorting the integrity of the skin grafts in the neovagina.

In the surgical procedure we have described, we did not have to suture the labia in the midline to prevent the vaginal mold from falling out as is done in the McIndoe method. This reduced the postoperative pain usually encountered in McIndoe because of the sutured labia hence our patient was able to ambulate early and recovery was faster. We also removed the vaginal stent after 10 days compared to the 12 to 14 days mentioned in the McIndoe method hence reducing on the period of hospital stay of the patient.

Our modified procedure is less superior when compared to the Vacchietti laparoscopic technique in regard to anatomical and functional outcome of the newly created vagina [7, 8]. But in this part of the world, laparoscopy is not readily available making the Vacchietti procedure inappropriate for a hospital in this type of setting. This makes our modified procedure ideal for our hospital in a low resource setting.

Conclusion

In patients with vaginal agenesis in low resource settings, a modification of the McIndoe method where a cylinder of a 60cm^3 syringe acts as a stent/vaginal mold for 10 days without suturing the labia to keep it in place can be done successfully with little chance of vaginal restenosis in the future.

The postoperative pain and length of stay in hospital associated with this method is less when compared to the conventional McIndoe procedure.

Acknowledgements
The authors are grateful to the operating room staff plus ward staff of Mbarara Regional Referral Hospital who participated in the management of this patient before, during and after the operation.
Special thanks to Medled medical missions USA and UNFPA for all the material and financial support offered that helped to organize the surgical camp in which this patient was operated upon.

Funding
There are no sources of funding to be declared for this study.

Authors' contributions
MK, NJ and TM did the clinical evaluation of the patient, came to a diagnosis and operated on the patient using the technique described above. MK, PK and NJ did the follow-up of the patient. MK, PK wrote all the versions of the manuscript and revised it critically for important intellectual content. All authors read and approved the final manuscript to be published. All authors agreed to be accountable for all aspects of the work.

Competing interests
The authors declare that they have no competing interests.

Author details
[1]Faculty of Medicine, Mbarara University of Science and Technology, P.O. BOX 1410 Mbarara, Uganda. [2]Department of Obstetrics and Gynecology, Mbarara Regional Referral Hospital, P.O. BOX 40 Mbarara, Uganda. [3]United Nation Fund for Population Activities, Kampala, Uganda. [4]Department of Obstetrics and Gynecology, University of California, Los Angeles, USA. [5]Medled Medical Missions, Burlingame, California, USA.

References
1. Evans TN, Poland L, Boving RL. Vaginal malformations. Am J Obstet Gynecol. 1981;141(8):910–20.
2. McIndoe AH. The treatment of congenital absence and obliterative conditions of the vagina. Br J Plast Surg. 1950;2(4):254–64.
3. Laufer MR. Congenital absence of the vagina: in search of the perfect solution. When, and by what technique, should a vagina be created? Curr Opin Obstet Gynecol. 2002;14(5):441–2.
4. McIndoe AH, Banniser JB. An operation for the cure of congenital absence of the vagina. J Obstet Gynecol Br Emp. 1938;45:490–4.
5. Wheeless CR, Roenneburg ML. McIndoe vaginoplasty for neovagina, online Atlas of Pelvic surgery. 1995.
6. Vecchietti G. Creation of an Artificial Vagina in Rokitansky–Kster–Hauser Syndrome. Attual Ostet Ginecol. 1965;11:131–47.
7. Fedele L, Bianchi S, Tozzi L, Borruto F, Vignali M. A New Laparoscopic Procedure for Creation of a Neovagina in Rokitansky–Küster–Hauser Syndrome. Fertil Steril. 1996;66:854–7.
8. Borruto F, Chasen ST, Chervenak FA, Fedele L. The Vecchietti procedure for surgical treatment of vaginal agenesis: comparison of laparoscopy and laparotomy. Int J Gynaecol Obstet. 1999;64(2):153–8.
9. Beksac MS, Salman MC, Dogan NU. A New Technique for Surgical Treatment of Vaginal Agenesis Using Combined Abdominal-Perineal Approach. Case Rep Med. 2011;2011:6 Article ID 120175.

18

Combined bladder neck preservation and posterior musculofascial reconstruction during robotic assisted radical prostatectomy: effects on early and long term urinary continence recovery

Riccardo Bartoletti[1,3]*(iD), Andrea Mogorovich[1], Francesco Francesca[2], Giorgio Pomara[2] and Cesare Selli[1]

Abstract

Background: To evaluate the effects of combined bladder neck preservation and posterior reconstruction techniques on early and long term urinary continence in patients treated by robotic assisted radical prostatectomy (RARP).

Methods: Two-hundred ninety-two patients who previously underwent radical prostatectomy were retrospectively selected for a case-control study, excluding those with anastomotic strictures and significant perioperative complications and re-called for a medical follow-up visit after their consent to participate the study. They were divided in 3 different groups according to the surgical technique previously received: radical retropubic prostatectomy (RRP) combined with bladder neck preservation (BNP), RARP with bladder neck resection, and RARP combined with BNP and posterior musculofascial reconstruction (PRec).
Functional and oncologic outcomes evaluation were integrated by a questionnaire on urinary continence status, abdominal ultrasound scan, uroflowmetry and post-void urine volume measurement.
Urinary continence definition included the terms "no pad" or "safety pad".

Results: Two hundred thirty-two patients responded to the phone call interview and were enrolled in the study. They presented comparable age, prostate volume and BMI. Differences in comorbidities, ASA score and medications, did not influence the postoperative functional results, focused on continence outcome.
Early urinary continence was achieved in 49.38% and 24.73% of patients who previously underwent RARP + BNP + PRec and simple RARP respectively ($p = 0.000$)as well as late 12-months urinary continence was obtained in 92.59% and 79.56% of patients.($p = 0.01$). Late urinary continence in the RRP + BNP group was comparable to the result obtained in the simple RARP group. The potential effects of nerve sparing technique on urinary continence have not been evaluated.

Conclusions: The combined technique of RARP + BNP + PRec seems to be effective to determine early and long term significant effects on urinary continence of patients with comparable body mass index, age and prostate volume. No statistically significant differences were found between the simple RARP and the RRP + BNP groups.

Keywords: Prostate cancer surgery, Robot assisted radical prostatectomy, Bladder neck preservation, Posterior musculofascial reconstruction, Urinary continence

* Correspondence: riccardo.bartoletti@hotmail.com
[1]Urology Unit University of Pisa, Pisa, Italy
[3]Urology University Unit, Cisanello Hospital, Via Paradisa 2, 56124 Pisa, Italy
Full list of author information is available at the end of the article

Background

Postoperative urinary continence recovery after laparoscopic robotic assisted radical prostatectomy (RARP) is related to multiple factors such as patient and disease characteristics, surgical skill and experience and techniques used for surgical demolition and reconstruction.

Previous studies have been conducted by several authors with conflicting results while meta-analysis studies were mainly based on observational retrospective data rather than prospective comparative randomized clinical trials.

Fifty-one articles regarding case series and comparative studies were recently analyzed by Ficarra et al. [1]. Considering the "no pad" or "safety pad" conditions as the continence definition, they found a prevalence of urinary continence after RARP ranging from 89 to 92%. Age, body mass index, lower urinary tract symptoms and prostate volume were the most relevant preoperative predictors of urinary incontinence. The possible role of different surgical techniques was also evaluated in comparative studies. [2–6]. In particular, anterior and posterior reconstructions before the urethro-vesical anastomosis were evaluated in five different studies including 2234 patients. Moreover better early and long term continence rates were found in patients who underwent bladder neck preservation (BNP) and RARP in comparison to those treated by bladder neck resection and reconstruction as also previously reported by other authors [7, 8]. Ficarra et al. concluded that the prevalence of urinary incontinence after RARP is mainly influenced by several factors such as preoperative patient characteristics, surgeon experience but not adjunctive reconstruction techniques. Posterior musculofascial reconstruction seems to offer a slight advantage in terms early continence recovery in comparison with the "no-reconstruction" group. [1].

Walz et al. recently underlined the relevant role of surgical anatomy of the prostate and the adjacent tissues involved in radical prostatectomy, stating that the anatomy varies in each patient, and the approach should be individualized according with cancer and patient characteristics to improve oncologic and functional results at the same time [9].

None of the previous studies evaluated the combination of bladder neck sparing and posterior musculofascial reconstruction despite the variability of different parameters related with both the disease and the patient characteristics.

The aim of the present study was to compare the combination of two different surgical techniques such as bladder neck preservation (BNP) and posterior bladder neck reconstruction (PRec) in patients who underwent RARP for prostate cancer treatment.

Methods

Two-hundred ninety-two patients who previously underwent radical prostatectomy for prostate cancer were enrolled in a retrospective case-control observational study to assess the urinary continence outcomes according the STROBE statement and in accordance with the Declaration of Helsinki. The study was conducted in the same medical center by two different urological teams.

Patients were selected consecutively in order to obtain comparable preoperative predictors of urinary continence such as BMI and prostate volume. Informed consent to participate the study was collected from all the re-called subjects. Patients with anastomotic strictures and significant perioperative complications were excluded.

The patient selection was performed along a period of 7 years from 2009 to 2016. The RRP + BNP procedure was predominantly performed during the first 3 years while the RARP was more frequently adopted during the following 4 years. The surgical procedure choice was determined by the availability of slots for robotics. During the first 3 years the Da Vinci robot was seldom available in a multidisciplinary robotic centre. During the following 4 years it was routinely used despite the number of patients candidate to radical prostatectomy was greater of that included in the robotic slots. The patients have been divided into three different groups. The first included patients treated by RRP according to Walsh [10], BNP and urethro-vesical anastomosis with interrupted sutures. The urinary catheter removal was always done two weeks after the surgery and retrograde cystography control. Urinary continence was investigated 12 months after surgery. The second group included a series of patients who previously underwent RARP (Montsouris technique) and standard urethro-vesical anastomosis according to Van Velthoven [11, 12]. The third group included patients who previously underwent RARP with BNP, posterior urethrovesical reconstruction (PRrec) according to Rocco modified by Coelho and urethrovesical anastomosis according to Van Velthoven [12–14]. The present study includes only patients who did not require bladder neck reduction due to wide caliber (grade 1-2 according to Lee et al.). [15].

The catheter removal was done seven days after the surgery. Continence was retrospectively investigated in the two groups treated with RARP before surgery, immediately after the urethral catheter removal and 3,6 and 12 months respectively.

Patients operated with RARP and standard anastomosis and those treated with open radical retropubic prostatectomy and bladder neck sparing technique represented the two control groups of our retrospective case control study.

All the patients were re-called for a medical follow up visit.

The medical follow up included the evaluation of oncologic and functional outcomes and was integrated with abdominal ultrasound scan, uroflowmetry and post-void urine volume measurement. Moreover a questionnaire regarding the pre and post operative continence was administered as follows:

- Which urinary symptoms did you present prior of the surgery?
- Did you receive other prostate surgeries prior the radical prostatectomy procedure?
- Did you get immediate urinary continence after urinary catheter removal?
- If not, how long did you wait for a satisfactory urinary continence after the radical prostatectomy procedure?
- How many pads do you use in a day?
- Did you receive urethral dilations or surgeries after the urinary catheter removal?

Complete urinary continence definition was described as "no pad" or "safety pad" according with Ficarra et al. [1]. Slight/moderate incontinence has been defined as "no more than 2 pads a day" although this concept may be considered as arbitrary due to the individual perception of "the need to feel oneself clean". More than 2 pads a day was classified as "severe incontinence".

Statistical analysis was conducted by comparing the different groups of patients with the Fisher test according the following layout in order to discriminate the potential role of BNP, robotic approach and PRec in the continence recovery in a series of patients with comparable preoperative predictors such as age, BMI and prostate volume between the 3 groups:

- 1) RARP + BNP + PRec vs RARP
- 2) RARP vs RRP + BNP
- 3) RARP + BNP + PRec vs RRP + BNP

Present data are recorded on a dedicated database which includes each single patient clinical but not personal information except for age and BMI. This is the reason because data can't be shared in a proper repository.

Median values and standard deviations were calculated in each of the series. The power of the study was considered at 80% with a 95% confidence interval.

Results

The median age and the BMI of patients operated by RRP procedure were 65.7 ± 6.5 years and 27.14 ± 2.40 respectively while that of patients operated by RARP were 69 ± 6.91 years and 26.31 ± 3.19 respectively. ($p = 0.4$).

Differences in comorbidities, ASA score and medications, did not influence the postoperative functional results, focused on continence outcome.

Seventy-nine point 45 % of patients responded to the phone recall and received the medical monitoring. All the others (20.55%) were considered as drop out from the study: 6 patients deceased for unrelated diseases and 54 refused to come to the Hospital or receive a telephone interview. The patient selection is described in Table 1.

Two-hundred thirty-two patients responded the phone recall and participated the medical monitoring outpatient visit.

One-hundred sixty one patients (69.8%) had urinary symptoms prior of the surgery. About 30% of them presented urgency properly treated by anticholinergics. No urinary incontinence was reported. No previous surgeries on the prostate gland have been performed on the 3 series of patients.

Median age and BMI were not statistically different between the groups as well as prostate volume except for the study group (RARP + BNP + PRec) where patients with a smaller prostate volume were less represented than in the two other groups.

Preoperative PSA values and Gleason scores of all patients were mainly included in the low risk group (PSA <10 ng/ml and Gleason score ≤ 6) while overstaging and overgrading were found at pathological analysis in particular in the RARP group. Patient characteristics are described in Table 1. Four experienced urologic surgeons have been involved in the present study. (C.S., A.M., F.F., G.P.). Robotic procedures were initiated in 2007 and by 2009 the learning curve was over. Initially there was limited access to robotics and the great majority of cases were underwent open surgery. Subsequently two additional robots have been acquired and the percentage of robotic procedures increased significantly.

Patients with urgency have been individually evaluated by urine culture with antibiotics administration in case of infection and anticholinergics in case the urine culture did not result as positive. Asymptomatic bacteriuria in uncomplicated patients was not treated by antibiotic therapy.

The mean follow-up time for the RARP and the RRP groups was 26.2 and 51.2 months respectively.

Early continence within 14 days from catheter removal was achieved in 49.38% and 24.73% of patients who previously underwent RARP + BNP + PRec. and RARP respectively ($p = 0.000$). Urinary continence improved progressively in both groups. Late 12- months full continence was obtained in 92.59% of the RARP + BNP + PRec. group and 79.56% of the simple RARP group ($p = 0.01$) (Table 2).

Table 1 Patients selection and patient characteristics

	RARP BNP + PRec. n (%)	RARP(no BNP+ no PRec.) n (%)	Open RRP + BNP n(%)	Total n(%)
Selected patients	105	125	62	292
Enrolled patients	81	93	58	232
Age (median) ± SD	69 ± 6.91		65.7 ± 6.5	
BMI Kg/m^2(median) ± SD	26.31 ± 3.19		27.14 ± 2.40	
Prostate volume				
< 50 cm^3	4 (5)	18 (19.3)	13 (22.4)	35 (15)
> 50 cm^3	77 (95)	75 (80.7)	45 (77.6)	197 (85)
Phone call drop out -Pts deceased for unrelated causes	24 (29.6)	32 (34.4)	4 (6.9)	60 (25)
	3	2	1	6
-Pts. who refused to respond the questionnaire or participate the visit	21	30	3	54
Preoperative clinical data	*n(%)*	*n(%)*	*n(%)*	*n(%)*
PSA <10 10–20 > 20	69(85.18) 12(14.81) 0 (0)	67(72.04) 23(24.73) 3(3.3)	42 (72.41) 13 (22.41) 3 (5.17)	178 (76.72) 48 (20.68) 6 (2.58)
Gleason score Low risk Intermediate risk High risk	66 (81.48) 11 (13.58) 4 (4.93)	68 (73.11) 18 (19.35) 7 (7.52)	35 (60.34) 17 (29.31) 6 (10.34)	169 (72.84) 46 (19.82) 17 (7.32)
Postoperative pathological data	*n(%)*	*n(%)*	*n(%)*	*n(%)*
Stage				
T1-T2 T3	70 (86.41) 11 (13.58)	69 (85.18) 24 (25.80)	47 (81.03) 11 (18.96)	186 (80.17) 46 (19.82)
Gleason score				
Low risk Intermediate risk High risk	39 (48.14) 31 (38.27) 11 (13.58)	41 (44.08) 38 (40.86) 14 (15.05)	24 (41.37) 26 (44.82) 8 (13.79)	104 (44.82) 95 (40.94) 33 (14.22)

RARP = robot assisted radical prostatectomy, *BNP* = bladder neck preservation, *PRec.* =posterior reconstruction

Similarly complete continence was achieved by 75.86% of patients who previously underwent RRP + BNP and compared to those treated by RARP + BNP + PRec. (p = 0.01) (Table 3). Due to this reason no statistically significant differences were found between the simple RARP and the RRP + BNP groups (Table 4) .

Severe urinary incontinence was found just in about 5% of patients in the RARP + BNP + PRec. group but in 15% of patients treated with simple RARP despite BMI and patients age were comparable in both groups as well as pathological stage and Gleason score, while prostate volume was greater in the first group.

Adjuvant radiotherapy was performed 13.7%, 30% and 12.3% of patients in the RRP + BNP, RARP, RARP + BNP + PRec groups respectively, at least six months after surgery. The continence status was unaffected by adjuvant

Table 2 Urinary continence comparative results between the two groups of patients who underwent to RARP

	RARP BNP + PRec. n/%	RARP(no BNP+ no PRec.) n/%	p value
Severe incontinence (12 months)	4 (4.93)	14 (15.05)	0.03
Slight/Moderate incontinence (12 months)	2 (2.46)	5 (5.37)	n.s.
Socially acceptable continence (no pads)			
Early	40 (49.38)	23 (24.73)	0.000
At 3 months	63 (77.77)	44 (47.31)	
At 6 months	69 (85.18)	60 (64.51)	
At 12 months	75 (92.59)	74 (79.56)	0.01

Early as well as long term socially acceptable continence was obtained in the patients who underwent to the combined BNP + PRec surgical technique

Table 3 Urinary continence comparative results between patients who underwent to RARP + BNP + PRec vs those treated by RRP + BNP

	RARP BNP + PRec.	OPEN RRP + BNP	p value
	n/%	n/%	
Severe incontinence (12 months)	4 (4.93)	8 (13.79)	n.s.
Slight/Moderate incontinence (12 months)	2 (2.46)	6 (10.34)	n.s.
Socially acceptable continence (no pads)			
Early	40 (49.38)		
At 3 months	63 (77.77)		
At 6 months	69 (85.18)		
At 12 months	75 (92.59)	44 (75.86)	0.01

radiotherapy in comparison with that observed after surgery.

Patients with moderate/severe incontinence were all counseled and treated by rehabilitation and medical therapy as the first step, then advised to undergo surgical treatments such as sling or artificial urinary sphincter placement.

No patients presented urethral or urethro-vesical anastomosis complications in the RARP groups while 5 (8.6%) patients who underwent to RRP presented strictures of the urethro-vesical junction. Two patients were treated by one step urethral dilation while three underwent trans-urethral incision without further recurrences or complications. These five patients presented long term slight/moderate urinary incontinence.

Discussion

BMI, prostate volume and patient's age have been considered as independent predictors of urinary continence recovery by several authors, despite some results seem to be conflictual [16–18].

Comparative continence rates between normal, overweight and obese patients who previously underwent to radical prostatectomy have been recently found by Gozen [19]. Conversely Kumar demonstrated a significantly higher continence rate in a group of patients with none of the risk factors such as age > 70 years, BMI > 35 Kg/m^2, prostate weight > 80 g. [18]. This is the reason why consecutive patients with comparable risk factors have been selected in the present series in order to exclude possible biases, except for few subjects older than

70 years who demonstrated an increased risk of developing postoperative urinary incontinence.

Konety already provided detailed information regarding the relationship between prostate size and urinary continence after radical prostatectomy, by using the CaPSURE data base which included 2097 evaluable patients. They differentiated 3 different group of patients according to prostate volume (<25, 25–50 and >50 cm^3.) and found that patients with volume larger than 50 cm^3 had lower rates of continence. [17]. This is the reason why our patients were classified by discriminating prostate volume less or more than 50 cm^3.. Patients with lower prostate volume were mainly represented in the simple RARP and the RRP groups despite the group treated by combined RARP and BNP + PRec. demonstrated the best urinary continence rate.

Other relevant variables that have to be considered to obtain the best results in terms of urinary continence include the surgical skill and the surgical technique adopted.

Surgical skill remains one of the most critical issues in urologic surgery and particularly the use of different techniques such as RRP, laparoscopic radical prostatectomy and RARP. All the surgeons participating the study had sufficient experience regarding both the utilized surgical techniques with at least 100 procedures either for RRP or RARP.

The surgical technique adopted may vary in relation with the previously described independent predictors of urinary continence and the disease extension. Other significant parameters such as the prostate gland morphology and the presence of a large third lobe in particular

Table 4 Urinary continence comparative results between patients who underwent to RARP vs those treated by RRP + BNP

	RARP	OPEN RRP + BNP	p value
	n/%	n/%	
Severe incontinence (12 months)	14 (15.05)	8 (13.79)	n.s.
Slight/Moderate incontinence (12 months)	5 (5.37)	6 (10.34)	n.s.
Socially acceptable continence (no pads)			
At 12 months	74 (79.56)	44 (75.86)	n.s.

and/or the abnormal anatomy of the prostate apex may also be related with the long term functional results but were not evaluated in the present study [20, 9].

BNP represents a significant step during the surgical demolitive approach to the prostate. The risk of developing surgical positive margins seems to be very low and related to those cancers originated from the gland's transition zone [21]. None of our patients who received BNP presented positive surgical margins at the prostate base.

Gu et al. recently described the results obtained on a series of 233 patients who previously underwent to RARP with BNP. Early urinary continence with "no pads" was achieved by 69.1% of evaluable patients. [8]. Stolzenburg reported similar results on a retrospective series of 240 patients. [22]. On the other hand, Nyarangi-Dix found significantly higher early and overall continence rates in a randomized controlled trial on 208 patients treated with BNP during radical prostatectomy independently from the open or robotic approach. [21].

Patients treated by RRP + BNP demonstrated comparable results in terms of urinary continence as those who underwent simple RARP. As a consequence the hypothesized advantages of BNP may be substantially undervalued if used in the open RRP approach other than the simple RARP. The robot-assisted technique helps in the surgical field magnification and improvement of anatomical dissection as well as the use of Van Velthoven's vs interrupted suture. This analysis has been also confirmed by Ficarra that found 11.3% and 7.5% absolute risk of urinary incontinence in patients who previously underwent to RRP and RARP respectively (RARP OR: 1.53; $p = 0.03$). [1]. In our study BNP during RRP likely helped to cover the urinary continence gap between the two surgical techniques.

Similarly the effects of posterior reconstruction introduced by Rocco seems to have more advantages in the early urinary continence recovery other than the long term continence rates. [1, 23]. Urinary continence assessment after reconstruction of the peri-prostatic tissues in patients undergoing RARP was conducted in a controlled trial on a series of 116 consecutive patients prospectively randomized. There was no statistically significant difference in continence recovery between the two groups. [2]. Conversely Hurtes described substantial advantages of the reconstructive group in a series of 72 randomized patients prospectively collected during a period of two years. [5]. The simple RARP group presented an increased number of patients with long term severe incontinence (15.05%) when compared to the combined BNP + PRec. group (4.93%) despite the number of patients with prostate volume lower than 50 cm^3. was about five times larger in the first of the two groups. This phenomenon may be justified by the larger number of pT3 patients in the simple RARP group (25.8%) in comparison to the other one (13.5%).

The innovative use of the combined technique BNP + PRec. demonstrated significant effects on both the early and the long term urinary continence recovery in comparison with the other two groups. In particular the progressive urinary continence rate recovery between the two groups of patients treated by RARP along a 12 months period, demonstrated an early, mid and long term improvement of continence in favour of the combined BNP/PRec. technique.

To our knowledge this is the first study demonstrating the possible effects of such combined demolitive/reconstructive surgical techniques, although prospective randomized clinical trials should be properly designed to obtain definitive results.

We recognize that the present study has several limitations. This was a retrospective analysis of series of patients who underwent radical prostatectomy along a period of seven years and operated according to different surgical techniques. An objective assessment of baseline continence status was not performed to obtain effective comparable results. The use of pads was arbitrary taken as a proxy for the assessment of postoperative continence status other than the use of validated questionnaires. Finally the effect of nerve sparing technique on urinary continence was not evaluated.

Conclusions

In conclusion our findings suggest that the combined surgical technique of RARP plus BNP and PRec according to Coelho, provide early and long term statistically significant effect on urinary continence in patients without subjective increased risk of incontinence due to insisting factors such as large prostate volume, high body mass index and age > 70 years.

Abbreviations
BMI: body mass index; BNP: bladder neck preservation; PRec: posterior musculofascial reconstruction; RARP: robotic assisted radical prostatectomy; RRP: retropubic radical prostatectomy

Acknowledgments
The corresponding author certifies that.
All persons who have made substantial contributions to the work reported in this manuscript but who do not fulfill the authorship criteria are named with their specific contributions in an Acknowledgment in the manuscript. All persons named in the Acknowledgment have provided written permission to be named.
If an acknowledgment section is not included, no other persons have made substantial contributions to the manuscript.

Competing interests:
The authors declare that they have no competing interests.

Funding
No funding was obtained for this study.

shared in a proper repository. Data are however available from the authors upon reasonable request and with permission of the Hospital General Director.

Authors' contributions
The corresponding author certifies that each author has met all criteria indicated below and hereunder indicates each author's general and specific contributions by listing his/her name nest to the relevant section. The corresponding author certifies that the manuscript represents original and valid work and that neither this manuscript nor one with similar content under my authorship has been published elsewhere. Each author has given final approval of the submitted manuscript. Each author has participated sufficiently in the work to take public responsibility for all of the content. Each author qualifies for authorship by listing his/her name on the appropriate line of the categories of contributions listed below. RB: Conception and design. AM, GP: Acquisition of data. RB, AM: Analysis and interpretation of data. RB: Drafting the manuscript. CS, FF: Critical revision for intellectual content. GP: Statistical analysis. None: Obtaining funding. RB: Supervision. FF, GP, CS, AM: Surgery.

Ethics approval and consent to participate
Verbal informed consent to participate in the study was collected from all the re-called subjects because follow up was conducted via phone call. The ethics approval was unnecessary for observational studies according to national regulations (AIFA Guidelines on observational studies. GU 31 march 2008). A notification letter was sent to the Local Ethical Committee in Pisa (CEAVNO) and the committee confirmed no ethical approval was required for this retrospective observational study.

Author details
[1]Urology Unit University of Pisa, Pisa, Italy. [2]Urology Unit AOUP, Pisa, Italy. [3]Urology University Unit, Cisanello Hospital, Via Paradisa 2, 56124 Pisa, Italy.

References
1. Ficarra V, Novara G, Rosen RC, Artibani W, Carroll PR, Costello A, Menon M, Montorsi F, Patel VR, Stolzenburg JU, Van der Poel H, Wilson TG, Zattoni F, Mottrie A. Systematic review and meta-analysis of studies reporting urinary continence recovery after robot-assisted radical prostatectomy. Eur Urol. 2012;26:405–17.
2. Menon M, Muhletaler F, Campos M, Peabody JO. Assessment of early continence after reconstruction of the periprostatic tissues in patients undergoing computer assisted (robotic) prostatectomy: results of a 2 group parallel randomized controlled trial. J.Urol. 2008;180:1018–23.
3. Sammon JD, Muhletaler F, Peabody JO, Diaz-Insua M, Satyanaryana R, Menon M. Long term functional urinary outcomes comparing single vs double-layer urethrovesical anastomosis: two year follow up of a two-group parallel randomized controlled trial. Urology. 2010;76:1102–7.
4. Koliakos N, Mottrie A, Buffi N, De Naeyer G, Willemsen P, Fonteyne E. Posterior and anterior fixation of the urethra during robotic prostatectomy improves early continence rates. Scand J Urol Nephrol. 2010;44:5–10.
5. Hurtes X, Roupret M, Vaessen C. Anterior suspension combined with posterior reconstruction during robot-assisted laparoscopic prostatectomy improves early return of urinary continence: a prospective randomized multicentre trial. BJU Int. 2012;110(6):875–83.
6. Tan G, Srivastava A, Grover S. Optimizing vesicourethral anastomosis healing after robot-assisted laparoscopic radical prostatectomy: lessons learned from three techniques in 1900 patients. J.Endourol. 2010;24:1975–83.
7. Friedlander DF, Alemozaffar M, Hevelone ND, Lipsitz SR, Hu JC. Stepwise description and outcomes of bladder neck sparing during robot-assisted laparoscopic prostatectomy. J.Urol. 2012;188:1754–60.
8. Gu X, Araki M, Wong C. Continence outcomes after bladder neck preservation during robot-assisted laparoscopic prostatectomy (RALP). MinInv Ther and AllTechnol. 2015;24(6):364–71.
9. Walz J, Epstein JI, Ganzer R, Graefen M, Guazzoni G, Kaouk J, Menon M, Mottrie A, Myers RP, Patel V, Tewari A, Villers A, Artibani W. A critical analysis of the current knowledge of surgical natomy of the prostate related to optimization of cancer control and preservation of continence and erection in candidates for radical prostatectomy: an update. Eur Urol. 2016;70:301–11.
10. Walsh PC, Jewett HJ. Radical surgery for prostatic cancer. Cancer. 1980; 45(suppl.7):1906–11.
11. Guillonneau B, Vallancien G. Laparoscopic radical prostatectomy: the Montsouris technique. J Urol. 2000 Jun;163(6):1643–9.
12. Freire MP, Weinberg AC, Lei Y, Soukup JR, Lipsiz SR, Prasad SM, Korke SF, Lin T, JC H. Anatomic bladder neck preservation during robotic-assisted laparoscopic radical prostatectomy: description of technique and outcome. Eur Urol. 2009;56:972–80.
13. VanVelthoven RF, Ahlering TE, Peltier A, Skarecky DW, Clayman RV. Technique for laparoscopic running urethra vesical anastomosis: the single knot method. Urology. 2003;61:699–702.
14. Coelho RF, Chauhan S, Orvieto MA, Sivaraman A, Palmer K, Coughlin G, Patel VR. Influence of modified posterior reconstruction of the rhabdosphyncter on early recovery of continence and anastomotic leakage rates after robot-assisted radical prostatectomy. Eur Urol. 2011;59:72–80.
15. Lee Z, Sehgal SS, Graves RV, Sue YK, Llukani E, Monahan K, Mac Gill A, Eun D, Lee DI. Functional and oncological outcomes of graded bladder neck preservation during robot-assisted radical prostatectomy. J.Endourol. 2014;28:48–55.
16. Kim JJ, Ha YS, Kim JH, Jeon SS, Lee DH, Kim WJ, Kim IY. Independent predictors of recovery of continence 3 months after robot assisted laparoscopic radical prostatectomy. JEndourol. 2012;26:1290–5.
17. Konety BR, Sadetsky N, Carroll PR. Recovery of urinary continence following rdical prostatectomy: the impact of prostate-volume analysis of data from the CaPSURE data base. JUrol. 2007;177:1423–6.
18. Kumar A, Samavedi S, Bates AS, Coelho RF, Rocco B, Palmer K, Patel VR. Continence outcomes of robot-assisted radical prostatectomy in patients with adverse urinary risk factors. BJUInt. 2015;116:764–70.
19. Gozen AS, Akin Y, Ozden E, Ates M, Hruza M, Rassweiler J. Impact of body mass index on outcomes of laparoscopic radical prostatectomy with long term follow up. Scand JUrol. 2015;49:70–6.
20. Ki Jo J, Kyu Hong S, Byun SS, Zargar H, Autorino R, Lee SE. Urinary continence after robot-assisted laparoscopic radical prostatectomy: the impact of intravesical prostatic protrusion. Yonsei MedJ. 2016;5:1145–51.
21. Nyarangi-Dix JN, Radtke JP, Hadaschik B, Pahernik S, Hohenfellner M. Impact of complete bladder neck preservation on urinary continence. Quality of life and surgical margins after radical prostatectomy: a randomized,controlled, single blind trial. J.Urol. 2013;189:891–8.
22. Stolzenburg JU, Kallidonis P, Hicks J, Do M, Dietel A, Sakellaropoulos G, Al-Aown A, Liatsikos E. Effects of bladder neck preservation during endoscopic extraperitoneal radical prostatectomy on urinary continence. Urol Int. 2010; 85:135–8.
23. Rocco F, Carmignani L, Acquati P, Gadda F, Dell'Orto P, Rocco B, Bozzini G, Gazzano G, Morabito A. Restoration of posterior aspect of rhabdosphincter shortens continence time after radical retropubic prostatectomy. J Urol. 2006;175(6):2201–6.

19

The surgical technique and initial outcomes of Anatolian neobladder: a novel technique of ileal neobladder after radical cystectomy

Z. Talat, B. Onal, B. Cetinel, C. Demirdag, S. Citgez*⬥ and C. Dogan

Abstract

Background: We describe a detailed novel step-by-step approach for creation of an ileal neobladder and compare the outcomes with standart neobladder.

Methods: Between August 2009 and January 2016, 36 consecutive patients with bladder cancer underwent radical cystectomy and orthotopic urinary diversion with an ileal neobladder. A novel technique of ileal neobladder construction, called the Anatolian neobladder, was designed by a single surgeon (ZT). Demographics and clinical data were collected. Perioperative, oncologic, and functional outcomes were reported. Complications were graded as early or late. These outcomes were compared with patients who underwent standard neobladder during this period in our center.

Results: The operation was technically successful in all cases. Early postoperative complications occurred in 33.3% of the patients. Daytime continence was achieved successfully in 83.3% of the patients. No patient had severe metabolic acidosis. Six patients (16.6%) died during follow-up, five due to metastatic bladder cancer and one due to a cardiac problem. There was no any statistically significant difference between novel technique and standard neobladder for oncological and functional outcomes.

Conclusions: The Anatolian ileal neobladder is as feasible and safe as standard neobladder technique for urinary diversion in patients with bladder cancer undergoing radical cystectomy.

Keywords: Bladder cancer, Orthotopic neobladder, Radical cystectomy, Ileal neobladder

Background

Orthotopic neobladders are constructed for urinary diversion after radical cystectomy. An orthotopic neobladder should achieve several normal bladder characteristics, including a continence mechanism, adequate capacity at a low pressure, and an antireflux mechanism for preventing upper urinary tract dilatation [1].

Camey first described an orthotopic neobladder in which a small tubular bowel segment was used as a bladder substitute by anastomosing it directly to the urethra without detubularization [2]. Since this version was described, many different types of orthotopic neobladders have been described, consisting of different gastrointestinal segments [3–5]. Intestinal detubularization plays an important role in the formation of low pressure and

adequate bladder volume. Based on this, various techniques have been acceptable using different types of bowel segments (ileum, ileo-colon, colon, sigmoid) and uretero-intestinal anastomosis. Studer et al. reported use of a detubularized ileal pouch as a bladder substitute in patients with an intact urethra after cystectomy [6]. There is no agreement on the significant advantage of a single technique over another, despite the description of each technique by the investigators.

We present our experience with a new surgical technique for ileal neobladder creation using 45 cm of ileum. The neobladder is constructed in a simple triangular configuration without a chimney. A spherical apex segment forms the neourethra at the bottom, which provides a sufficient part for anastomosis. The surgical technique, perioperative complications, and medium-term results, including cancer control and continence, are described.

* Correspondence: drsinharib@yahoo.com
Department of Urology, Istanbul University-Cerrahpasa, Cerrahpasa Medical Faculty, Fatih, 34098 Istanbul, Turkey

The outcomes of were compared with patients who underwent standard neobladder in our center.

Methods

Patients

A total of 52 patients (36 with novel technique, 16 with standard neobladder) with a preoperative diagnosis of invasive bladder cancer who were treated at our center between August 2009 and January 2016 were studied (Table 1). All patients underwent radical cystectomy and urinary diversion with creation of an orthotopic neobladder made of terminal ileum. Their charts were reviewed for preoperative (age, sex, disease status, creatinine level), perioperative (operative time, complications, morbidity), and postoperative (imaging methods, laboratory results, continence, complications, morbidity) data. Patients followed for less than 1 year were not included.

Measurements

The patients had high-grade recurrent stage T1, T2, or T3 bladder cancer. Preoperative imaging studies, including chest x-ray, and abdominal and pelvic computerized tomography (CT), indicated node-negative disease with no evidence of distant metastases in all patients. We used seftriaxone + metronidazol for antibiotic prophylaxis in patients. Single J stents were removed at postoperative 8th–10th days. Foley catheter was removed at postoperative 21st day after cystogram was performed. Patients were evaluated initially 4 weeks postoperatively and then at three-month intervals. CT and laboratory investigations were performed at each visit. We used routine cystogram postoperative 2. month to see the bladder capacity and check if there is any reflux. Complications were graded as early (grouped based on the modified Clavien system) or late (defined as those occurring more than 1 month postoperatively) [7]. Patients with complications underwent additional imaging studies, including excretory urography, voiding cystourethrography or renal scan, as needed. Continence was evaluated by patient self-report during the

follow-up visits and International Consultation on Incontinence Questionnaire Short Form (ICIQ-SF). If the patient uses more than 1 pad per day, he/she is considered to be an incontinent. Urodynamic evaluation was performed in patients with daytime incontinence. The outcomes were compared with standard neobladder [6].

Statistical analysis

Statistical analysis was done with SPSS for Windows 10.0 (SPSS, Inc., Chicago, IL, USA). Continuous and non-continuous numeric variables were described as median (Range). The Mann-Whitney U test was used to compare continuous and non-continuous numeric variables. Kaplan Meier analysis was used to calculate overall survival (OS). $P < 0.05$ was considered statistically significant.

Surgical technique

A 45 cm ileal segment was separated, starting at an appropriate point 15 to 20 cm from the ileocecal junction to avoid gastrointestinal problems postoperatively (Fig. 1). The intestinal continuity was rebuilt by an end-to-end anastomosis with surgical staplers (Fig. 2). The whole separated ileal segment was cut at the antimesenteric border for detubularization. Proximal and distal sides of the ileal loop were anastomosed side-to-side and a bagel-shaped detubularized ileal segment was formed (Figs. 3 and 4). Three identical points, starting from the medial border of the anastomosis segment, were identified and united at the center. Then, the medial edges of the ileal loop were

Table 1 The preoperative findings

	Novel technique (Anatolian neobladder) (n = 36)	Standard technique (Studer neobladder) (n = 16)	p
Age, years, mean ± SD	54.7 ± 11.6	58.0 ± 4.9	0.16
Sex			> 0.999
-Male	34 (94.4%)	15 (93.7%)	
-Female	2 (5.6%)	1 (6.3%)	
ASA	2 (1–3)	2 (1–3)	0.77
Chemotherapy			
-Neo-adjuvant	9 (25%)	4 (25%)	> 0.99
-Adjuvant	2 (5.5%)	1 (6.2%)	> 0.99

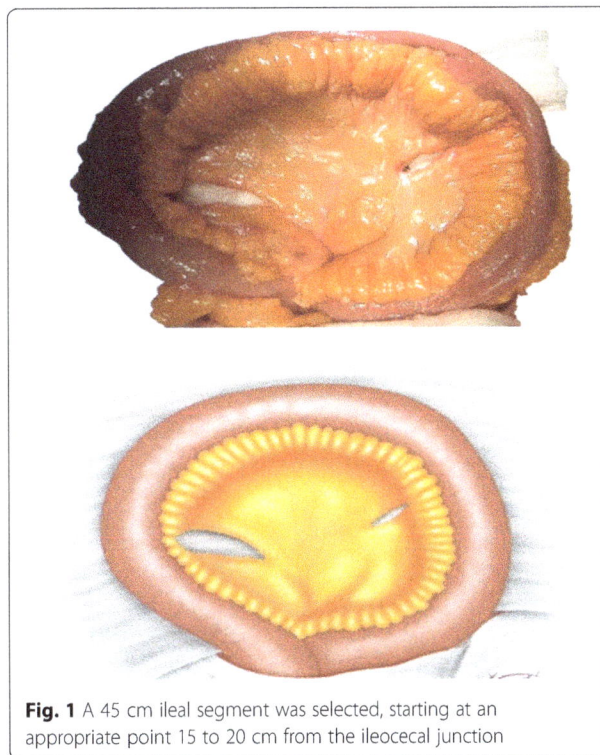

Fig. 1 A 45 cm ileal segment was selected, starting at an appropriate point 15 to 20 cm from the ileocecal junction

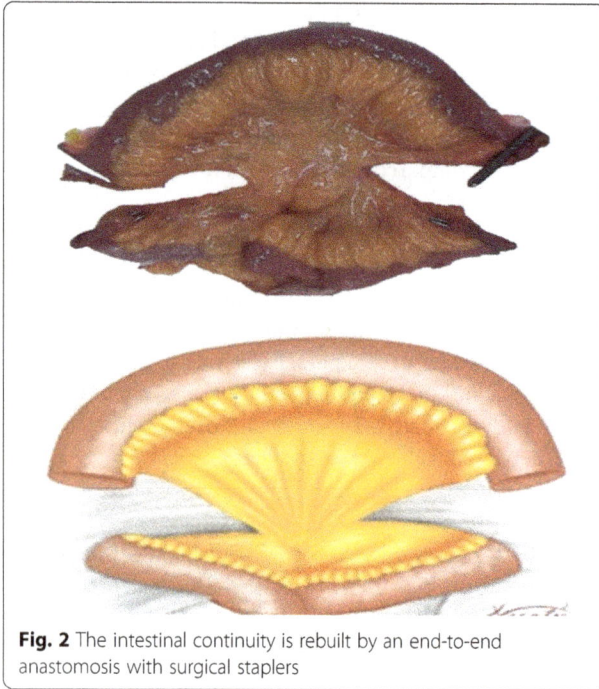

Fig. 2 The intestinal continuity is rebuilt by an end-to-end anastomosis with surgical staplers

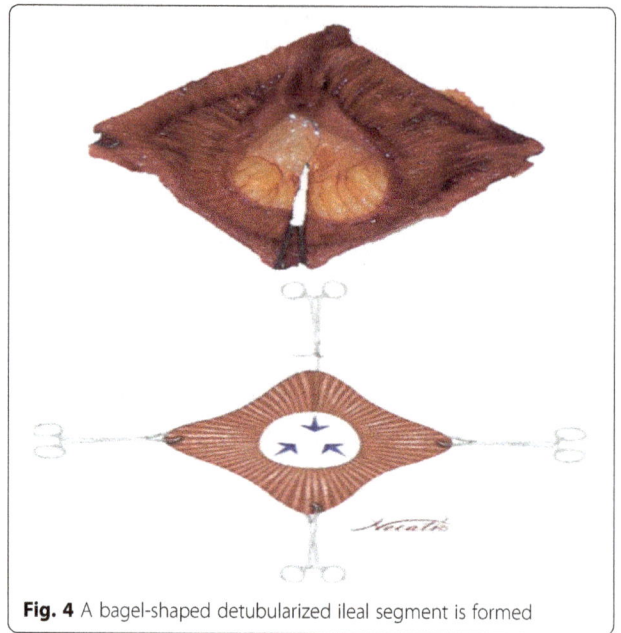

Fig. 4 A bagel-shaped detubularized ileal segment is formed

joined by a running through-and-through suture of 3–0 polyglactin continuously, resulting in a goosefoot image in the centrum (Fig. 5). After this stage, a triangular configuration was formed. Also, three points from the lateral side of the detubularized ileal loop were identified and united at the center, and the lateral edges of the ileal loop were sutured continuously with 3–0 polyglactin, leaving the lower part of the reservoir open for the urethroileal anastomosis. Both ureters were spatulated and anastomosed end-to-side to the neobladder over appropriate single J stents with an antireflux mechanism (Fig. 6). The ureteral

stents were fixed to the ileal mucosa and taken out of the pouch by stabbing the anterior wall of the reservoir (Fig. 7). The urethroileal anastomosis was performed over a transurethral 22-French catheter with six to eight 3–0 polyglactin sutures. The pelvis was drained with a 28-French tube drain.

Results

Median follow-up was 44 months (range, 12–85 months). The operation was technically successful in all cases. There were no intraoperative or perioperative deaths. Mean operative time was 5.5 h (range, 4–6.5 h) and 5.6 h (4–7 h) for novel technique and standard technique, respectively ($p < 0.001$). There were no severe intraoperative complications. Mean amount of blood loss was 550 mL (350–1700 mL) and 580 mL (300–1800 mL), for novel technique and standard technique, respectively ($p = 0.22$). The perioperative and postoperative outcomes were given in Table 2. Kaplan Meier analysis of overall survival (OS) for two techniques was showed in Fig. 8.

Early postoperative complications were occurred in 33.3% and 31.2% of the patients, for novel technique and standard technique, respectively ($p = 0.55$). According to the Clavien classification of surgical complications, a Grade 2 urinary infection occurred in 5 patients (13.8%) and 2 patients (12.5%) for novel technique and standard technique, respectively, all of whom improved with antibiotic treatment. Grade 2 paralytic ileus occurred in 3 patients (8.3%) and 1 patient (6.2) for novel technique and standard technique, respectively; however, open surgery was not required in any patient. Late complications were noted in 6 patients (16.6%) and 3 patients for novel

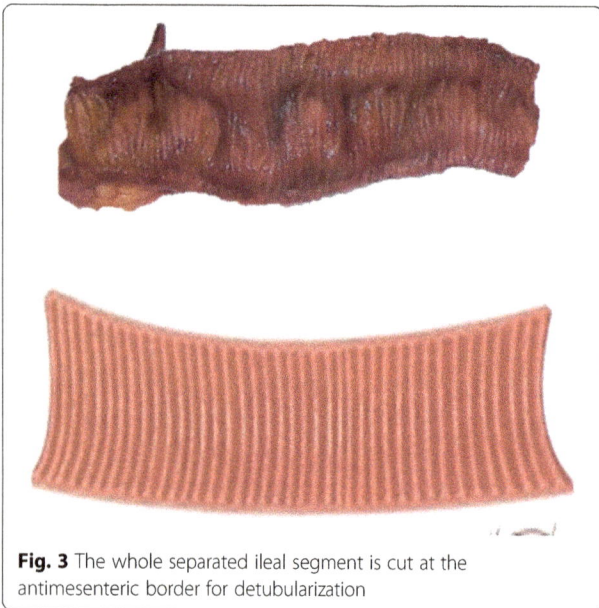

Fig. 3 The whole separated ileal segment is cut at the antimesenteric border for detubularization

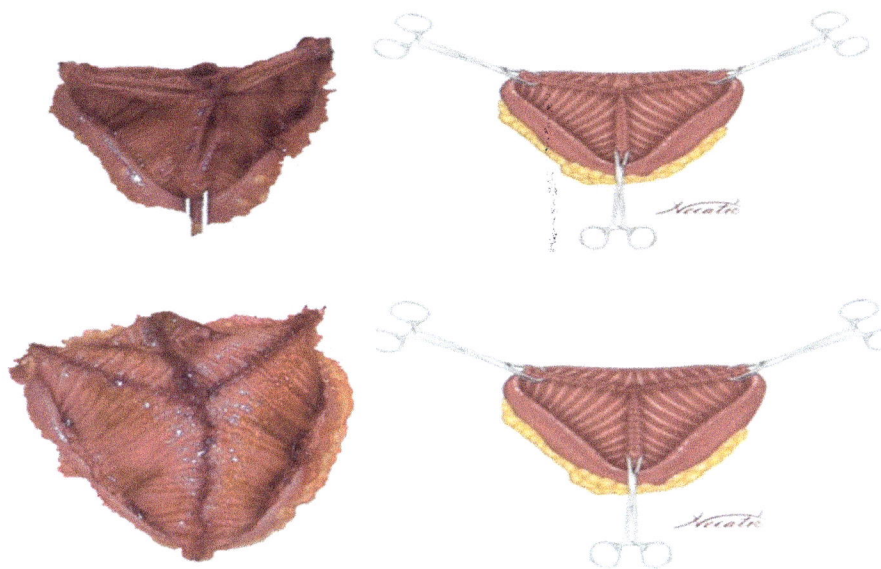

Fig. 5 Three identical points, starting from the medial border of the anastomosis segment, are identified and united at the center, and the medial edges of the ileal loop are joined

technique and standard technique, respectively; urinary infection in three (8.3%) for novel technique and 1 patient for standard technique, and incisional hernia in one (2.7%) for novel technique. The latter patient required additional surgical treatment. Stenosis of the ureterointestinal anastomosis in one patient (2.7%) for novel technique and 1 patient (6.2%) for standard technique were repaired with open surgery. There were no metabolic complications. An intravenous pyelogram (IVP) was performed when necessary (Fig. 9). Ureteral stenosis in one patient (2.7%) for novel technique and 1 (6.2%) for standard neobladder were treated endoscopically. The perioperative admission rate

was found 27.7% and 25% for novel technique and standard technique, respectively. Six patients (16.6%) in novel technique and 3 patients (18.7%) in standard technique died during follow-up. Five of them in novel technique died because of recurrent bladder cancer and one of unrelated cancer. Also, 2 of them in novel technique died because of recurrent bladder cancer and one of unrelated cancer.

Continence improved by stages with time and most patients became continent within a mean of 3.5 months (range, 1–12 months) postoperatively for both two techniques. Self-catheterization was performed before bedtime to improve nighttime continence until patients regained

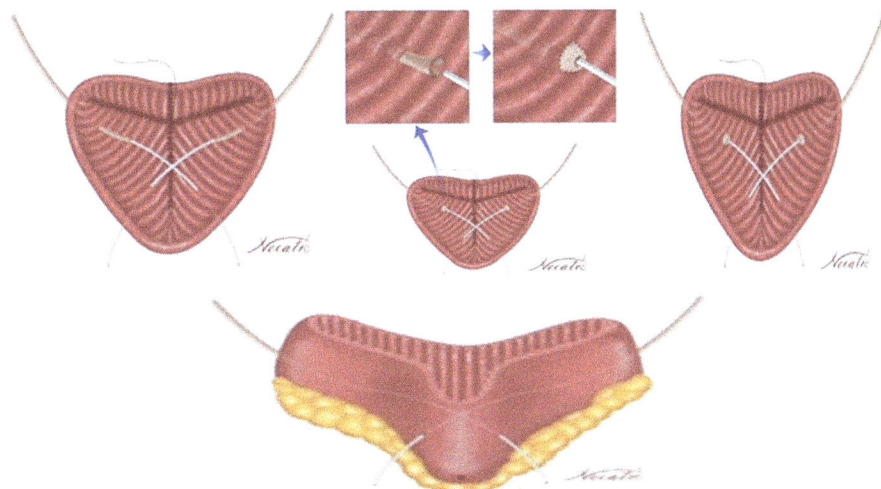

Fig. 6 Both ureters are spatulated and anastomosed end-to-side to the neobladder over appropriate single J stents with an antireflux mechanism

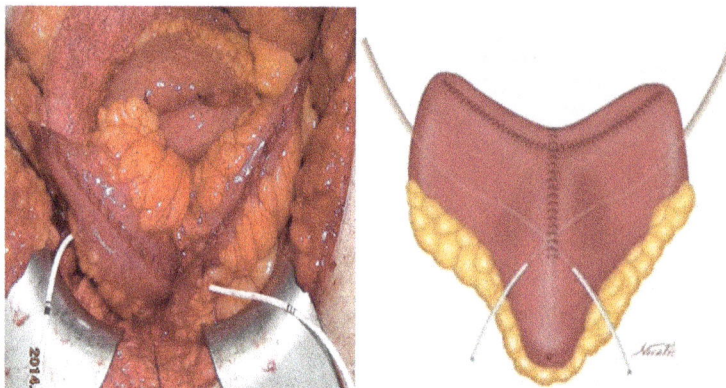

Fig. 7 The triangular-shaped Anatolian pouch is formed. The ureteral stents are fixed to the ileal mucosa and taken out of the pouch by stabbing the anterior wall of the reservoir. The urethroileal anastomosis is performed over a transurethral 22-French catheter with six to eight 3–0 polyglactin sutures

continence. Complete daytime continence was achieved in 32 of the 36 patients (88.8%) and 14 of the 16 patients (87.5%) for novel technique and standard technique, respectively ($p = 0.89$). Nighttime continence was achieved in 20 (55.5%) and 9 (56.2%) patients, for novel technique and standard technique, respectively ($p = 0.96$). Urodynamic evaluation was performed in four patients of novel technique (Fig. 10) and revealed urodynamic stress incontinence in two and low pressure low flow in two.

Discussion

Various types of orthotopic neobladders are used as a method of urinary diversion after radical cystectomy. Although new neobladder techniques have been described, it is still controversial as to how best to shape it. A normal neobladder should be safe and easy to create. Ideally, it should have low pressure. It should also be of the appropriate capacity. There should be no reflux in the upper urinary tract and the development of stricture

Table 2 The perioperative and postoperative outcomes

	Novel technique (Anatolian Neobladder) (n = 36)	Standard technique (Studer neobladder) (n = 16)	p
Bleeding (ml)	550 (350–1700)	580 (300–1800)	0.22
Operation time (h)	5.5 (4–6.5)	5.6 (4–7)	< 0.001
Hospitalization time (day)	7.3 (6–20)	7.3 (5–14)	0.80
Early postoperative complications	12 (33.3%)	5 (31.2%)	0.55
-Urinary infection (Grade 2[a])	5 (13.8%)	2 (12.5%)	
-Paralytic ileus (Grade 2[a])	3 (8.3%)	1 (6.2%)	
-Skin infection (Grade 2[a])	4 (11.1%)	2 (12.5%)	
Late postoperative complications	6 (16.6%)	3 (18.7%)	0.65
-Urinary infection	3 (8.3%)	1 (6.2%)	
-Incisional hernia	1 (2.7%)	–	
-Urethro-neobladder stenosis	1 (2.7%)	1 (6.2%)	
-Uretero-neobladder stenosis	1 (2.7%)	1 (6.2%)	
Survival time (months) (95%CI)	71.6 (62.6–80.6)	69.1 (53.9–84.1)	0.72
Perioperative admission rate	27.7%	25.0%	0.84
Postmictuonal residual urine (mL) 2. month	34.7	34.4	0.80
Postoperative ICIQ-SF score	2.7 (0–21)	2.6 (0–21)	0.72
Continence improved			
-Daytime continence	32/36 (88.8%)	14/16 (87.5%)	0.89
-Nighttime continence	20/36 (55.5%)	9/16 (56.2%)	0.96

[a]According to the Clavien classification of surgical complications

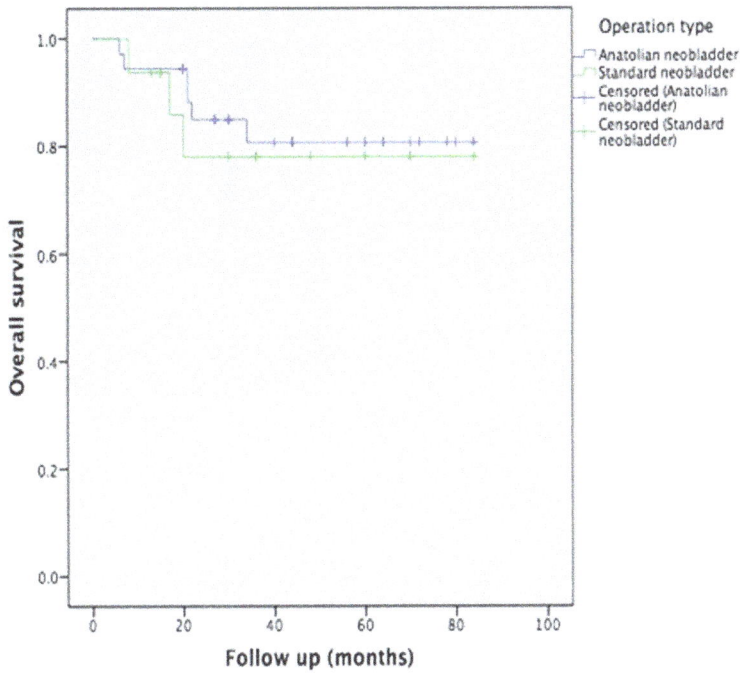

Fig. 8 Kaplan Meier analysis of overall survival (OS)

in the ureters should be prevented. In addition, day- and nighttime continence should be ensured [8]. The Studer neobladder and other ileo-colonic neobladder techniques which are known for long term outcomes are the most frequently performed methods [5, 6, 9–11]. The Studer technique has these characteristics and has significant advantages [6]. Generally, surgeons adopt one or two techniques that are suitable for them. As surgeons perform a significant number of these reconstructive techniques per year, it is reasonable for them to adopt a technique that is appropriate, easy to perform and long-term results are known. Our clinic is a high volume center for radical cystectomy (> 25) and a mean of 30 patients underwent this operation within a year. These reasons prompted us to design a new neobladder construction. In our novel technique, the operative time is acceptable. The main advantage of this technique is that a simple shape, like an original bladder configuration, is constructed. The ileal segment used for the ureteroileal anastomosis is formed spontaneously and the ureters are anastomosed to the bottom of the neobladder without creating a chimney (Fig. 7). Residual urine volume was not significant in patients due to the bladder configuration. In the Anatolian neobladder, we fixed both upper

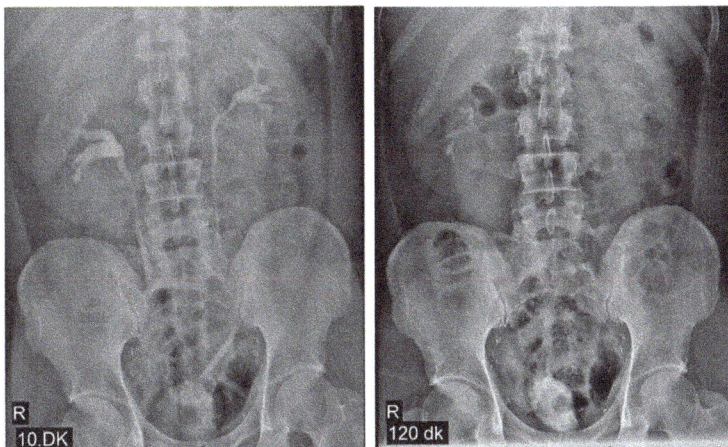

Fig. 9 IVP shows no dilatation of the upper urinary tract system

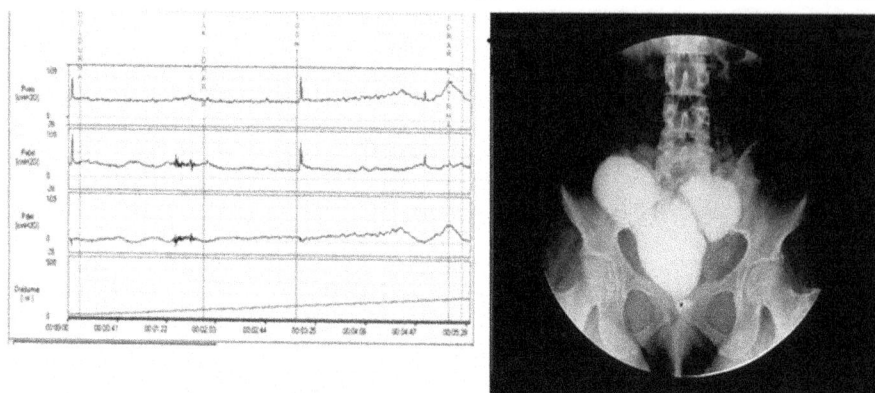

Fig. 10 Urodynamic evaluation was performed in a patient with daytime incontinence during follow-up. The cystometric image also is seen in the Figure

corners of the ileal pouch to the psoas muscles. In our opinion, this was another factor that led to good emptying of the neobladder.

The ureters were anastomosed to the neobladder according to the technique of Abol-Eneim and Ghoneim [12]. We anastomosed the spatulated end of the ureters to the intestinal mucosa using a direct mucosa-to-mucosa and inverted ureteral nipple technique. Use of an isoperistaltic limb of ileum as an antireflux mechanism offers the advantage of an easily constructed ureterointestinal anastomosis with a low incidence of reflux and confusion of the upper tracts. To date, of 72 renal units, there is no confusion of any renal unit. This rate of upper tract preservation is acceptable. Before removing the Foley catheters postoperatively, we routinely perform cystography to demonstrate no reflux in the renal units.

There were no severe intraoperative complications in our study. Mean blood loss was 550 mL (range, 350–1700) and 580 mL (300–1800 mL), for novel technique and standard technique, respectively and there were no statistically significant differences between two techniques ($P = 0.22$). Protection of the upper urinary tract is a critical point during orthotopic neobladder reconstructions. In our study, urinary infection occurred in eight patients (22.2%), all of whom improved with medical treatment. Rogers and Scardino used a modification of the Studer technique and reported acute pyelonephritis in two of 20 patients (10%) [13]. In another study, Yoneda et al. used a modified Studer technique and reported acute pyelonephritis in 27% of the patients [14]. Our series had a similar rate of pyelonephritis and there was no statistically difference for postoperative urinary infection rates between novel technique and standard neobladder in this study. Paralytic ileus occurred in three patients (8.3%) for novel technique and in 1 (6.2%) for standard neobladder, but open surgery was not required in any patient. Incisional hernia in one patient required additional surgery. No other late complications occurred.

Stenosis of the uretero-neobladder anastomosis in one patient (2.7%) for novel technique and 1 patient for standard technique (6.2%), were treated by additional open surgery. Ureterointestinal anastomosis should prevent stenosis and obstruction [15]. Stenosis of the urethra in one patient (2.7%) for novel technique and 1 patient (6.2%) for standard technique, were treated endoscopically. Authors should remember that the rate of complications after radical cystectomy and orthotopic urinary diversion is not to be underestimated. In the review published by Faba et al., they stated that the complications were significant after cystectomy and orthotopic urinary diversion and they were not as low as in previous publications [16]. It was emphasized that complications were encountered in the 20th year after the operation and therefore follow-up should be done.

In our study, there were no metabolic complications. Use of the terminal ileum was not advocated because of the potential risk of vitamin B12 and bile acid malabsorption, and resultant diarrhea [17]. Exclusion of the ileocecal valve from the normal alimentary tract and interference with feces transit time also may account for diarrhea in these patients. There are several reports of metabolic acidosis occurring in patients during follow-up [5, 6]. Hautmann et al. reported that 48% of patients with an ileal neobladder required alkalizing treatment for acidotic imbalance [5]. Gakis et al. described the advantages of using a terminal ileal segment for orthotopic urinary diversion [17]. Metabolic consequences due to bowel wall secretion and urinary reabsorption from the intestinal reservoir can be compensated best in the terminal ileum or jejunum. As a result, the terminal ileal segment is the most ideally suited bowel segment for orthotopic urinary diversion. There were no metabolic complications in our patients during the early follow-up period. We routinely evaluated laboratory values and replaced vitamin B and sodium bicarbonate if necessary during long-term follow-up.

Complete daytime continence was achieved in 32 of the 36 patients (88.8%) and 14 of the 16 patients (87.5%) for novel technique and standard technique, respectively ($p = 0.89$). Also, nighttime continence was achieved in 20 (55.5%) and 9 (56.2%) patients, for novel technique and standard technique, respectively ($p = 0.96$) and there was no statistically significant difference between two techniques. Parekh et al. reported that patients with bladder substitution achieved daytime control more rapidly than those who underwent radical prostatectomy, and stress urinary incontinence was rare [18]. Also, patient adaptation and mental capacity to understand the new bladder are important factors for achieving continence. Our success rate for achieving continence was similar to that of other studies [5, 6, 13, 15]. In addition, there was no statistically difference between our novel technique and standard technique in this study.

Finally, the complication rate was acceptable, and there was no perioperative mortality for novel technique and standard technique, in this study. In addition, this bladder substitute of novel technique appears to be technically easier and safe. However, there are several limitations to our study. One limitation was that our data were collected retrospectively. Consecutively, 36 patients were included in this study and compared with 16 patients who underwent standard neobladder. However, the number of patients was limited and long-term results were not known. This might have decreased the power of the study. However, the functional results and postoperative morbidity rates in our series were acceptable. Future studies including larger series of patients should be designed prospectively to overcome existing limitations.

Conclusions

Our study demonstrated the feasibility of novel technique (Anatolian neobladder) in the treatment of bladder cancer after radical cystectomy. It can be an alternative to other ileal neobladder techniques. Further prospective and randomized controlled comparative studies including large series of patients are needed.

Abbreviations
CT: Computerized tomography; ICIQ-SF: International Consultation on Incontinence Questionnaire Short Form; OS: Overall survival

Acknowledgements
We would like to thank Ahmet Necati Sanli, for making the illustration of our technique.

Funding
No funding was obtained for this study.
Also, we would like to thank Eren Esen, for performing statistical analysis of this study.

Authors' contributions
ZT, BO, BC, SC, CD1 made substantial contributions to conception and design, analysis and interpretation of data, he gave final approval of the version to be published. BO, SC, CD2 and BC made substantial contributions to conception and design, and acquisition of data. BO, BC, SC, CD1 and CD2 made substantial contributions to conception and design, was involved in drafting the manuscript and revising it critically for important intellectual content. ZT, SC, CD1, BO, BC and CD2 made substantial contributions to acquisition of data, analysis and interpretation of data, and was a major contributor in writing the manuscript. All authors above have read and approved of the final manuscript.

Competing interests
The authors declare that they have no competing interests.

References
1. Benson MC, Seaman EK, Olsson CA. The ileal ureter neobladder is associated with a high success and a low complication rate. J Urol. 1996;155:1585–8.
2. Lilien OM, Camey M. 25-year experience with replacement of the human bladder (Camey procedure). J Urol. 2017;197(2S):173–9.
3. Light JK, Marks JL. Total bladder replacement in the male and female using the ileocolonic segment (LeBag). Br J Urol. 1990;65(1):467–72.
4. Melchior H, Spehr C, Knop-Wagemann I, Persson MC, Junemann KP. The continent ileal bladder for urinary tract reconstruction after cystectomy: a survey of 44 patients. J Urol. 1988;139(4):714–8.
5. Hautmann RE, Miller K, Steiner U, Wenderworth U. The ileal neobladder: 6 years of experience with more than 200 patients. J Urol. 1993;150(1):40–5.
6. Studer UE, Danuser H, Hochreiter W, Springer JP, Turner WH, Zingg EJ. Summary of 10 years' experience with an ileal lowpressure bladder substitute combined with an afferent tubular isoperistaltic segment. World J Urol. 1996;14:29–39.
7. Dindo D, Demartines N, Clavien PA. Classification of surgical complications: a new proposal with evaluation in a cohort of 6336 patients and results of a survey. Ann Surg. 2004;240:205.
8. McDougal WS. Use of intestinal segments and urinary diversion. In: Walsh PC, Retik AB, Vaughan ED, Wein AJ, editors. Campbell's Urology, 8th edn. Philadelphia: Saunders, 2002, Vol 4, Chap 10, 3745–3788.
9. Meyer JP, Blick C, Arumainayagam N, Hurley K, Gillatt D, Persad R, Fawcett D. A three-Centre experience of orthotopic neobladder reconstruction after radical cystectomy: revisiting the initial experience, and results in 104 patients. BJU Int. 2009;103:680–3.
10. Thuroff JW, Alken P, Riedmiller H, Jacobi GH, Hohenfellner R. 100 cases of Mainz pouch: continuing experience and evolution. J Urol. 1988;140:283–8.
11. Marshall FF, Mostwin JL, Radebaugh LC, Walsh PC, Brendler CB. Ileocolic neobladder post-cystectomy: continence and potency. J Urol. 1991;145:502–4.
12. Abol-Eneim H, Ghoneim MA. A novel uretero-ileal reimplantation technique: the serous lined extramural tunnel. A preliminary report. J Urol. 1995;151:1193–7.
13. Rogers E, Scardino PT. A simple ileal substitute bladder after radical cystectomy. Experience with a modification of the Studer pouch. J Urol. 1995;153:1432–8.
14. Yoneda T, Igawa M, Shiina H, Shigeno K, Urakami S. Postoperative morbidity, functional results and quality of life of patients following orthotopic neobladder reconstruction. Int J Urol. 2003;10:119.
15. Studer UE, Spiegel T, Casanova GA, Springer J, Gerber E, Ackermann DK, Gurtner F, Zingg EJ. Ileal bladder substitute: antireflux nipple or afferent tubular segment? Eur Urol. 1991;20(4):315–26.
16. Faba OR, Tyson MD, Artibani W, et al. Update of the ICUD-SIU International consultation on bladder Cancer 2018: urinary diversion. World J Urol. 2018. https://doi.org/10.1007/s00345-018-2484-3.
17. Gakis G, Stenzi A. Ileal neobladder and its variants. Eur Urol Suppl. 2010;9:745–53.
18. Parekh DJ, Gilbert WB, Smith JA Jr. Functional lower urinary tract voiding outcomes after cystectomy and orthotopic neobladder. J Urol. 2000;163:56–9.

20

Percutaneous nephrolithotomy versus retrograde intrarenal surgery for the treatment of kidney stones up to 2 cm in patients with solitary kidney

Yunjin Bai[†], Xiaoming Wang[†], Yubo Yang, Ping Han and Jia Wang[*]

Abstract

Background: To compare the treatment outcomes between percutaneous nephrolithotomy (PCNL) and retrograde intrarenal surgery (RIRS) for the management of stones larger than 2 cm in patients with solitary kidney.

Methods: One hundred sixteen patients with a solitary kidney who underwent RIRS ($n = 56$) or PCNL ($n = 60$) for large renal stones (>2 cm) between Jan 2010 and Nov 2015 have been considered. The patients' characteristics, stone characteristics, operative time, incidence of complications, hospital stay, and stone-free rates (SFR) have been evaluated.

Results: SFRs after one session were 19.6% and 35.7% for RIRS and PCNL respectively ($p = 0.047$), but the SFR at 3 months follow-up comparable in both groups (82.1% vs. 88.3%, $p = 0.346$). The calculated mean operative time for RIRS was longer ($p < 0.001$), but the mean postoperatively hospital stay was statistically significantly shorter ($p < 0.001$) and average drop in hemoglobin level was less ($p = 0.040$). PCNL showed a higher complication rate, although this difference was not statistically significant.

Conclusions: Satisfactory stone clearance can be achieved with multi-session RIRS in the treatment of renal stones larger than 2 cm in patients with solitary kidney. RIRS can be considered as an alternative to PCNL in selected cases.

Keywords: Solitary kidney, Retrograde intrarenal surgery, Percutaneous nephrolithotomy

Background

Renal calculi, especially large stone, are very dangerous for patients with solitary kidney. They may cause urinary tract infection, anuria, renal insufficiency or sepsis [1]. Therefore, stones in patients with solitary kidney need active treatment. The management of stones in this cohort as yet remains a challenging scenario, complete removal of the stone and protection of the renal function through safely surgical treatments is critical [1, 2].

Percutaneous nephrolithotomy (PCNL) is the mainstay of management for large (> 2 cm) or complicated renal stones [3]. Although this technique affords high success rates and accelerated stone clearance, regardless of stone composition and size [4], it is an aggressive treatment with severe complications for patients with solitary kidney. These patients are likely to have increased thickness of the renal parenchyma as a consequence of the compensatory hypertrophy, thus they are more likely to suffer bleeding when be treated with PCNL than patients with bilateral kidneys [5]. In addition, significant bleeding in these patients means potential acute renal failure due to urinary obstruction by blood clots and the absence of supplementary renal function of the other kidney [6]. Perhaps anatomically oriented access can be made so that the risk of this complication is minimized, but cannot be totally avoided.

* Correspondence: wangjiawch@163.com
[†]Equal contributors
Department of Urology, Institute of Urology, West China Hospital, Sichuan University, Chengdu, China

In the past few years, improvements in endoscopy technology make retrograde intrarenal surgery (RIRS) more attractive, even for special circumstances, which has been used as an alternative option to PCNL for renal stones with a low complication rate [3]. In patients contraindicated for PCNL and with unfavorable treatment characteristics, such as morbid obesity, advanced vertebral deformities, serious cardiopulmonary diseases or those receiving anticoagulant treatment, RIRS is a reliable choice [3]. Which is a preferable treatment method for preserving functioning renal parenchyma [2], and this is crucial to the management of patients with solitary kidney [1]. Unfortunately, RIRS cannot be recommended as first-line treatment due to which stone-free rate (SFR) showed a negative correlation with stone size [7]. SFR after RIRS was achieved in 30% of patients with >2 cm stones and usually needed re-treatment; however, overall complication rates not related to stone sizes [7]. Therefore, patients with >2 cm stones should be counseled individually as staged procedures often required to remove calculi from the kidney without compromising the safety of RIRS. In addition, one concern about performing RIRS in a solitary kidney is the risk of renal function injury. Recently, Kuroda and coworkers [1] have shown that no significant difference was found in term of the change in glomerular filtration rate after RIRS between patients with solitary kidney and bilateral kidneys.

Current guidelines do not provide clear recommendations concerning the management of renal stones in patients with solitary kidney. Selecting the optimal management strategies for this cohort can be challenging, as each treatment modality has unique advantages and disadvantages. In the present study, we compared the efficacy and safety features between PCNL and RIRS with a flexible ureteroscope in the treatment of > 2 cm renal stones in patients with solitary kidney.

Methods

After approval was obtained from the Institutional Review Board, the data of 116 consecutive patients with solitary kidney underwent PCNL or RIRS with a flexible ureteroscopy for kidney stones between January 2010 and November 2015 at our institution were retrospectively reviewed. Solitary kidney is identified as patients with either functional or anatomical solitary kidney. Solitary functional kidney is defined as patients whose preoperative evaluation showed a contralateral kidney function is < 5% in split renal function on a 99mTc-labeled dimercaptosuccinic acid single-photon emission computed tomography or drip infusion pyelography showed the contralateral kidney was significantly atrophic and had no urine secretion. The decision to perform PCNL or flexible ureteroscopy was based on individual surgeon discretion and patient selection.

Patient assessment before surgery included history-taking, clinical examination, laboratory examination, ultrasonography, plain radiograph of kidney-ureter-bladder (KUB), and non-contrast computed tomography (CT). Grade of hydronephrosis was categorized as none, mild, moderate, or severe, based on the appearance of the pelvis on ultrasonography and the presence of calices and/or parenchymal atrophy. Stone size was measured preoperatively and calculated as the sum of the largest axis of each stone on CT.

The operation time was defined as the time from the start of the first procedure to the termination of the surgical operation. For PCNL and RIRS, it was started with the puncture for an access tract and placement of flexible ureteroscope, respectively. The duration of hospitalization was defined as the time from the day of surgery to discharge for each session. Stone-free status was assessed by ultrasonography and/or a KUB, and was defined as the absence of any stones. Complications were classified using the Clavien-Dindo classification system [8].

PCNL technique

Under general anesthesia and prone position, an 18 gauge needle was placed into proper calyx under C-arm fluoroscopy guidance. After a guidewire was inserted and fixed, dilation was performed serially with a fascial dilator up to 24 F and a 26 F sheath was placed through the tract. With using 8/9.8 F rigid ureteroscope, stone disintegration was performed using holmium laser and fragments were removed by flushing or forceps. An 18 F nephrostomy tube was placed at the end of the operation in all cases and usually removed on the fourth day after surgery, provided that there was no complication or the nephrostomy tube is draining clear urine.

RIRS technique

Generally, a 6 F ureteral stent was placed 10–14 days before RIRS to relieve acute obstruction and infection, or to dilate the ureter for passage of the ureteroscope. Under general anesthesia, patients were positioned in lithotomy position. After two guidewires were advanced to the renal pelvis, a ureteral access sheath was implanted and a 7.5F flexible ureteroscope was inserted along the guidewires. Fragmentation of the stone burden was accomplished with a 4–12 W Holmium laser and then removed using stone basket. If operative time exceeded 90 min, we discontinued the procedure to minimize perioperative complications. At the end of the operation, a double-J stent was implanted in the pelvis routinely. KUB was taken on the first day after RIRS to assessed the residual stones and the location of the stents. Patients were reevaluated on the first and third postoperative month with laboratory examination, and KUB or CT scan. The double-J stent was removed under local anesthesia, as appropriate.

Statistical method

The SPSS 19.0 software was used for all data analyses. Categorical variables were presented as number of subjects (n) and percentage (%), and analyzed using the Chi-squared or Fisher's exact test as appropriate. The continuous data were presented as mean ± standard deviation and analyzed using the independent samples t test of variance. A two-sided $p < 0.05$ was considered to be statistically significant.

Results

Patients' characteristics and stone parameters are listed in Table 1. The groups were similar at baseline in terms of age, sex ratio, size and location distribution of stones, etiologies of the solitary kidney, comorbidities, and prevalence and grade of hydronephrosis (Table 1). Nineteen patients in PCNL and 55 in RIRS group were received double-J stent placement before surgery. Preoperative stenting and nephrostomy were carried out in 12 cases because of pyelonephritis in PCNL group. In RIRS group, a ureteral stent had been placed preoperatively to relieve acute obstruction and infection, or to dilate the ureter for passage of the ureteroscope.

Perioperative and postoperative variables are presented in Table 2. The operation time in the RIRS group (99.46 ± 31.08 min) was significantly longer ($p < 0.001$) than that in the PCNL group (78.95 ± 29.81 min), and a substantial number of patients with RIRS required reoperation. The postoperative hospital stay was significantly longer in PCNL group ($p < 0.001$). Kidney function as evaluated by serum creatinine level was stable for both approaches.

The initial SFR were 19.6% and 35.7% of the RIRS and PCNL groups, respectively ($p = 0.047$). Among patients with residual stones, 6 patients required second PCNL and 12 patients required RIRS in the PCNL group. In RIRS group 2 patients required PCNL, 27 patients required second RIRS. Other auxiliary procedures (shock wave lithotripsy, SWL) included 7 (11.7%) patients in PCNL group and 19 (33.9%) in RIRS group. After the auxiliary treatments, the final SFR at 3 months follow-up increased to 88.3% for PCNL group and 82.1% for RIRS group ($p = 0.346$).

Complications in both approaches are displayed in Table 2. The majority complications were graded I and II. Overall complication rate in the PCNL group was higher (31.7% vs. 25% in the PCNL and RIRS groups, respectively; $p = 0.426$). The infectious-related complications including fever and urinary

Table 1 Clinical data of patients in PCNL and RIRS groups

	PCNL ($n = 60$)	RIRS ($n = 56$)	P
Age, yr	52.22 ± 10.56	48.84 ± 11.27	0.098
Gender, n (%)			0.395
Male	44 (73.3)	37 (66.1)	
Female	16 (26.7)	19 (33.9)	
Laterality, left, n (%)	33 (55.0)	27 (48.2)	0.465
Stone size, mm(range)	29.6 ± 5.7 (20–44)	27.7 ± 4.7 (20–39)	0.052
Site of stone, n (%)			0.438
Pelvis	10 (16.7)	17 (30.4)	
Lower calyx	15 (25.0)	12 (21.4)	
Middle calyx	1 (1.7)	2 (3.6)	
Upper calyx	1 (1.7)	1 (1.8)	
Multiple	33 (55.0)	24 (42.9)	
Hydronephrosis, n (%)			0.054
None or mild	29 (48.3)	37 (66.1)	
Moderate or severe	31 (51.7)	19 (33.9)	
Preoperative double-J stent, n (%)	9 (15.0)	55 (98.2)	<0.001
Preoperative nephrostomy, n (%)	3 (5.0)	0	-
Recurrent stone former, n (%)	26 (43.3)	30 (53.6)	0.270
Comorbidities, n(%)			
Diabetes mellitus	9 (15.0)	7 (12.5)	0.696
Hypertension	13 (21.7)	9 (16.1)	0.442
Heart diseases	4 (6.7)	2 (3.6)	0.739
Renal insufficiency	13 (21.7)	9 (16.1)	0.442
Etiology of solitary kidney, n (%)			0.764
Contralateral nephrectomy	26 (43.3)	28 (50.0)	
Congenital	1 (1.7)	1 (1.8)	
Functional	33 (55.0)	27 (48.2)	
Stone composition, n (%)			0.307
Calcium based	45 (75.0)	39 (69.6)	
Uric acid	6 (10.0)	11 (19.6)	
Infection	9 (15.0)	6 (10.7)	

tract infection requiring additional antibiotics were comparable between the two groups. Every group had one patient developed sepsis. The mean drop in the postoperative hemoglobin concentration in PCNL group was significantly higher than that in RIRS group ($p = 0.004$), and blood transfusions were required in 7 (11.7%) patients in the PCNL group. No nephrectomy or angioembolization was required. There was no significant difference between the two groups in stone compositions ($p = 0.307$).

Table 2 Perioperative and Postoperative Data

	PCNL (n = 60)	RIRS (n = 56)	P
Operation time, min (range)[a]	78.75 ± 27.0 (42–141)	99.1 ± 29.5 (45–157)	<0.001
Postoperative hospitalization time, d (range)[a]	5.9 ± 1.5 (4–9)	2.0 ± 1.0 (1–5)	<0.001
Drop in Hb level in g/dl (range)	13.3 ± 6.6 (1.1–37.4)	10.2 ± 4.4 (2.8–21.3)	0.004
Initial stone-free, n (%)	25 (35.7)	11 (19.6)	0.047
Auxiliary procedures, n (%)			
PCNL	6 (10.0)	2 (3.6)	0.318
RIRS	12 (20.0)	27 (48.2)	0.001
Shock wave lithotripsy	7 (11.7)	19 (33.9)	0.004
Final stone-free rate, %	53 (88.3)	46 (82.1)	0.346
Preoperative serum creatinine in umol/L (range)	110.6 ± 38.1 (40.5–212.9)	113.8 ± 44.5 (18–263.4)	0.675
Postoperative serum creatinine in umol/L (range)	131.7 ± 57.4 (28.4–308.7)	136.6 ± 56.8 (28.8–305.5)	0.647
Complications (Clavein classification), %	19 (31.7)	14 (25.0)	0.426
Fever (G I)(%)	7 (11.7)	9 (16.1)	0.492
Urinary tract infection requiring additional antibiotics (G II) (%)	3 (5.0)	2 (3.6)	1.000
Urine leakage < 12 h(G II) (%)	1 (1.7)	0	-
Transfusion (G II) (%)	7 (11.7)	0	-
Steinstrasse (G IIIa) (%)	0	2 (3.6)	-
Sepsis (G IVa) (%)	1 (1.7)	1 (1.8)	1.000

[a]initial procedure plus auxiliary procedure

Discussion

Nowadays, the surgical management of renal stones has been dramatically changed because of tremendous reformation in endoscopy technology. As increased risk of perioperative complications and impairment of renal function for patients with solitary kidney during surgical management [6], thus, which surgical approach use continues to be of significant concern. In the era of minimally invasive surgery, RIRS and PCNL are two major surgical techniques for removing large renal stones [3], and PCNL has become the standard treatment with which all other approaches should be compared. A number of pertinent questions remain without conclusive answers, despite various studies reported in the literature, such as: how safe are PCNL or RIRS? What are the factors that portend a poor outcome with PCNL? How do complications compare PCNL with RIRS? Our results suggested that both PCNL and RIRS can safely be carried out for patients with solitary kidney. Final SFRs were similar in both groups. The main advantage of the RIRS over PCNL seems to be the less of mean decrease in the hemoglobin level. However, RIRS often required auxiliary treatment.

The primary concern of PCNL in solitary kidneys was the risk to develop complication such as severe uncontrollable bleeding that may cause an anephric state. The over complications after PCNL in these patients was 30.6%, of which 5.6% required blood transfusion [9]. Risk factors for serious bleeding include upper calix puncture,

large stone, multiple tracts, inexperienced surgeon, and solitary kidney [5]. It was reported that the need for blood transfusion and the risk of severe bleeding were higher after PCNL in solitary kidneys compared to bilateral kidneys [5]. Hosseini and colleagues performed PCNL on 412 patients with solitary kidney, 19 (4.6%) patients encountered bleeding requiring transfusion, but none of them required nephrectomy [10]. Compensatory hypertrophy is common in solitary kidneys with increasing thickness of the renal parenchyma. It was speculated that access through such thick renal parenchyma may increase the risk of bleeding [5].

Continuous improvements in instruments and techniques of PCNL have helped urologists to perform this procedure with high levels of safety and efficacy in challenging cases such as stones in solitary kidneys [10]. Previous study reported that PCNL is a safe and efficient treatment for patients with solitary kidney despite the lower SFR (82.1% vs. 83.5%; $p = 0.970$) and increased morbidity (21.5% vs. 17.3%; $p = 0.287$) compared to patients with bilateral kidneys [11]. A recent systematic review confirmed the efficacy of PCNL for stones in patients with solitary kidney with initial and overall SFRs of 78.1% and 86.8% respectively [9]. It is surprising that PCNL for renal stones in these patients provided significant improvement in renal function [12]. In another study, Zeng and colleagues [2] compared the treatment outcomes between minimally invasive PCNL and RIRS for stones larger than 2 cm in patients with solitary kidney. They found SFRs after a single procedure were 71.7% in the minimally invasive PCNL group and 43.4% in the RIRS group ($p = 0.003$), and both groups with similar complications rates. Our single-session SFR in both groups was relatively low (35.7% vs 19.6% in the PCNL and RIRS groups, respectively). This may be related with that majority patients in our center had more complicated stones. In addition, the main reason for PCNL had a higher initial SFR than RIRS is that larger fragments fall back to the lower calix during RIRS.

Although SFR of RIRS is inferior to that of PCNL [13], considering patients with solitary kidney have the potential to encounter serious systemic disease, RIRS should always be considered at any time due to its efficacy and minimally invasive. Good outcomes of RIRS in terms of morbidity rate may be outweighed by its SFR in some cases, which is not neglected, especially in patients with solitary kidney. Bryniarski et al. [14] assessed outcomes after RIRS and PCNL. They found that transfusion required in 13 of PCNL patients and no transfusion in the RIRS patients. Gao et al.[15] have reported 26.6% (12/45) patients of RIRS encountered complications and 20% (9/45) were identified as I Clavien grade and no patients required blood transfusions. For our study, no major complications occurred and minor complications often were experienced. In our series, a 6 F stent had been routinely placed 10–14 days before RIRS to relieve acute obstruction and infection, which may be account for the infectious complications were also comparable between the two groups.

RIRS has been frequently considered in the treatment of larger renal stones as an alternative to PCNL. Although hemorrhagic diseases are often regarded as contraindications for both PCNL and SWL, RIRS demonstrated pretty safety in these patients [16]. Furthermore, with the increasing numbers of obese and morbid obese patients, the status of PCNL for renal stones may face challenges because great skin-kidney distance in these patients may lead to the puncture needle cannot reach the kidney. Fortunately, RIRS can be executed without limited outcomes for obese patients [17].

Stones in solitary kidney represent a management dilemma for the urologists. PCNL and RIRS are widely known to decrease surgery-related morbidity, while complete removal of calculi in solitary kidney from a single percutaneous or nature tract was difficult. Zhong et al [18] reported that combined use the two techniques can extract the calculi quickly, shorten operation time, make a high SFR. In addition, combined therapy can reduce the need for the number of tracts and then reduce the loss of blood and potential complications related to multiple tracts. Therefore, combined therapy can be used as a feasible treatment option for large renal stones in patients with solitary kidney.

RIRS is often performed as an ambulatory surgery in the Western countries. For patients and hospitals, they will choose RIRS as it is a less invasive treatment with less length of hospital stay. Under the culture background and the health insurance policy in China, both PCNL and RIRS were done as inpatient surgical procedure. Our patients are usually unwilling to discharge with the nephrostomy tube in place, thus, the hospital stay was longer in the both groups in our country. In addition, the solitary kidney patients in our series with large stones, treatment should be more careful and postoperative observation period needs to be extended. Our results are in line with other researches on RIRS or PCNL for large stone in China in term of hospitalization time [2, 15].

Our study has several limitations. First, this study was a retrospective design undertaken at a single center with a limit number of patients, we cannot eliminate the potential selection bias. Additionally, PCNL or RIRS in solitary kidney is a relative uncommon surgery and prospective design is challenging to be performed. Furthermore, the follow-up period of 3 months was quite short. We might not have detected the longer-term complications such as hypertension, renal impairment or ureteral stenosis.

Conclusions
For larger than 2 cm renal stones in patients with solitary kidneys, PCNL offers initial SFRs superior to those of RIRS. However, satisfied outcomes can be acquired with multisession RIRS. Furthermore, hospital stay and complications of PCNL can be significantly reduced with RIRS. Therefore, RIRS represents a good alternative treatment to PCNL in well selected cases with larger renal stones in patients with solitary kidneys.

Abbreviations
CCS: Case-control study; CI: Confidence interval; LPL: Laparoscopic pyelolithotomy; MD: Mean difference; NOS: Newcastle-Ottawa Scale; OR: Odds ratio; PCNL: Percutaneous nephrolithotomy; RCT: Randomized controlled trial; SFR: Stone-free rate; UTI: Urinary tract infection

Acknowledgments
Not applicable.

Funding
This work was collectively supported by grant (National Natural Science Foundation of China (No. 81270841)).

Authors' contributions
Conceived and designed the experiments: PH and JW. Analyzed the data: JYB and XMW. Contributed reagents/materials/analysis JYB and XMW. Wrote

Percutaneous nephrolithotomy versus retrograde intrarenal surgery for the treatment of kidney stones up...

137

the manuscript: JYB. Designed the software used in analysis: YBY. All authors read and approved the final manuscript.

Competing interests

The authors declare that they have no competing interests.

References

1. Kuroda S, Fujikawa A, Tabei T, Ito H, Terao H, Yao M, Matsuzaki J. Retrograde intrarenal surgery for urinary stone disease in patients with solitary kidney: A retrospective analysis of the efficacy and safety. Int J Urol. 2016;23:69–73.
2. Zeng G, Zhu W, Li J, Zhao Z, Zeng T, Liu C, Liu Y, Yuan J, Wan SP. The comparison of minimally invasive percutaneous nephrolithotomy and retrograde intrarenal surgery for stones larger than 2 cm in patients with a solitary kidney: a matched-pair analysis. World J Urol. 2015;33:1159–64.
3. Turk C, Petrik A, Sarica K, Seitz C, Skolarikos A, Straub M, Knoll T. EAU Guidelines on Interventional Treatment for Urolithiasis. Eur Urol. 2016;69: 475–82.
4. Unsal A, Resorlu B, Atmaca AF, Diri A, Goktug HN, Can CE, Gok B, Tuygun C, Germiyonoglu C. Prediction of morbidity and mortality after percutaneous nephrolithotomy by using the Charlson Comorbidity Index. Urology. 2012; 79:55–60.
5. El-Nahas AR, Shokeir AA, El-Assmy AM, Mohsen T, Shoma AM, Eraky I, El-Kenawy MR, El-Kappany HA. Post-percutaneous nephrolithotomy extensive hemorrhage: a study of risk factors. J Urol. 2007;177:576–9.
6. Giusti G, Proietti S, Cindolo L, Peschechera R, Sortino G, Berardinelli F, Taverna G. Is retrograde intrarenal surgery a viable treatment option for renal stones in patients with solitary kidney? World J Urol. 2015;33:309–14.
7. Skolarikos A, Gross AJ, Krebs A, Unal D, Bercowsky E, Eltahawy E, Somani B, de la Rosette J. Outcomes of Flexible Ureterorenoscopy for Solitary Renal Stones in the CROES URS Global Study. J Urol. 2015;194:137–43.
8. de la Rosette JJ, Zuazu JR, Tsakiris P, Elsakka AM, Zudaire JJ, Laguna MP, de Reijke TM. Prognostic factors and percutaneous nephrolithotomy morbidity: a multivariate analysis of a contemporary series using the Clavien classification. J Urol. 2008;180:2489–93.
9. Jones P, Aboumarzouk OM, Rai BP, Somani BK. Percutaneous Nephrolithotomy (PCNL) for Stones in Solitary Kidney: evidence from a systematic review. Urology. 2016. doi:10.1016/j.urology.2016.10.022.
10. Hosseini MM, Yousefi A, Hassanpour A, Jahanbini S, Zaki-Abbasi M. Percutaneous nephrolithotomy in solitary kidneys: experience with 412 cases from Southern Iran. Urolithiasis. 2015;43:233–6.
11. Saltirov I, PK PT. Percutaneous nephrolithotripsy in patients with solitary kidneys: A single-center experience. Eur Urol Suppl. 2013;12:e1352.
12. El-Tabey NA, El-Nahas AR, Eraky I, Shoma AM, El-Assmy AM, Soliman SA, Shokeir AA, Mohsen T, El-Kappany HA, El-Kenawy MR. Long-term functional outcome of percutaneous nephrolithotomy in solitary kidney. Urology. 2014;83:1011–5.
13. De S, Autorino R, Kim FJ, Zargar H, Laydner H, Balsamo R, Torricelli FC, Di Palma C, Molina WR, Monga M, De Sio M. Percutaneous nephrolithotomy versus retrograde intrarenal surgery: a systematic review and meta-analysis. Eur Urol. 2015;67:125–37.
14. Resorlu B, Unsal A, Ziypak T, Diri A, Atis G, Guven S, Sancaktutar AA, Tepeler A, Bozkurt OF, Oztuna D. Comparison of retrograde intrarenal surgery, shockwave lithotripsy, and percutaneous nephrolithotomy for treatment of medium-sized radiolucent renal stones. World J Urol. 2013;31:1581–6.
15. Gao X, Peng Y, Shi X, Li L, Zhou T, Xu B, Sun Y. Safety and efficacy of retrograde intrarenal surgery for renal stones in patients with a solitary kidney: a single-center experience. J Endourol. 2014;28:1290–4.
16. Turna B, Stein RJ, Smaldone MC, Santos BR, Kefer JC, Jackman SV, Averch TD, Desai MM. Safety and efficacy of flexible ureterorenoscopy and holmium:YAG lithotripsy for intrarenal stones in anticoagulated cases. J Urol. 2008;179:1415–9.
17. Hyams ES, Munver R, Bird VG, Uberoi J, Shah O. Flexible ureterorenoscopy and holmium laser lithotripsy for the management of renal stone burdens that measure 2 to 3 cm: a multi-institutional experience. J Endourol. 2010;24:1583–8.
18. Zhong W, Zhao Z, Wang L, Swami S, Zeng G. Percutaneous-based management of Staghorn calculi in solitary kidney: combined mini percutaneous nephrolithotomy versus retrograde intrarenal surgery. Urol Int. 2015;94:70–3.

21

How to perform the dusting technique for calcium oxalate stone phantoms during Ho:YAG laser lithotripsy

Jeong Woo Lee[1], Min Gu Park[2] and Sung Yong Cho[3*]

Abstract

Background: To determine the most efficacious setting of Holmium:yttrium-aluminum-garnet (Ho:YAG) laser with a maximum power output of 120 W with in vitro phantom-stone dusting technique.

Methods: A laser was used to treat two $4 \times 3 \times 3$ mm^3 sized phantom stones in 5 mL syringes with 1 mm-sized holes at the bottom. According to the pulse width (short 500, middle 750, long pulse 1000 µsec), maximal pulse repetition rates from 50 to 80 Hz were tested with pulse energy of 0.2, 0.4, 0.5, and 0.8 J. Six times of the mean dusting times were measured at each setting. Dusting was performed at continuous firing of the laser until the stones become dusts < 1 mm.

Results: The mean Hounsfield unit of phantom stones was 1309.0 ± 60.8. The laser with long pulse generally showed shorter dusting times than short or middle pulse width. With increasing the pulse energy to 0.5 J, the dusting time decreased. However, the pulse energy of 0.8 J showed longer dusting times than those of 0.5 J. On the post-hoc analysis, the pulse energy of 0.5 J, long pulse width, and the repetition rates of 70 Hz demonstrated significantly shorter dusting times than other settings.

Conclusions: The results suggest that long pulse width with 0.5 J and 70 Hz would be the most efficacious setting for dusting techniques of plaster stone phantoms simulating calcium oxalate stones using the 120 W Ho:YAG laser.

Keywords: Calcium oxalate, Dusting, Energy, Ho:YAG laser, Lithotripsy

Background

Laser lithotripsy has remained the first-line treatment option for urinary stones with technical advancements in dedicated endoscopes, instruments, and accessories [1–3]. Recent investigations demonstrated high success rates and low complication rates of the minimally invasive surgical techniques using the Holmium:yttrium-aluminum-garnet (Ho:YAG) laser, especially in miniaturized percutaneous nephrolithotomy and retrograde intrarenal surgery [4–7]. The pulsed Ho:YAG laser has become one of the main lithotripters along with the ultrasonic or pneumatic lithotripter [2].

Laser efficacy during lithotripsy is essential to obtain the maximal surgical efficacy and excellent surgical outcome.

The efficacy of Ho:YAG laser-mediated stone fragmentation is better with increased energy per pulse and reduced pulse width, but not consistently with pulse repetition rates with a power output of 10~20 W [8–10]. Meanwhile, stone dusting with low pulse energy and high pulse repetition rates reduces the size of fragmented stones until they become dusts, which improves stone clearance [8]. This is because the Ho:YAG laser produces less retropulsion from the fiber tip in the lower power energy, which affects the surgical efficacy.

The recent development of the high-power output 120 W Ho:YAG laser system has provided surgeons with additional options for stone dusting, courtesy of increased pulse repetition rates from 50 to 80 Hz and three different options of pulse width from 500 to 1000 µsec. However, there is no consensus of the optimal laser setting for stone dusting. To provide clarity, we investigated the impact of pulse energy, width, and

* Correspondence: kmoretry@daum.net

[3]Department of Urology, Seoul Metropolitan Government-Seoul National University Boramae Medical Center, Seoul National University College of Medicine, 20, Boramae-ro 5-Gil, Dongjak-gu, Seoul 156-707, Republic of Korea
Full list of author information is available at the end of the article

repetition rates on the dusting efficacy of phantom stones in vitro using the 120 W Ho:YAG laser system. The aim was to determine the most efficacious laser setting for stone dusting.

Methods

The authors sought to determine the influence on the dusting efficacy according to each setting value of the hand-held optical fiber of Ho:YAG laser pulse energy (pulse width) and the repetition rate based on each pulse width.

Laser system and parameters

The experiments were performed using a 2.1 μm emitting Lumenis VersaPulse PowerSuite Holmium (Ho:YAG) surgical laser 120H® (Lumenis Ltd., Israel) with a maximum power output of 120 W for fibers with core diameters of 200 μm. Pulse widths were short (500 μsec), middle (750 μsec), and long (1000 μsec). The maximal pulse repetition rates were 50, 70, and 80 Hz. The pulse energies were 0.2, 0.4, 0.5, and 0.8 J. The maximal repetition rates differed according to the pulse width and pulse energy.

Stone sample preparation

The molded plaster phantom stones were obtained from SINI Inc. (Ui-Wang, Gyeonggi-do, Korea) (Fig. 1). The stone density mimics the hardness of human calcium oxalate monohydrate calculi, consistent with a prior study [4]. Two calculi were used for each laser experiment. The stone size was cut up into equal cubical pieces of $4 \times 3 \times 3$ mm^3.

Hand-held dusting techniques

Only freshly cleaved 200 μm fibers were used. The fiber tip was positioned 1 to 2 mm from the phantom stone by the investigator (Cho SY). The 5 ml syringes had a 1 mm-sized hole at the bottom where stone dust exited the syringe into a pan (Fig. 2). The irrigation pressure was set to 40 cmH$_2$O from the phantom stones. Dusting was performed with continuous firing of the laser until the stones became a dust with a particle size < 1 mm. The dusting time was defined from the initiation of laser firing to the formation of this dust.

Statistical analyses

All parameters represented the mean value ± standard deviation (percentage). Comparative results were analyzed using independent t-test or Mann-Whitney U test between the two groups and Kruskal-Wallis test among the groups. Post-hoc analysis with Tukey's honestly significant difference test was performed. Categorical variables were analyzed by Chi-square and Fisher's exact test. Statistical significance was considered at $P < .05$. Statistical analyses were performed by the statistical software SPSS version 20 (IBM, Armonk, NY) and R version 3.0.1 (http://www.r-project.org).

Results

The mean Hounsfield unit was 1309.0 ± 60.8. The mean dusting time was determined from six measurements of each study criterion given. The results are summarized in Table 1. The highest repetition rate was 70 Hz with long and middle pulse widths and pulse energies of 0.2, 0.4, and 0.5 J, and 80 Hz with short pulse width and pulse energies from 0.2 to 0.5 J. The highest repetition

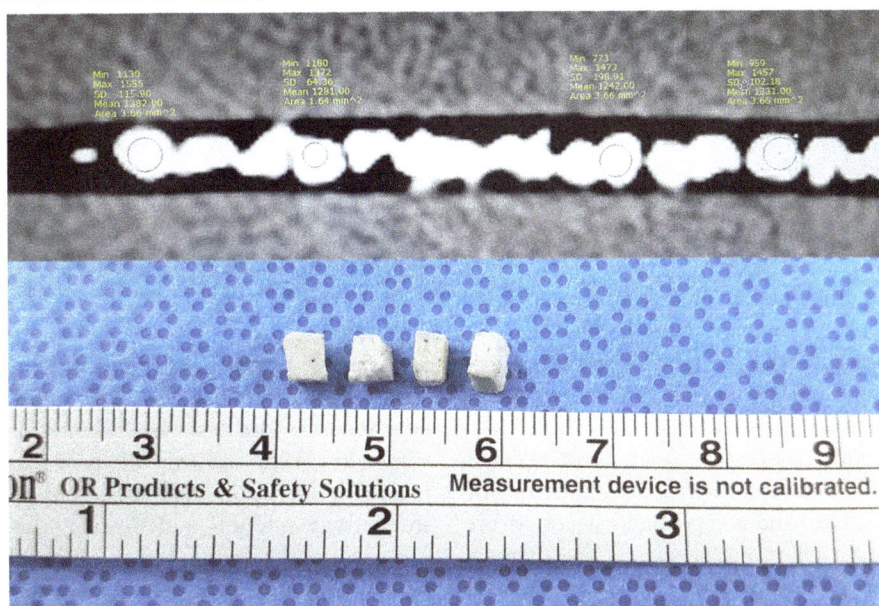

Fig. 1 a Stone density measured in the computed tomography scan images. b Each cubical stone of 4x3x3 mm^3

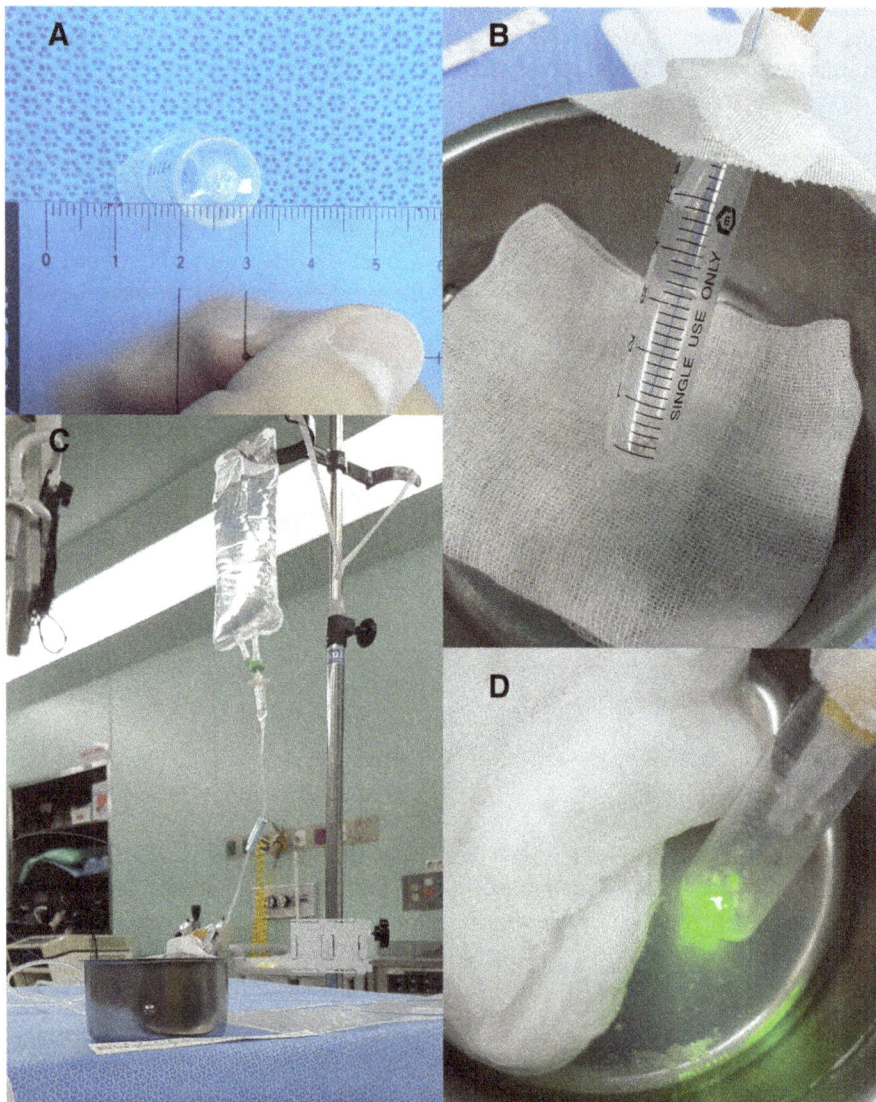

Fig. 2 a A 1 mm-sized hole at the bottom of the syringe for fragmented particles to go out. **b** A laser fiber was positioned 1–2 mm away from the phantom stones when the dusting technique starts. **c** Irrigation fluid at the height of 40cmH$_2$O to mimic the real practice situation. **d** Dusts < 1 mm went out of the syringe during laser firing. When the all particles disappear in the syringe, the duration of dusting was checked by a stop-watch

rate was 50 Hz for 0.8 J of pulse energy for each pulse width.

The long pulse width generally produced shorter dusting times than short or middle pulse widths. As the pulse energy increased to 0.5 J, the dusting time decreased. However, the pulse energy of 0.8 J produced a longer dusting time than pulse energy of 0.5 J.

Figure 3 depicts results of a post-hoc analysis of the mean dusting time measured at each setting. Pulse energy of 0.5 J, a long pulse width, and a repetition rate of 70 Hz proved to be the most efficacious dusting setting (Group A). Group B included pulse energy of 0.5 J (middle and short pulse widths) and 0.4 J or 0.8 J (long pulse width). Group C included pulse energies of 0.4 J and 0.8 J with middle or short pulse width. Group D comprised pulse energy of 0.2 J regardless of pulse width and repetition rate.

Discussion

The pulsed Ho:YAG laser is used predominantly with flexible ureterorenoscopic and miniaturized percutaneous devices. This laser has become the preferred lithotripter in clinical use over the past two decades [2]. The maximal efficacy of laser lithotripsy techniques, mainly stone fragmentation and dusting, are essential to improve surgical outcomes. The efficacy of lithotripsy obtained using the Ho:YAG laser depends on laser settings that include energy per pulse, pulse width, and pulse repetition rates [8]. Factors that favor the fragmentation

Table 1 Dusting time (sec) according to each laser setting

Dusting time (sec)	Hz	Test	0.2 J	Hz		0.4 J	Hz		0.5 J	Hz		0.8 J
Short pulse	80	1	1120	80	1	720	80	1	540	50	1	600
		2	1080		2	800		2	660		2	780
		3	1560		3	750		3	900		3	720
		4	1440		4	960		4	540		4	910
		5	1350		5	1000		5	600		5	800
		6	1470		6	750		6	580		6	760
	Mean ± S.D		1336.7 ± 195.6	Mean ± S.D		830.0 ± 119.7	Mean ± S.D		636.7 ± 136.5	Mean ± S.D		761.7 ± 101.7
Middle pulse	70	1	1140	70	1	780	70	1	360	50	1	780
		2	1250		2	900		2	480		2	700
		3	1080		3	820		3	400		3	650
		4	1360		4	990		4	500		4	660
		5	1240		5	800		5	420		5	590
		6	1180		6	700		6	410		6	660
	Mean ± S.D		1208.3 ± 97.7	Mean ± S.D		831.7 ± 100.9	Mean ± S.D		428.3 ± 52.3	Mean ± S.D		673.3 ± 63.1
Long pulse	70	1	1140	70	1	540	70	1	300	50	1	540
		2	1260		2	600		2	350		2	500
		3	1050		3	480		3	280		3	620
		4	1300		4	580		4	320		4	600
		5	1220		5	600		5	350		5	500
		6	1200		6	900		6	300		6	480
	Mean ± S.D		1195.0 ± 89.4	Mean ± S.D		616.7 ± 146.1	Mean ± S.D		316.7 ± 28.8	Mean ± S.D		540.0 ± 58.0

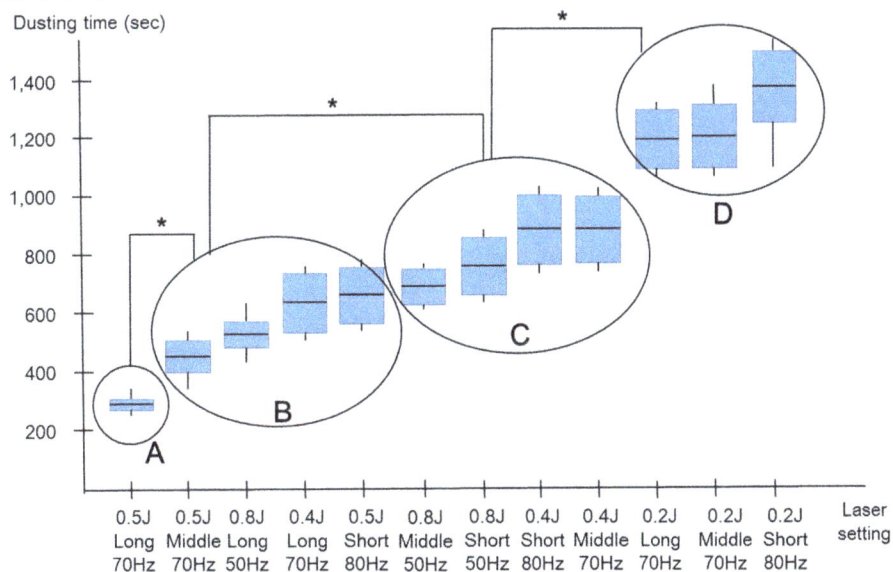

Fig. 3 Post-hoc analysis to compare the mean dusting time per each setting and across the groups **a** (0.5 J, a long pulse width, and 70 Hz), **b** (0.5 J (middle and short pulse widths), **c** (0.4 and 0.8 J, middle or short pulse width), and **d** (0.2 J groups)

efficacy of the Ho:YAG laser with a power output of 10~ 20 W are increased pulse energy and reduced pulse width [8–10]. Stone dusting is a recently established outcome of Ho:YAG laser use. Dusting is routinely performed with a low pulse energy and high pulse repetition rate to obtain maximum stone clearance. A Ho:YAG laser system with a maximum power output of 120 W was recently developed, which enables the surgeon to choose increased pulse repetition rates of 50 Hz or 80 Hz according to the pulse energy. Additionally, this new device has three different options of pulse width (short, middle, and long pulse of 500, 750, and 1000 μsec, respectively). Few investigations have assessed the optimal settings of this laser system. The present study involving in vitro reproducible experiments with phantom stones was done to define the most efficient laser setting for stone dusting.

The ideal for stone dusting during Ho:YAG lithotripsy is to use a setting that produces maximal fragmentation efficacy. The aim is to transform stone fragments into dust particles < 1 mm in size. Previous investigations explored the effect of various pulse energy of the Ho:YAG laser for stone fragmentation [11–13]. Increased pulse energy increases fragmentation power but increases retropulsion for the fragmented stones. Increased retropulsion may induce less energy transmission to stones and lower repetition rates, which may result in less fragmentation efficacy [14]. Low pulse energy (0.2 J) produces small fragment debris and less retropulsion at a slower fragmentation rate [11]. Presently, a pulse energy of 0.5 J and 70 Hz repetition rate with a long pulse was the most appropriate setting for stone dusting of plaster stones representing calcium oxalate monohydrate stones. This may be because retropulsion is significant in determining stone dusting efficacy. A low pulse energy of 0.2 or 0.4 J may be not efficacious to fragment phantom stones with a mean Hounsfield unit of 1309.0.

The association between pulse width and stone fragmentation efficacy has been studied in vitro [8, 9, 14–17]. In one study, short pulse width (120–190 μsec) produced equivalent fragmentation effectiveness, but more retropulsion compared to long pulse width (210–350 μsec) [15]. A ureter and caliceal model was used to demonstrate that a pulse width of 700 μsec provided less retropulsion and more effective stone fragmentation compared to a pulse width of 350 μsec [14]. In contrast, in an in vitro impacted and immobile phantom stones model, reduction of the pulse width from 700 to 350 μsec increased the fragmentation effectiveness of a Ho:YAG system with 10 W power [9]. In the present study, the mean dusting time decreased with increasing pulse width from 500 to 1000 μsec. The long pulse width (1000 μsec) provided the most effective stone dusting at a pulse energy ≥0.4 J.

Pulse repetition rates may not be critical to fragmentation efficacy [10, 11]. In these studies, the mean dusting time did not differ significantly at a pulse repetition rate of 70 and 80 Hz. These findings support the view that energy per pulse and pulse width, rather than pulse repetition rate, are more closely associated with stone fragmentation and stone dusting.

The present results might support the following 'ideal' settings of the Ho:YAG laser in stone dusting. The energy should be as low as possible to minimize retropulsion, while being powerful enough to break down the targeted stones. A longer pulse width is better than a shorter width. Higher repetition rates may be better than the lower ones.

Evidence about the dusting efficacy during stone surgery with the 120 W Ho:YAG laser system is limited. During laser lithotripsy, dusting technique usually needs the laser setting of low-pulse energy and high frequency [18]. A recent investigation assessed surgical outcomes of dusting technique in 82 renal units of 71 patients utilizing 120 W Ho:YAG laser with 200-μm fibers [19]. The mean stone size was 12.5 ± 8.7 mm and the mean Hounsfield unit was 993 ± 353. The laser setting for hard stones (> 1000 HU) during dusting technique was pulse energy of 0.3 J, 70 Hz repetition rates and short pulse width mode. For soft stones (< 1000 HU), the laser setting was pulse energy of 0.2 J, 80 Hz repetition rates and short pulse width mode. Although there were no direct comparative results between short and long pulse width modes, the complete stone free rate was 39% and < 2 mm residual fragments were identified in 69%. Another important point is the heat generation during laser lithotripsy. There have been few studies on thermal effects in terms of injury to adjacent organs during dusting technique with the 120 W Ho:YAG laser system. The authors did not measure fluid temperature during continuous firing of the laser. However, continuous irrigation with cool normal sline prevented overgeneration of heat during experiments. Further laboratory studies or clinical trials are needed to confirm the most efficacious and safe setting for dusting technique with the 120 W Ho:YAG laser system.

This study has some limitations. The experiments were not performed to mimic minor calyces of the human kidneys. So, the results do not reflect the situation in which a fragmented stone might migrate from one to another calyx. Phantom stones were previously reported to provide an adequate model to evaluate efficacy of stone fragmentation and retropulsion of Ho:YAG laser setting [8–17]. The authors used a single kind of phantom stone, which mimicked human calcium oxalate monohydrate calculi. The optimal stone fragmentation can be achieved according to helical/snail schema and the present study could not show the effect of stone retropulsion. In addition, only straightened laser fibers of 200 μm were used. Further studies are needed to determine the appropriate laser settings for other clinically possible situations including different kinds of stones.

Conclusions

In vitro reproducible experiments with phantom stones mimicking calcium oxalate monohydrate calculi demonstrates that a pulse energy of 0.5 J, long pulse width, and a repetition rate of 70 Hz provides the most efficacious dusting with the high-power output 120 W Ho:YAG laser in combination with a 200-μm fiber. The findings do not apply to other types of human calculi, but still have value in clinical practice.

Abbreviation

Ho:YAG: Holmium:yttrium-aluminum-garnet

Acknowledgements
None.

Funding
This research was supported by the Materials and Components Technology Development Program of MOTIE/KEIT, Republic of Korea (10067258, Development of a holmium/thulium laser resonator for treatment of prostatic hyperplasia).

Authors' contributions
LJW: analysis and interpretation of data, statistical analysis, drafting of the manuscript. PMG: conception and design, acquisition of data, supervision. CSY: conception and design, acquision of data, obtaining funding, administrative, technical, or material support, supervision. All authors read and approved the final manuscript.

Author details
¹Department of Urology, Dongguk University Ilsan Hospital, Dongguk University College of Medicine, 27, Dongguk-ro, Ilsandong-gu, Goyang-si, Gyeonggi-do 410-773, Republic of Korea. ²Department of Urology, Seoul Paik Hospital, Inje University College of Medicine, 9, Mareunnae-ro, Jung-gu, Seoul 100-032, Republic of Korea. ³Department of Urology, Seoul Metropolitan Government-Seoul National University Boramae Medical Center, Seoul National University College of Medicine, 20, Boramae-ro 5-Gil, Dongjak-gu, Seoul 156-707, Republic of Korea.

References
1. Bader MJ, Eisner B, Porpiglia F, Preminger GM, Tiselius HG. Contemporary management of ureter stones. Eur Urol. 2012;61:764–72.
2. Blackmon RL, Irby PB, Fried NM. Comparison of holmium:YAG and thulium fiber laser lithotripsy: ablation thresholds, ablation rates, and retropulsion effects. J Biomed Opt. 2011;16:071403.
3. Lee SH, Kim TH, Myung SC, et al. Effectiveness of flexible ureteroscopic stone removal for treating ureteral and ipsilateral renal stones: a single-center experience. Korean J Urol. 2013;54:377–82.
4. Lee JW, Park J, Lee SB, Son H, Cho SY, Jeong H. Mini-percutaneous nephrolithotomy vs retrograde intrarenal surgery for renal stones larger than 10 mm: a prospective randomized controlled trial. Urology. 2015;86:873–7.
5. Kumar A, Kumar N, Vasudeva P, Kumar Jha S, Kumar R, Singh H. A prospective, randomized comparison of shock wave lithotripsy, retrograde intrarenal surgery and miniperc for treatment of 1 to 2 cm radiolucent lower calyceal calculi: a single center experience. J Urol. 2015;193:160–4.
6. Kirac M, Bozkurt ÖF, Tunc L, Guneri C, Unsal A, Biri H. Comparison of retrograde intrarenal surgery and mini-percutaneous nephrolithotomy in management of lower-pole renal stones with a diameter of smaller than 15 mm. Urolithiasis. 2013;41:241–6.
7. Sabnis RB, Jagtap J, Mishra S, Desai M. Treating renal calculi 1-2 cm in diameter with minipercutaneous or retrograde intrarenal surgery: a prospective comparative study. BJU Int. 2012;110:E346–9.
8. Bader MJ, Pongratz T, Khoder W, et al. Impact of pulse duration on ho:YAG laser lithotripsy: fragmentation and dusting performance. World J Urol. 2015; 33:471–7.
9. Wezel F, Häcker A, Gross AJ, Michel MS, Bach T. Effect of pulse energy, frequency and length on holmium:yttrium-aluminum-garnet laser fragmentation efficiency in non-floating artificial urinary calculi. J Endourol. 2010;24:1135–40.
10. Chawla SN, Change MF, Chang A, Lenoir J, Bagley DH. Effectiveness of high-frequency holmium:YAG laser stone fragmentation: the "popcorn effect". J Endourol. 2008;22:645–50.
11. Sea J, Jonat LM, Chew BH, et al. Optimal power settings for holmium:YAG lithotripsy. J Urol. 2012;187:914–9.
12. Spore SS, Teichman JM, Corbin NS, Champion PC, Williamson EA, Glickman RD. Holimium: YAG lithotripasy: optimal power settings. J Endourol. 1999;13:559–66.
13. Corbin NS, Teichman JM, Nguyen T, et al. Laser lithotripsy and cyanide. J Endourol. 2000;14:169–73.
14. Finley DS, Petersen J, Abdelshehid C, et al. Effect of holmium:YAG laser pulse width on lithotripsy retropulsion in vitro. J Endourol. 2005;19:1041–4.
15. Kang HW, Lee H, Teichman JM, Oh J, Kim J, Welch AJ. Dependence of calculus retropulsion on pulse duration during Ho: YAG laser lithotripsy. Lasers Surg Med. 2006;38:762–72.
16. Lee HJ, Box GN, Abraham JB, et al. In vitro evaluation of nitinol urological retrieval coli and ureteral occlusion device: retropulsion and holmium laser fragmentation efficiency. J Urol. 2008;180:969–73.
17. Marguet CG, Sung JC, Springhart WP, et al. In vitro comparison of stone retropulsion and fragmentation of the frequency doubled, double pulse nd: yag laser and the holmium:yag laser. J Urol. 2005;173:1797–800.
18. Patel AP, Knudsen BE. Optimizing use of the holmium:YAG laser for surgical management of urinary lithiasis. Curr Urol Rep. 2014;15:397.
19. Tracey J, Gagin G, Morhardt D, Hollingsworth J, Ghani KR. Ureteroscopic high-frequency dusting utilizing a 120-W holmium laser. J Endourol. 2018; 32:290–5.

22

The effect of surgery report cards on improving radical prostatectomy quality: the SuRep study protocol

R. H. Breau[1,2], R. M. Kumar[1]*⬤, L. T. Lavallee[1,2], I. Cagiannos[1,2], C. Morash[1,2], M. Horrigan[2], S. Cnossen[2], R. Mallick[2], D. Stacey[2,3], M. Fung-Kee-Fung[2], R. Morash[4], J. Smylie[4], K. Witiuk[2] and D. A. Fergusson[2]

Abstract

Background: The goal of radical prostatectomy is to achieve the optimal balance between complete cancer removal and preserving a patient's urinary and sexual function. Performing a wider excision of peri-prostatic tissue helps achieve negative surgical margins, but can compromise urinary and sexual function. Alternatively, sparing peri-prostatic tissue to maintain functional outcomes may result in an increased risk of cancer recurrence. The objective of this study is to determine the effect of providing surgeons with detailed information about their patient outcomes through a surgical report card.

Methods: We propose a prospective cohort quasi-experimental study. The intervention is the provision of feedback to prostate cancer surgeons via surgical report cards. These report cards will be distributed every 3 months by email and will present surgeons with detailed information, including urinary function, erectile function, and surgical margin outcomes of their patients compared to patients treated by other de-identified surgeons in the study. For the first 12 months of the study, pre-operative, 6-month, and 12-month patient data will be collected but there will be no report cards distributed to surgeons. This will form the pre-feedback cohort. After the pre-feedback cohort has completed accrual, surgeons will receive quarterly report cards. Patients treated after the provision of report cards will comprise the post-feedback cohort. The primary comparison will be post-operative function of the pre-feedback cohort vs. post-feedback cohort. The secondary comparison will be the proportion of patients with positive surgical margins in the two cohorts. Outcomes will be stratified or case-mix adjusted, as appropriate. Assuming a baseline potency of 20% and a baseline continence of 70%, 292 patients will be required for 80% power at an alpha of 5% to detect a 10% improvement in functional outcomes. Assuming 30% of patients may be lost to follow-up, a minimum sample size of 210 patients is required in the pre-feedback cohort and 210 patients in the post-feedback cohort.

Discussion: The findings from this study will have an immediate impact on surgeon self-evaluation and we hypothesize surgical report cards will result in improved overall outcomes of men treated with radical prostatectomy.

Keywords: Prostate cancer, Radical prostatectomy, Surgeon feedback, Surgical report cards, Audit and feedback, Knowledge translation

* Correspondence: rkuma015@uottawa.ca
[1]Division of Urology, Department of Surgery, The Ottawa Hospital, University of Ottawa, Ottawa, ON, Canada
Full list of author information is available at the end of the article

Background

Prostate cancer and the side effects of treatment are major public health issues, since the disease is diagnosed in approximately 18% of men [1]. The vast majority of patients diagnosed currently have localized disease that can be cured surgically with radical prostatectomy [2–4]. Since the prostate is in close proximity to the urethral sphincter and nerves that facilitate erections for sexual function, these structures are often inadvertently injured or purposefully resected during tumour resection. Consequently, approximately 0.3–12.5% of men suffer permanent urinary incontinence after a radical prostatectomy, and up to 30% of men use incontinence pads [5–8]. It is also estimated that 75% of patients will suffer from temporary or permanent erectile dysfunction following a radical prostatectomy [9, 10]. Maintenance of urinary and erectile function is related to surgical technique, and significant differences in function following radical prostatectomy have been observed between surgeons [11–13].

Positive surgical margins occur in approximately 11–38% of patients [14, 15]. A positive surgical margin can be an indication of locally-advanced disease, but is also a reflection of surgical technique. Surgical margin rate has been highlighted as an indicator of surgical quality that should be monitored prospectively [16] Significant variability exists in positive margin rates between surgeons [2, 11, 17, 18]. The surgical margin status of a patient is important because this outcome is highly associated with increased need for secondary salvage treatments and lower overall survival [19–21].

In a 2006 provincial pathology audit, positive surgical margins were found in 33% of patients who had tumours that did not extent outside the prostate (pathologic stage T2) in Ontario, Canada (population 12,160,282). In 2008, a Cancer Care Ontario expert clinician panel set a provincial goal to reduce the incidence of positive surgical margins to less than 25% [22]. Since that time, Cancer Care Ontario has been providing feedback to clinicians on the incidence of positive surgical margins in their patients. As of 2011, the incidence of pT2 positive surgical margins in Ontario had dropped to 21% [23]. This finding supported the hypothesis that prospective reporting and feedback can affect surgeon behaviour, resulting in improvement. The findings in Ontario are consistent with randomized trials that show feedback to clinicians generally result in practice improvement [24].

A potential negative consequence of surgical margin scrutiny by Cancer Care Ontario is that surgeons may be performing a wider excision of peri-prostatic tissue, purposely sacrificing erectile nerve tissue to lower the risk of a positive margin, and as a result compromise urinary and sexual function. Clearly, a balance must be struck between ensuring complete cancer removal and preservation of a patient's urinary and sexual function. Isolated critical evaluation of surgical margin rates may have had the unintended effect of increasing long term side effects that are important to patients. Ideally, all clinically important outcomes should be assessed when evaluating surgical quality, not only surgical margin status.

The primary purpose of this study is to determine if providing prostate cancer surgeon feedback on their patients' improves overall surgical quality as measured by surgical margin rates and patient reported functional outcomes.

Methods

Study design and setting

This is a prospective cohort quasi-experimental before-and-after study at The Ottawa Hospital. The Ottawa Hospital is an academic hospital affiliated with the University of Ottawa. The Ottawa Hospital serves the Champlain Local Health Integration Network (LHIN), which is a geographic boundary that contains a population of approximately 1.3 million people [25]. Approximately 80% of prostate cancer patients in the Champlain LHIN who receive a radical prostatectomy are treated by one of eight prostate cancer surgeons at the Ottawa Hospital. The intervention in this study is the provision of feedback to prostate cancer surgeons via surgical report cards. These report cards will be distributed every 3 months by email. The report card will present surgeons with outcomes of their patients compared to patients treated by other de-identified surgeons in the study.

Study participants

All prostate cancer surgeons will participate in this study. While all surgeons will use a common clinical pathway and provide consistent information, the surgical technique is not mandated by the study. All patients undergoing radical prostatectomy by each surgeon will be eligible, regardless of tumour stage, histology and previous pelvic treatments including surgery or radiation. Extent of planned and performed neurovascular bundle preservation will not be mandated, but will be prospectively collected from the operating surgeon. Surgeons will report their nerve spare intent prior to surgery and their perceived nerve spare achieved following surgery. All surgical approaches (open, laparoscopic, and robotic assisted laparoscopic) will be included. Given that patients are contacted for assessment of symptoms, consent will be obtained from each patient. Patients will be excluded if they 1) decline or are incapable of providing consent; 2) are less than 18 years of age; or 3) are being treated outside of The Ottawa Hospital. Patient information and outcomes will be collected prior to surgery and 6- and 12-months following surgery. Approximately 230 radical prostatectomy procedures are performed annually at The Ottawa Hospital.

Assessment and data collection

Pre-surgery

Prior to treatment, patients will complete two functional assessments that were selected based on content validity, common use in clinical practice, and availability in English and French: (1) The Expanded Prostate Cancer Index Composite (EPIC), and (2) the EQ-5D. EPIC is a 50-item robust and comprehensive prostate cancer-specific instrument that measures a broad spectrum of urinary, bowel, sexual, and hormonal symptoms. The EPIC has been widely validated and used in prostate cancer clinical trials and treatment quality initiatives [26] and will serve as the basis for urinary and erectile function assessment. EQ-5D is a simple, easy to use assessment of overall health status and provides a descriptive profile and a single index value for reporting [27]. The EQ-5D is valid and reliable across a broad range of clinical settings and languages.

Other pre-operative baseline characteristics will be collected, including patient age, height, weight, clinical tumour stage, tumour grade, and prostate specific antigen (PSA) concentration. This information is available from the standardized pre-operative pathway documents and will be abstracted by study personnel.

Time of surgery

Synoptic reporting will be used by surgeons and pathologists to aid with data collection. Surgeons will document planned and achieved preservation of neurovascular bundles. Pathology reports will be used to determine cancer stage, tumour grade, tumour size, location of extraprostatic tumour extention (if applicable), extent of extraprostatic tumour extension (if applicable), location of a positive surgical margin (if applicable), and extent of a positive surgical margin (if applicable).

Post-surgery

At 6 and 12 months post-operative, patients will be mailed the same quality-of-life and functional assessment questionnaires that were completed prior to surgery. Study personnel will contact patients who do not return the questionnaires to facilitate completion or to determine why the patient does not wish to participate. This duration of follow-up was chosen because functional outcomes improve over time and most outcomes have generally stabilized by 12 months post-surgery [28]. Post-operative interventions that could confound results will be determined by asking patients if they currently use erectile function aids, have had urinary continence procedures, received pelvic radiation, or received androgen deprivation. All post-operative PSA values will be documented.

Surgical report card intervention and control

Descriptive baseline, pathological, and follow-up information will be summarized and tabulated. The primary measures of surgical quality on the surgeon report cards will be: post-operative urinary continence, post-operative erectile function (stratified by baseline function and tumour stage), and rate of positive surgical margins (stratified by tumour stage). An example of a surgical report card is displayed in Additional file 1. Urinary continence will be defined as requiring no continence pads (i.e. score of 0 on question 5 of the EPIC questionnaire), and potency will be defined as a firm enough erection for intercourse (score of 4 on question 18 of the EPIC questionnaire). Changes in patients' overall health status will also be summarized.

For the pre-feedback cohort, pre-operative, 6-month, and 12-month patient data will be collected but there will be no report cards distributed to surgeons. This will form the pre-feedback cohort. When accrual to the pre-feedback cohort is complete (anticipated to be 12 months from initiation of the study), surgeons will begin receiving report cards. Patients treated after the provision of report cards will form the post-feedback cohort for analyses. A summary of the study timeline is presented in Fig. 1.

Outcomes

The primary outcomes will be post-operative function of the patient cohort before surgeon feedback (pre-feedback cohort) compared to post-operative function of the patient cohort after surgeon feedback (post-feedback cohort). The secondary comparison will be the proportion of patients with positive surgical margins in the pre-feedback cohort compared to post-feedback cohort. Outcomes will be stratified or adjusted by important co-variates such as patient age, tumour stage, tumour grade, pre-operative PSA, baseline urinary function, baseline sexual function, and nerve preservation status.

Analysis and sample size

The comparison between pre-and post-feedback functional outcomes will be done by using generalized linear model that treats the intervention as an effect that is either present or absent for a patient (absent for the pre-feedback cohort and present the post-feedback cohort). In the analysis the surgeons will be considered as clusters to account for repeated measurements. In the model other covariates like patient age, tumour stage, tumour grade, pre-operative PSA, baseline urinary function, baseline sexual function, and nerve preservation status will be used. An estimate of the difference between pre-feedback and post-feedback potency or continence will be obtained from the above model.

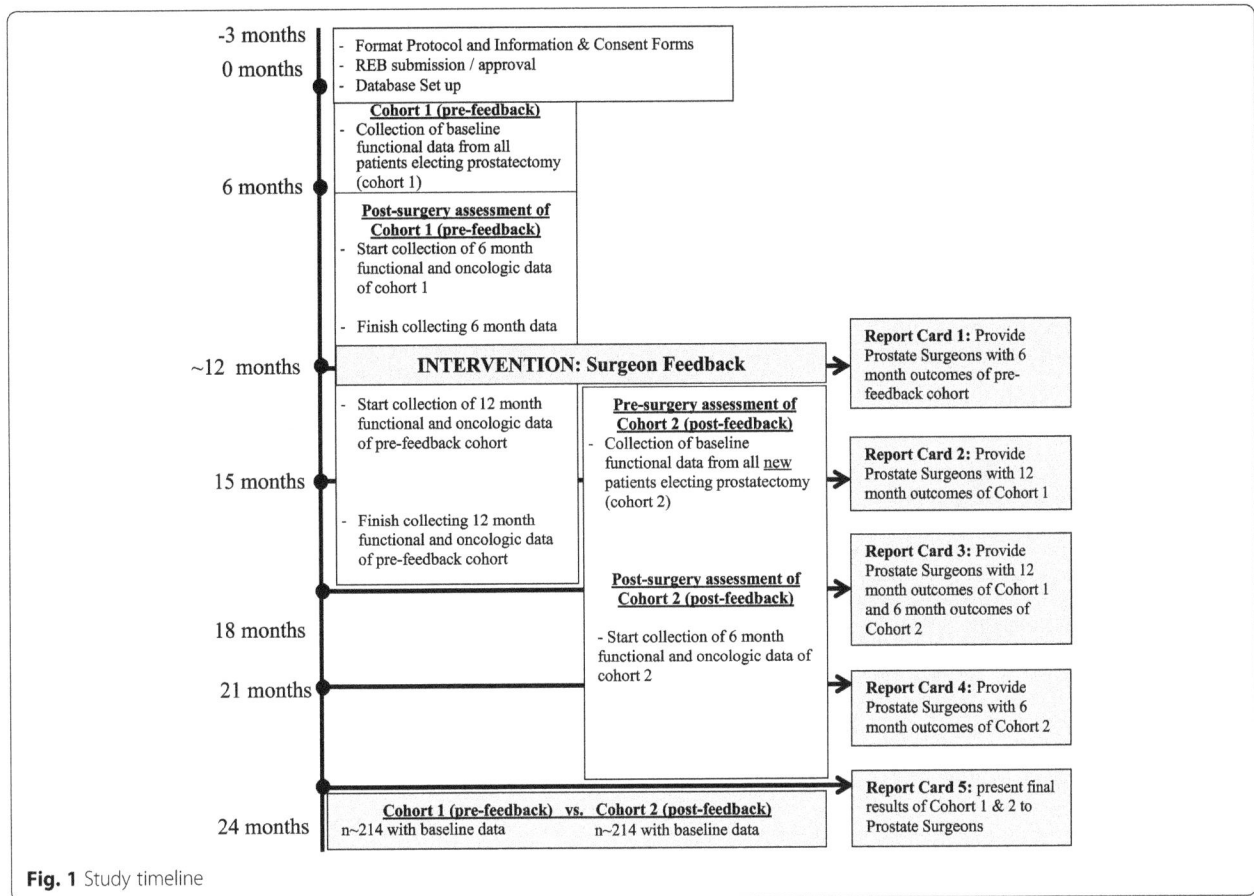

Fig. 1 Study timeline

An overall improvement of 10% in potency or incontinence following the surgeon feedback intervention (post-intervention cohort) will be considered clinically significant. Assuming a baseline potency of 20% and a baseline continence of 70%, 294 patients would be required for 80% power at an alpha of 5%. Assuming as much as a 30% lost to follow up, we will require a minimum of 210 patients in the pre-feedback cohort and 210 patients in the post-feedback cohort.

Discussion

As a result of improved survival due to early detection of prostate cancer, side effects of radical prostatectomy that affect long term quality-of-life are of paramount importance to patients. However, there are no proven methods to improve surgical quality in these domains. Furthermore, initiatives to lower margin rates may compromise these outcomes if they are not considered. This proposal is innovative and significant because, to the best of our knowledge, it will be the first prospective study that provides feedback to surgeons about oncological and functional outcomes in men treated with radical prostatectomy. Furthermore, it will allow us to assess whether providing feedback to surgeons results in improvement in surgical quality.

The findings from this initiative will have an immediate impact on surgeon self-evaluation, and we hypothesize this will result in improved overall outcomes and satisfaction for men treated with radical prostatectomy at our institution. In addition to the immediate benefits to patient counseling, this study is designed so it can be freely available and transferable for use in any hospital or region that aims to monitor and improve prostate cancer treatment quality.

Funding
Funded in part by Prostate Cancer Canada (Discovery 2014 D2014–2), The Ottawa Hospital Academic Medical Organization, and the Prostate Cancer Fight Foundation & TELUS Ride For Dad. All statements in this report are solely those of the authors.

Trial status
The trial is in the recruiting phase at the time of manuscript submission.

Authors' contributions
RHB designed the study and drafted the manuscript, RMK acquired data and drafted the manuscript, LTL contributed to the design and drafting of the manuscript. IC, CM, SC, DS, MFKF, RMorash, JS, KW, and DA contributed to the design and revised the manuscript. MH acquired data and contributed to manuscript revisions. RMallick contributed to the

design, drafted the analytic plan, and revised the manuscript. All authors read and approved the final manuscript. All authors are accountable for all aspects of the work.

Competing interests

The authors declare that they have no competing interests.

Author details

[1]Division of Urology, Department of Surgery, The Ottawa Hospital, University of Ottawa, Ottawa, ON, Canada. [2]Ottawa Hospital Research Institute, Ottawa, ON, Canada. [3]Faculty of Health Sciences, University of Ottawa, Ottawa, ON, Canada. [4]The Ottawa Hospital Cancer Program, Ottawa, Canada.

References

1. Klein EA, Platz EA, Thompson IM. In: Wein AJ, et al., editors. Epidemiology, Etiology, and Prevention of Prostate Cancer, in Campbell-Walsh Urology. Philadelphia: Saunders; 2006. p. 2854–73.
2. Hull GW, et al. Cancer control with radical prostatectomy alone in 1,000 consecutive patients. J Urol. 2002;167(2 Pt 1):528–34.
3. Bill-Axelson A, et al. Radical prostatectomy versus watchful waiting in early prostate cancer. N Engl J Med. 2011;364(18):1708–17.
4. Schroder FH, et al. Screening and prostate-cancer mortality in a randomized European study. N Engl J Med. 2009;360(13):1320–8.
5. Nitti VW. In: Walsh PC, et al., editors. Postprostatectomy Incontinence, in Campbell-Walsh Urology. New York: Saunders; 2002. p. 1053–72.
6. Fowler FJ Jr, et al. Patient-reported complications and follow-up treatment after radical prostatectomy. The National Medicare Experience: 1988-1990 (updated June 1993). Urology. 1993;42(6):622–9.
7. Oefelein MG. Prospective predictors of urinary continence after anatomical radical retropubic prostatectomy: a multivariate analysis. World J Urol. 2004; 22(4):267–71.
8. Hollabaugh RS Jr, et al. Preservation of putative continence nerves during radical retropubic prostatectomy leads to more rapid return of urinary continence. Urology. 1998;51(6):960–7.
9. Walz J, et al. A critical analysis of the current knowledge of surgical anatomy related to optimization of cancer control and preservation of continence and erection in candidates for radical prostatectomy. Eur Urol. 2010;57(2):179–92.
10. Kundu SD, et al. Potency, continence and complications in 3,477 consecutive radical retropubic prostatectomies. J Urol. 2004;172(6 Pt 1):2227–31.
11. Eastham JA, et al. Variations among individual surgeons in the rate of positive surgical margins in radical prostatectomy specimens. J Urol. 2003; 170(6 Pt 1):2292–5.
12. Wilson A, et al. Radical prostatectomy: a systematic review of the impact of hospital and surgeon volume on patient outcome. ANZ J Surg. 2010; 80(1–2):24–9.
13. Wilt TJ, et al. Association between hospital and surgeon radical prostatectomy volume and patient outcomes: a systematic review. J Urol. 2008;180(3):820–8 discussion 828-9.
14. Yossepowitch O, et al. Positive surgical margins in radical prostatectomy: outlining the problem and its long-term consequences. Eur Urol. 2009;55(1): 87–99.
15. Preston MA, et al. The prognostic significance of capsular incision into tumor during radical prostatectomy. Eur Urol. 2011;59(4):613–8.
16. Grossfeld GD, et al. Impact of positive surgical margins on prostate cancer recurrence and the use of secondary cancer treatment: data from the CaPSURE database. J Urol. 2000;163(4):1171–7 quiz 1295.
17. D'Amico AV, et al. The combination of preoperative prostate specific antigen and postoperative pathological findings to predict prostate specific antigen outcome in clinically localized prostate cancer. J Urol. 1998;160(6 Pt 1):2096–101.
18. Chun FK, et al. Surgical volume is related to the rate of positive surgical margins at radical prostatectomy in European patients. BJU Int. 2006;98(6): 1204–9.
19. Blute ML, et al. Use of Gleason score, prostate specific antigen, seminal vesicle and margin status to predict biochemical failure after radical prostatectomy. J Urol. 2001;165(1):119–25.
20. Thompson IM, et al. Adjuvant radiotherapy for pathological T3N0M0 prostate cancer significantly reduces risk of metastases and improves survival: long-term followup of a randomized clinical trial. J Urol. 2009; 181(3):956–62.
21. Bolla M, et al. Postoperative radiotherapy after radical prostatectomy: a randomised controlled trial (EORTC trial 22911). Lancet. 2005;366(9485):572–8.
22. Chin, J. et al. Guideline for Optimization of Surgical and Pathological Quality Performance for Radical Prostatectomy. Prostate Cancer Management. 2008. https://www.cancercareontario.ca/en/guidelines-advice/types-of-cancer/556. Assessed 29 Jan 2018.
23. Cancer Quality Council Ontario. Margin status in prostate Cancer surgery. 2010. http://www.cqco.ca/search/default.aspx?q=prostate%20margin&type= 0,89469-40484%7C-1,89613-78.
24. Ivers N, et al. Audit and feedback: effects on professional practice and healthcare outcomes. Cochrane Database Syst Rev. 2012;6:CD000259.
25. Champlain Local Health Integration Network. http://www.champlainlhin.on. ca/AboutUs/GeoPopHlthData/PopHealth.aspx. Accessed 3 Mar 2018.
26. Wei JT, et al. Development and validation of the expanded prostate cancer index composite (EPIC) for comprehensive assessment of health-related quality of life in men with prostate cancer. Urology. 2000;56(6):899–905.
27. Hurst NP, et al. Measuring health-related quality of life in rheumatoid arthritis: validity, responsiveness and reliability of EuroQol (EQ-5D). Br J Rheumatol. 1997;36(5):551–9.
28. Resnick MJ, et al. Long-term functional outcomes after treatment for localized prostate cancer. N Engl J Med. 2013;368(5):436–45.

23

Early post-operative serum albumin level predicts survival after curative nephrectomy for kidney cancer

Yongquan Tang[1†], Zhihong Liu[2†], Jiayu Liang[2], Ruochen Zhang[3], Kan Wu[2], Zijun Zou[4], Chuan Zhou[2], Fuxun Zhang[2] and Yiping Lu[2*] (iD)

Abstract

Background: Previous studies have shown that albumin-related systemic inflammation is associated with the long-term prognosis of cancer, but the clinical significance of an early (≤ 7 days) post-operative serum albumin level has not been well-documented as a prognostic factor in patients with renal cell cancer.

Methods: We retrospectively included patients hospitalized for kidney cancer from January 2009 to May 2014. First, the receiver operating characteristic analysis was used to define the best cut-off of an early post-operative serum albumin level in determining the prognosis, from which survival analysis was performed.

Results: A total of 329 patients were included. The median duration of follow-up was 54.8 months. Patients with an early post-operative serum albumin level < 32 g/L had a significantly shorter median recurrence-free survival (RFS; 49.1 versus 56.5 months, $P = 0.001$) and median overall survival (OS; 52.2 versus 57.0 months, $P = 0.049$) than patients with an early post-operative serum albumin level ≥ 32 g/L. After adjusting for age, BMI, tumor stage, post-operative hemoglobin concentration, and pre-operative albumin, globulin, and hemoglobin levels, multivariate Cox regression showed that an early post-operative serum albumin level < 32 g/L was an independent prognostic factor associated with a decreased RFS (HR = 3.60; 95% CI,1.05–12.42 [months], $P = 0.042$) and decreased OS (HR = 9.95; 95% CI, 1.81–54.80 [months], $P = 0.008$).

Conclusion: An early post-operative serum albumin level < 32 g/L is an independent prognostic factor leading to an unfavorable RFS and OS. Prospective trials and further studies involving additional patients are warranted.

Keywords: Kidney cancer, Survival, Hypoalbuminemia, Radical resection

Background

Kidney cancer is one of the most common malignancies involving the urogenital system [1]. The most important treatment for kidney cancer is surgical resection, but post-operative recurrences are common, especially for stage II and above. A number of risk factors have been reported; however, prognostication remains difficult [2, 3].

Notably, new prognostic factors have been described in recent years [4–7].

Several studies have reported that the early post-operative neutrophil-to-lymphocyte ratio may be a long-term prognostic factor for some cancers, including pancreatic, prostate, and bladder cancers [8–10]. This association may result from the potential anti-tumor effect of acute inflammation. Albumin is commonly used to evaluate nutritional status, but a recent study has shown that albumin is also involved in the inflammatory/stress reaction [11]. McMillan and colleagues [12] reported that the serum albumin level was positively correlated with the C-reactive protein level in 40 patients with lung or gastrointestinal cancer. Bozzetti

* Correspondence: yiping_luuro@163.com
†Yongquan Tang and Zhihong Liu contributed equally to this work.
²Department of Urology, Institute of Urology, West China Hospital, Sichuan University, Chengdu, China
Full list of author information is available at the end of the article

and colleagues [13] first reported the phenomenon of frequent hypoalbuminemia status in the early period after extensive surgery. Based on our previous data, the serum albumin level was < 35 g/L in > 50% of patients following curative nephrectomy ($P < 0.05$), then always recovered to the pre-operative level within 2 weeks. Some researchers have concluded that early post-operative hypoalbuminemia is associated with the pre-operative serum albumin level, age, and extent of surgery [12], while other studies have shown that post-operative hypoalbuminemia may lead to unfavorable short-term prognoses, such as acute kidney injury [13, 14], unbalanced substance metabolism [15–17], and surgical site infections [18, 19]. Such findings suggest that albumin has a role in immune-inflammatory reactions [11, 20].

Recent studies have revealed that albumin-related systemic inflammation is associated with the long-term prognosis in patients with advanced gastrointestinal cancer [11, 21, 22]. Cai and colleagues [23] found that hypoalbuminemia 3–5 weeks after initiation of tyrosine kinase inhibitors is independently associated with a significantly decreased progression-free survival (PFS) and overall survival (OS) in patients with advanced kidney cancer. Furthermore, when combined with the Memorial Sloan-Kettering Cancer Center (MSKCC) risk model, hypoalbuminemia improves the efficiency in predicting recurrence-free survival (RFS) and OS [23]. The current retrospective study determined the potential association between early (≤ 7 days) post-operative hypoalbuminemia with long-term prognosis after resection of kidney cancer.

Methods
Study population
In this retrospective single-center study we reviewed the electronic medical records of inpatients with kidney cancer who were admitted to the Department of Urology at West China Hospital of Sichuan University (Sichuan, China) between January 2009 and May 2014. All of the patients underwent curative surgery. The inclusion criteria included the following: > 18 years of age; a pathologic diagnosis of kidney cancer; and negative surgical margins. Negative surgical margin was defined as macroscopic evidence on surgical report or microscopic evidence on histopathologic report. The exclusion criteria were as follows: incomplete resection; history of other life-threatening diseases within 5 years before or after surgery; adjuvant or neoadjuvant treatment; and distant metastasis, with the exception of the adrenal gland. The study conformed to the Declaration of Helsinki and was approved by the Ethics Committee of West China Hospital.

Objectives
We primarily assessed the prognostic value of early post-operative hypoalbuminemia with respect to RFS and

OS in the curative resection of kidney cancer. We then determined the optimal cut-off point of the early post-operative serum albumin level in predicting the prognosis of kidney cancer. RFS was defined as the date of surgery to the date of recurrence, and OS was measured from the date of surgery to the date of death. For patients without a recurrence or who did not die, survival was censored at the date of the last follow-up evaluation. To distinguish confounding factors, subgroup analyses were performed.

Data collection
All data were obtained from medical records. The follow-up project adhered to the National Comprehensive Cancer Network (NCCN) clinical practice guidelines for kidney cancer [24]. Data were collected by two well-trained researchers. Any discrepancies in data interpretation were resolved by consensus of all authors. The data collected included demographic characteristics, date and type of surgery, clinical-pathologic TNM stage at the time of surgery, histopathologic characteristics, and date of recurrence and/or death if available or date of the last follow-up. TNM stage referred to the tumor size (T), local lymph node involvement (N), and remote metastasis (M), and was assessed according to imaging studies, surgical records, and histopathologic reports. TNM stage and anatomic stage/prognostic groups were also guided by the 2018 NCCN guidelines for kidney cancer [24]. Cancer recurrence was defined as unequivocal radiologic or biopsy evidence of emerging local or distant tumor lesions. In addition, we collated serum albumin, globulin, and hemoglobin data obtained pre- and post-operatively.

Statistics
All statistical analyses were carried out using Stata 14.0 (Stata Corp, College Station, TX, USA). The receiver operating characteristic (ROC) curve analysis was performed to determine the optimal cut-off point for the post-operative serum albumin level for use in the post-operative prognosis. Based on the cut-off point, we divided the patients into two groups, then survival curves were created using the Kaplan-Meier method and compared using the log-rank test. Gender, age, body mass index (BMI), stage, type of surgery, and pathologic pattern for both groups of patients were compared and tested one-by-one. Four-fold or R × C table data were analyzed with a chi-square test. The median of data with a non-normal distribution was designated as the average and analyzed with the Wilcoxon rank-sum test. The mean of data with a normal distribution was designated as the average and analyzed with a t-test [25]. A factor was entered into multivariate Cox regression analysis if a statistical difference existed in both groups of patients. The hazard ratio (HR) was adopted as the measurement. A P value < 0.05 indicated statistical significance.

Results

Patients and disease characteristics

A total of 694 patients were available in the database; 329 patients met the inclusion criteria. Among the 329 patients, 64% were male and the median age at the time of surgery was 56 years (range, 22–84 years). The median duration of follow-up was 54.8 months (range, 5.2–96.4 months). The mean pre- and post-operative serum albumin levels were 42.2 and 34.1 g/L, respectively ($P = 0.000$). ROC curve analyses showed that the optimal post-operative serum albumin cut-off level was 32 g/L (area under the curve [AUC] = 0.71) in predicting tumor recurrence (Fig. 1a) and 31 g/L (AUC = 0.80) in predicting death (Fig. 1b). Thus, we used 32 g/L as the cut-off point for grouping comparisons. A total of 99 patients had a serum albumin level < 32 g/L and 230 patients had a serum albumin level ≥ 32 g/L. The patient characteristics and laboratory test results for both groups are presented in Table 1. Age, BMI, tumor stage, post-operative hemoglobin concentration, and pre-operative albumin, globulin, and hemoglobin levels were statistically different (Table 1).

Survival analysis

No patients were lost to follow-up. The mean duration of follow-up in both groups was similar [58.5 (albumin < 32 g/L) and 59.9 (albumin ≥32 g/L) months, respectively; $P > 0.05$]. During follow-up, 30 patients (30.3%) had tumor recurrences and 24 patients (24.2%) did not survive in the group of patients with a post-operative serum albumin level < 32 g/L. Only 20 patients (8.7%) had tumor recurrences and 8 patients (3.5%) did not survive in the group of patients with a post-operative serum albumin level ≥ 32 g/L. The median RFS of patients with a post-operative serum albumin level < 32 g/L

was significantly less than patients with a post-operative serum albumin level ≥ 32 g/L (49.1 and 56.5 months, respectively; $P = 0.001$). The median OS of patients with a post-operative serum albumin level < 32 g/L was also significantly less than patients with a post-operative serum albumin level ≥ 32 g/L (52.2 and 57.0 months, respectively; $P = 0.049$). The group survival curves are shown in Fig. 2. The log-rank test revealed that the differences in group survival curves was significant ($P = 0.000$) for RFS (Fig. 2a) and OS (Fig. 2b).

Multivariate cox regression

Based on difference testing, age, BMI, tumor stage, post-operative hemoglobin concentration, and pre-operative albumin, globulin, and hemoglobin levels were entered into multivariate Cox regression analysis. An early post-operative serum albumin level < 32 g/L was shown to have an independent impact on the decreased RFS (HR = 3.60; 95% CI,1.05–12.42 [months]; $P = 0.042$) and OS (HR = 9.95; 95% CI, 1.81–54.80 [months]; $P = 0.008$). In addition, tumor stage was also an independent prognostic factor (Table 2). Therefore, subgroup analysis was performed based on tumor stage.

Sub-group analysis of stages II and III kidney cancer

The survival curves of patients grouped by tumor stage and relevant log-rank testing showed significant differences between stages I and II, and stages III and IV for RFS and OS, but not between stages II and III. Furthermore, after excluding patients with stages I and IV, the two groups had similar TNM stage distributions ($P = 0.995$). Survival analysis and log-rank testing showed that patients with a post-operative serum albumin level < 32 g/L had a significantly decreased RFS ($P = 0.036$) and decreased OS ($P = 0.012$) compared to patients with a post-operative

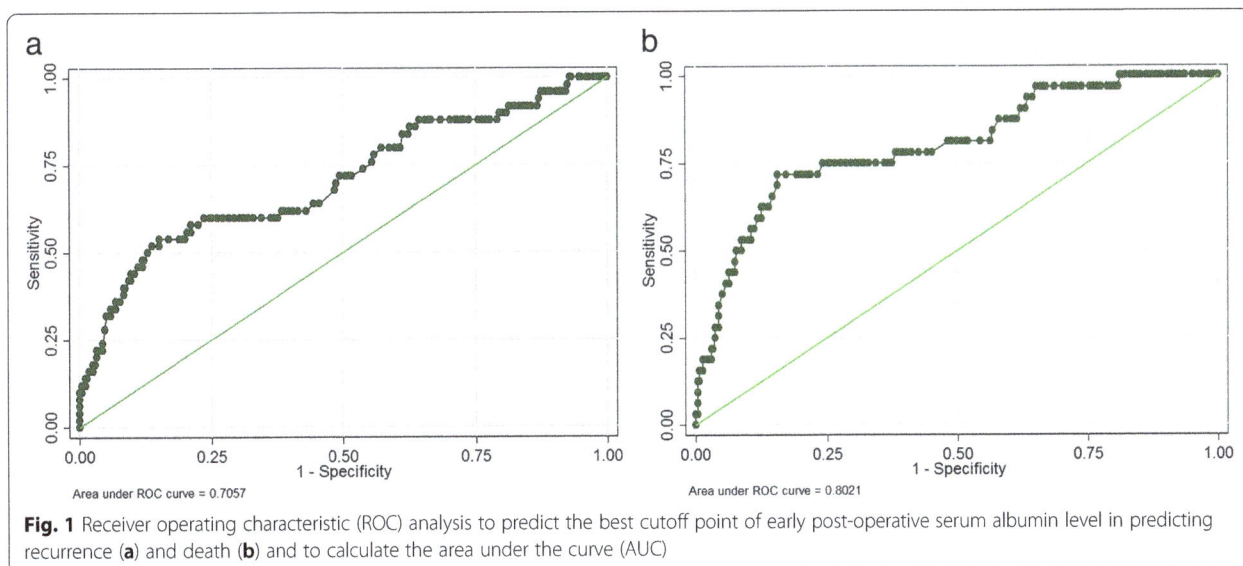

Area under ROC curve = 0.7057

Area under ROC curve = 0.8021

Fig. 1 Receiver operating characteristic (ROC) analysis to predict the best cutoff point of early post-operative serum albumin level in predicting recurrence (**a**) and death (**b**) and to calculate the area under the curve (AUC)

Table 1 The baseline and clinic-pathologic characteristics of patients grouped by post-operative serum albumin level

Variable	Serum albumin < 32 g/L (n = 99)	Serum albumin ≥ 32 g/L (n = 230)	P
Gender (%)			0.229
Male	59 (60)	153 (67)	
Female	40 (40)	77 (33)	
Age, y, median(range)	63 (22–82)	53 (24–84)	0.000*
BMI, Kg/m², mean ± SD	22.19 ± 0.38	23.84 ± 0.37	0.007*
Symptom (none/local/system)	(90/9/0)	(211/19/0)	0.805
ECOG-PS (0/1/2/3/4/5)	88/11/0/0/0	213/17/0/0/0	0.267
Stage (%)			0.000*
I	46 (46)	192 (83)	
II	18 (18)	13 (6)	
III	29 (29)	21 (9)	
IV	6 (6)	4 (2)	
Pathological type (%)			0.208
ccRCC	88 (89)	214 (93)	
nccRCC	11 (11)	16 (7)	
Type of surgery (%)			0.149
Radical nephrectomy	73 (74)	151 (66)	
Partial nephrectomy	26 (26)	79 (34)	
Fuhrman grade (%)			0.074
1–2	52 (53)	145 (63)	
3–4	47 (47)	85 (37)	
Preoperative, mean ± SD			
Alb, g/L	39.42 ± 0.43	43.43 ± 0.20	0.000*
Glb, g/L	29.20 ± 0.58	26.09 ± 0.25	0.000*
Hgb, g/L	128.09 ± 2.12	138.24 ± 1.06	0.000*
Post-operative, mean ± SD			
Alb, g/L	36.43 ± 0.19	28.77 ± 0.34	0.000*
Glb, g/L	24.27 ± 0.54	24.16 ± 0.24	0.834
Hgb, g/L	106.81 ± 1.78	123.71 ± 1.15	0.000*

*Significant
BMI body mass index, *SD* standard deviation, *ECOP-PS* Eastern Cooperative Oncology Group-performance status, *ccRCC* clear cell renal cell carcinoma, *nccRCC* non-clear cell renal cell carcinoma, *Alb* albumin, *Glb* globulin, *Hgb* hemoglobin

serum albumin level ≥ 32 g/L. Multivariate Cox regression analysis also showed that a early post-operative serum albumin level < 32 g/L was an independent prognostic factor associated with decreased RFS (HR = 6.76; 95% CI, 1.07–42.60; P = 0.042) and OS (HR = 26.92; 95% CI, 1.52–477.30; P = 0.025).

Sub-group analysis based on other factors

The histopathologic type of RCC is an important prognostic factor. Clear cell renal cell carcinoma (ccRCC) is the most common histopathologic type of kidney cancer.

There were 88 (89%) and 214 (93%) patients in the post-operative serum albumin levels < 32 g/L and ≥ 32 g/L, respectively. Survival analysis and log-rank testing showed that ccRCC patients with a post-operative serum albumin level < 32 g/L had a significantly decreased RFS (P = 0.00) and decreased OS (P = 0.00) than patients with a post-operative serum albumin level ≥ 32 g/L.

The type of surgical procedure is another important factor determining prognosis in patients with kidney cancer, especially in patients who undergo partial or radical nephrectomies. Of 329 patients, 224 and 105 underwent radical and partial nephrectomies, respectively. Log-rank testing showed that patients who underwent radical nephrectomies with post-operative serum albumin levels < 32 g/L had a significantly decreased RFS (P = 0.00) and decreased OS (P = 0.00) than patients with a post-operative serum albumin level ≥ 32 g/L. The RFS and OS among patients who underwent partial nephrectomies with a post-operative serum albumin level < 32 g/L were not significantly different compared with patients who had a post-operative serum albumin ≥32 g/L (P = 0.15 and 0.76, respectively).

Discussion

Despite radical resection of kidney cancer, local recurrence or distant metastasis is commonplace [26–28]. With the exception of known prognostic factors, such as tumor stage, pathologic type, and type of surgical procedure, other potential prognostic factors warrant further elucidation [2, 3, 29, 30]. In this retrospective study we report for the first time that an early post-operative serum albumin level is another long-term prognostic factor after radical resection of kidney cancer.

To prevent confounding factors as much as possible, we excluded patients who had incomplete tumor resections, other life-threatening diseases, and adjuvant and/or neoadjuvant treatment. We excluded patients without serum protein and cell testing post-operatively, but it is unlikely that bias was introduced because no guidelines specify laboratory testing early after surgery without an indication. In our medical center, all radical surgeries for kidney cancer were performed by well-trained clinicians. To ensure a sufficient duration of follow-up, we only included patients who underwent surgery prior to May 2014. Approximately 42% of the enrolled patients had a duration of follow-up > 5 years and 94% of the enrolled patients had a duration of follow-up > 3 years. The median duration of follow-up was nearly 5 years, and no patients were lost to follow-up.

The serum albumin level nearly returned to the pre-operative level in all patients who had repeat serum protein testing. A decrease in the serum albumin level may primarily result from exudation into the extravascular space and attenuation by perioperative bleeding and

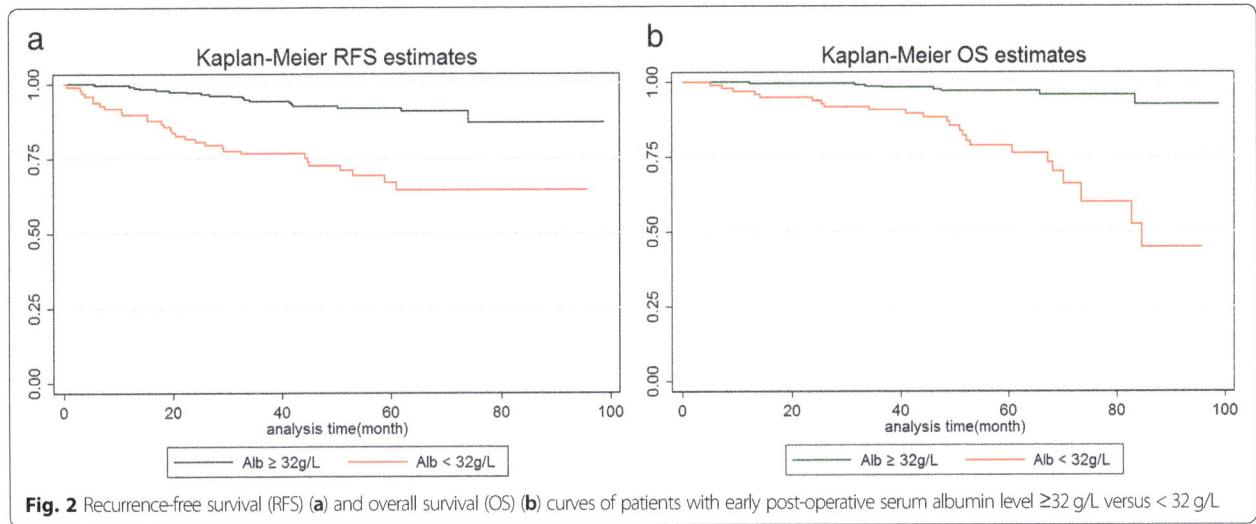

Fig. 2 Recurrence-free survival (RFS) (**a**) and overall survival (OS) (**b**) curves of patients with early post-operative serum albumin level ≥32 g/L versus < 32 g/L

fluid transfusion [11, 31]. We found a significant decrease in the hemoglobin concentration early after surgery coincident with the decrease in serum albumin level; however, the post-operative serum albumin level was significantly decreased compared with the serum albumin level regulated by the hemoglobin concentration (34.1 versus 37.0 g/L, P = 0.00), as follows: regulated serum albumin level ÷ pre-operative albumin level = post-operative hemoglobin concentration ÷ pre-operative hemoglobin concentration. This decrease is regarded as extravascular exudation. When the post-operative serum albumin level and extravascular exudation were entered into Cox regression, the results showed that the post-operative serum albumin level had a close association with RFS (HR = 0.85, P = 0.000) and OS (HR = 0.82, P = 0.000), unlike the

association between extravascular exudation and RFS (HR = 1.00, P = 0.113) and OS (HR = 0.99, P = 0.116).

For patients who underwent pathologic-complete resection of kidney cancer, we entered other universally-accepted prognostic factors before survival analysis, including gender, age, nutritional status (BMI), tumor stage, pathologic type, Fuhrman grade, and type of surgical procedure. Survival analysis showed that patients who had an early post-operative serum albumin level < 32 g/L had a significantly decreased RFS and OS. Although patients in the group of patients with a lower post-operative albumin level were older, had a lower BMI, and more than stage III cancer and some laboratory values differed, multivariate Cox regression analysis admitted all of these factors, and the results showed that an early post-operative serum albumin level < 32 g/L was an independent risk factor for a decreased RFS and OS. Positive results were obtained, even when patients were confined to stages II and III. In contrast, the log rank test did not reveal significant differences in RFS (P = 0.360) and OS (P = 0.814) between stages II and III in our patients. Sub-group analysis showed an association between the post-operative serum albumin level and long-term prognosis based on patients with ccRC who underwent radical nephrectomies versus partial nephrectomies; however, only 26 patients with a post-operative serum albumin level < 32 g/L underwent partial nephrectomies. Indeed, the negative result may reflect the limited sample size.

Limited by the potential retrospective bias, the prognostic value of an early post-operative serum albumin level warrants more high-quality studies for further elucidation. Based on good category power (AUC = 0.71–0.8), an early post-operative serum albumin level deserves more attention in predicting prognosis after radical resection of kidney cancer, especially combined with other prognostic factors. The mechanisms underlying the association remain unclear. In addition, whether or not transfusion of

Table 2 Effect of early post-operative plasma albumin level on recurrence-free survival and overall survival in multivariate Cox regression analyses adjusted by gender, age, body mass index (BMI), tumor stage and some other laboratory indexes

	Recurrence-free survival			Overall survival		
	HR	95% CI	P	HR	95% CI	P
Age	0.99	0.95–1.03	0.573	1.00	0.96–1.04	0.980
BMI	0.99	0.88–1.12	0.892	0.97	0.85–1.11	0.684
Stage	1.51	1.03–2.21	0.034*	1.40	0.90-2.17	0.136
Preoperative						
Alb	0.99	0.86–1.13	0.866	0.99	0.83–1.18	0.906
Glb	1.09	0.99–1.19	0.055	1.08	0.99–1.19	0.094
Hgb	1.01	0.98–1.05	0.420	1.00	0.96–1.05	0.816
Post-operative						
Alb < 32 g/L	3.60	1.05–12.42	0.042*	9.95	1.81-54.80	0.008*
Hgb	1.00	0.97-1.04	0.966	1.02	0.98–1.06	0.418

*Significant

HR hazard ratio, *CI* confidence interval, *Alb* albumin, *Glb* globulin, *Hgb* hemoglobin

albumin leads to decreased tumor recurrence and death after resection of kidney cancer should be investigated.

Conclusion

In patients after curative resection of kidney cancer, this retrospective study revealed that an early post-operative serum albumin level < 32 g/L is an independent risk factor associated with a decreased RFS and decreased OS. Prospective trials and further research in additional patients are needed.

Abbreviations

HR: Hazard Ratio; MSKCC: Memorial Sloan-Kettering Cancer Center; NCCN: National Comprehensive Cancer Network; OS: Overall Survival; RFS: Recurrence-free Survival; ROC: Receiver Operating Characteristic

Acknowledgements

Not applicable

Funding

This study is funded by the Department of Science and Technology of Sichuan Province, China (Grant No. 2017SZ0123 and 2014JY0183) and 1.3.5 project for disciplines of excellence, West China Hospital, Sichuan University.

Authors' contributions

YT and ZL contributed primarily to the conception and design, acquisition of data and analysis, interpretation of data and manuscript drafting; JL and RZ participated in the design, acquisition of data and analysis, interpretation of data and manuscript drafting. KW and ZZ involved in collecting data and drafting the manuscript; CZ and FZ have been involved in data analysis and manuscript drafting; YL mainly contributed to interpretation of data, revision in critical content, supervision and final approval of the version to be published. All authors have read and approved the manuscript, and ensure that this is the case.

Competing interests

The authors declare that they have no competing interests.

Author details

[1]Department of Pediatric Surgery, West China Hospital, Sichuan University, No. 37 of Guoxue Xiang, Chengdu 610041, China. [2]Department of Urology, Institute of Urology, West China Hospital, Sichuan University, Chengdu, China. [3]Department of Urology, Fujian Provincial Hospital, Fuzhou, China. [4]Department of Urology, the Third Affiliated Hospital, Sun Yat-sen University, Guangzhou, China.

References

1. Wein AJ, Kavouss LR, Partin AW, Novick AC, Peters CA: CAMPBELL-WALSH Urology, 10th Edition. Saunders 2012.
2. Dall'Oglio MF, Ribeiro-Filho LA, Antunes AA, Crippa A, Nesrallah L, Goncalves PD, Leite KR, Srougi M. Microvascular tumor invasion, tumor size and Fuhrman grade: a pathological triad for prognostic evaluation of renal cell carcinoma. J Urol. 2007;178(2):425–8 discussion 428.
3. Goncalves PD, Srougi M, Dall'lio MF, Leite KR, Ortiz V, Hering F. Low clinical stage renal cell carcinoma: relevance of microvascular tumor invasion as a prognostic parameter. J Urol. 2004;172(2):470–4.
4. Rabjerg M. Identification and validation of novel prognostic markers in renal cell carcinoma. Dan Med J. 2017;64(10):B5339.
5. Ha YS, Chung JW, Chun SY, Choi SH, Lee JN, Kim BS, Kim HT, Kim TH, Byun SS, Hwang EC, et al. Impact of preoperative thrombocytosis on prognosis after surgical treatment in pathological T1 and T2 renal cell carcinoma: results of a multi-institutional comprehensive study. Oncotarget. 2017;8(38): 64449–58.
6. Errarte P, Beitia M, Perez I, Manterola L, Lawrie CH, Solano-Iturri JD, Calvete-Candenas J, Unda M, Lopez JI, Larrinaga G. Expression and activity of angiotensin-regulating enzymes is associated with prognostic outcome in clear cell renal cell carcinoma patients. PLoS One. 2017;12(8):e0181711.
7. Cai W, Zhong H, Kong W, Dong B, Chen Y, Zhou L, Xue W, Huang Y, Zhang J, Huang J. Significance of preoperative prognostic nutrition index as prognostic predictors in patients with metastatic renal cell carcinoma with tyrosine kinase inhibitors as first-line target therapy. Int Urol Nephrol. 2017; 49(11):1955–63.
8. Tsujita E, Ikeda Y, Kinjo N, Yamashita YI, Hisano T, Furukawa M, Taguchi KI, Morita M, Toh Y, Okamura T. Postoperative neutrophil-to-lymphocyte ratio as a predictor of long-term prognosis after pancreatectomy for pancreatic carcinoma: a retrospective analysis. Am Surg. 2017;83(6):610–6.
9. Jang WS, Cho KS, Kim MS, Yoon CY, Kang DH, Kang YJ, Jeong WS, Ham WS, Choi YD. The prognostic significance of postoperative neutrophil-to-lymphocyte ratio after radical prostatectomy for localized prostate cancer. Oncotarget. 2017;8(7):11778–87.
10. Kang M, Jeong CW, Kwak C, Kim HH, Ku JH. The prognostic significance of the early postoperative neutrophil-to-lymphocyte ratio in patients with urothelial carcinoma of the bladder undergoing radical cystectomy. Ann Surg Oncol. 2016;23(1):335–42.
11. Nazha B, Moussaly E, Zaarour M, Weerasinghe C, Azab B. Hypoalbuminemia in colorectal cancer prognosis: nutritional marker or inflammatory surrogate? World J Gastrointest Surg. 2015;7(12):370–7.
12. Critselis E, Panagiotakos DB, Machairas A, Zampelas A, Critselis AN, Polychronopoulos E. Postoperative hypoproteinemia in cancer patients following extensive abdominal surgery despite parenteral nutritional support. Nutr Cancer. 2011;63(7):1021–8.
13. Manning RD Jr. Effects of hypoproteinemia on renal hemodynamics, arterial pressure, and fluid volume. Am J Phys. 1987;252(1 Pt 2):F91–8.
14. Sang BH, Bang JY, Song JG, Hwang GS. Hypoalbuminemia within two postoperative days is an independent risk factor for acute kidney injury following living donor liver transplantation: a propensity score analysis of 998 consecutive patients. Crit Care Med. 2015;43(12):2552–61.
15. Shao M, Wang S, Parameswaran PK. Hypoalbuminemia: a risk factor for acute kidney injury development and progression to chronic kidney disease in critically ill patients. Int Urol Nephrol. 2017;49(2):295–302.
16. Zhang T, Deng Y, He P, He Z, Wang X. Effects of mild hypoalbuminemia on the pharmacokinetics and pharmacodynamics of dexmedetomidine in patients after major abdominal or thoracic surgery. J Clin Anesth. 2015;27(8): 632–7.
17. Miwa A, Morioka I, Hisamatsu C, Fujioka K, Morikawa S, Shibata A, Yasufuku M, Yokoyama N, Matsuo M. Hypoalbuminemia following abdominal surgery leads to high serum unbound bilirubin concentrations in newborns soon after birth. Neonatology. 2011;99(3):202–7.
18. Sullivan SA, Van Le L, Liberty AL, Soper JT, Barber EL. Association between hypoalbuminemia and surgical site infection in vulvar cancers. Gynecol Oncol. 2016;142(3):435–9.
19. Lee JI, Kwon M, Roh JL, Choi JW, Choi SH, Nam SY, Kim SY. Postoperative hypoalbuminemia as a risk factor for surgical site infection after oral cancer surgery. Oral Dis. 2015;21(2):178–84.
20. Critselis E, Panagiotakos DB, Machairas A, Zampelas A, Critselis AN, Polychronopoulos E. Risk and predictive factors of hypoalbuminemia in cancer patients following extensive abdominal surgery despite total parenteral nutritional support. Int J Food Sci Nutr. 2012;63(2):208–15.
21. Crumley AB, Stuart RC, McKernan M, McMillan DC. Is hypoalbuminemia an independent prognostic factor in patients with gastric cancer? World J Surg. 2010;34(10):2393–8.
22. McMillan DC, Watson WS, O'Gorman P, Preston T, Scott HR, McArdle CS. Albumin concentrations are primarily determined by the body cell mass and the systemic inflammatory response in cancer patients with weight loss. Nutr Cancer. 2001;39(2):210–3.
23. Cai W, Zhang J, Chen Y, Kong W, Huang Y, Huang J, Zhou L. Association of post-treatment hypoalbuminemia and survival in Chinese patients with metastatic renal cell carcinoma. Chin J Cancer. 2017;36(1):47.

24. NCCN: NCCN clinical practice guidelines in oncology, kidney Cancer (version 2. 2017). https://www.nccn.org/professionals/physician_gls/default. aspx#kidney.
25. KANG L, Jia H, Shibao Y, Jun M. Medical statistics, 6th edition: People's medical publishing house. 2013.
26. Shum CF, Bahler CD, Sundaram CP. Matched comparison between partial nephrectomy and radical nephrectomy for T2 N0 M0 tumors, a study based on the National Cancer Database. J Endourol. 2017;31(8):800–5.
27. Kunath F, Schmidt S, Krabbe LM, Miernik A, Dahm P, Cleves A, Walther M, Kroeger N. Partial nephrectomy versus radical nephrectomy for clinical localised renal masses. Cochrane Database Syst Rev. 2017;5:Cd012045.
28. Demir O, Bozkurt O, Celik S, Comez K, Aslan G, Mungan U, Celebi I, Esen A. Partial nephrectomy vs. radical nephrectomy for stage I renal cell carcinoma in the presence of predisposing systemic diseases for chronic kidney disease. Kaohsiung J Med Sci. 2017;33(7):339–43.
29. Tsukamoto T, Kumamoto Y, Miyao N, Yamazaki K, Takahashi A, Satoh M. Regional lymph node metastasis in renal cell carcinoma: incidence, distribution and its relation to other pathological findings. Eur Urol. 1990; 18(2):88–93.
30. Cheigh JS, Kim H, Stenzel KH, Tapia L, Sullivan JF, Stubenbord W, Riggio RR, Rubin AL. Systemic lupus erythematosus in patients with end-stage renal disease: long-term follow-up on the prognosis of patients and the evolution of lupus activity. Am J Kidney Dis. 1990;16(3):189–95.
31. Ryan AM, Hearty A, Prichard RS, Cunningham A, Rowley SP, Reynolds JV. Association of hypoalbuminemia on the first postoperative day and complications following esophagectomy. J Gastrointes Surg. 2007;11(10): 1355–60.

Retroperitoneal laparoscopic partial nephrectomy with segmental renal artery clamping for cancer of the left upper calyx

Yajie Yu[1†], Chao Liang[1†], Meiling Bao[2], Pengfei Shao[1*] 🔟 and Zengjun Wang[1]

Abstract

Background: Currently, the standard treatment for renal pelvis carcinoma is radical nephroureterectomy with bladder cuff excision. To describe the feasibility of retroperitoneal laparoscopic partial nephrectomy with segmental renal artery clamping for cancer of renal pelvis, we report this special case for the first time.

Case presentation: A 67-year-old woman received this operation. Preoperative ureteroscopy revealed a papillary neoplasm with a pedicle in the upper calyx of the left kidney. After entering the retroperitoneal space and dissociating the renal artery and renal vein, the target artery was clamped beyond the final bifurcation before entering the parenchyma. After incision of the left renal parenchyma and exposure of the upper calyceal neck, the tumor was found confined to the upper calyx. Thereafter, the renal calyx and parenchyma were sutured successively after complete resection of the neoplasm. Postoperative pathological examination confirmed that the Grade I papillary carcinoma was confined to the mucosal layer. Thus far, there is no evidence of recurrence during the follow-up period for more than 42 months after surgery.

Conclusions: Retroperitoneal laparoscopic partial nephrectomy with segmental renal artery clamping of the kidney provides a feasible treatment modality for noninvasive tumors that are limited to the calyx.

Keywords: Laparoscopic partial nephrectomy, Retroperitoneal, Renal pelvis cancer, Segmental renal artery clamping, Upper calyx

Background

Upper tract urothelial carcinomas (UTUCs) are defined as tumors arising anywhere along the urothelial lining of the urinary tract from the renal calyces to the ureteral orifice. Currently, the standard treatment for renal pelvis carcinoma is radical nephroureterectomy with bladder cuff excision. In the current case, considering the fact that the patient had bilateral renal insufficiency and the tumor was localized, laparoscopic partial nephrectomy (LPN) with segmental renal artery clamping was eventually performed.

* Correspondence: spf_urology@sina.com
†Equal contributors
[1]Department of Urology, The First Affiliated Hospital of Nanjing Medical University, Nanjing 210029, China
Full list of author information is available at the end of the article

Case presentation

A 67-year-old woman who complained of gross hematuria for 3 days was admitted to our department on November 21, 2012. The patient reported hematuria without fever, and denied having low back pain or edema of lower limbs. She had been diagnosed with diabetes, but was not undergoing regular treatment. Her main laboratory examination and ancillary investigation results were as follows. Routine urine test showed occult blood in the urine, with ++ cells/μL. Biochemical examination showed a blood sugar level of 8.36 mmol/L. The serum creatinine (SCr) level and estimated glomerular filtration rate (eGFR) were 93.5 μmol/L and 60.78 ml/min/1.73 m^2, respectively. Urine cytology test showed the presence of tumor cells twice. Enhanced abdominal computed tomography (CT) revealed a soft tissue density in the upper calyx of the left

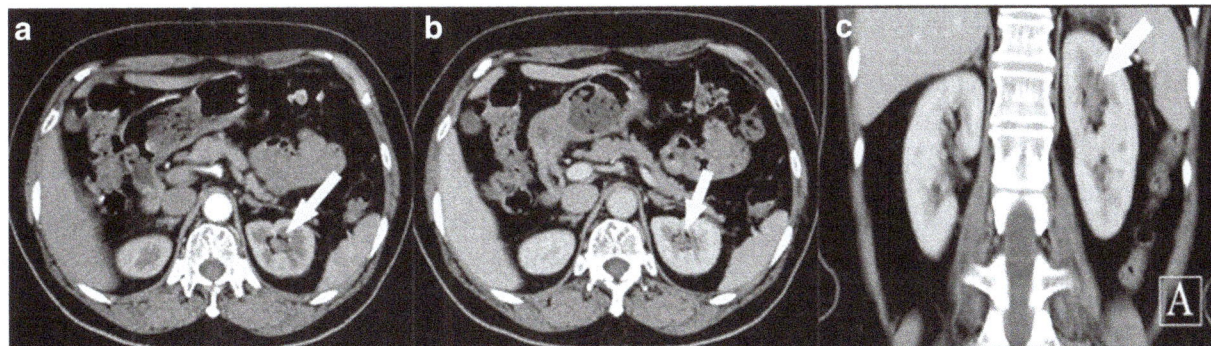

Fig. 1 Enhanced abdominal computed tomography revealing a soft tissue density (*white arrow*) in the upper calyx of the left kidney (**a**) Cross section, arterial phase (**b**) Cross section, venous phase (**c**) Coronal plane

kidney, suggesting pyelo-carcinoma (Fig. 1). Computed tomography angiography (CTA) identified the blood vessels that supply the tumor region (Fig. 2).

After admission, the patient received aggressive perioperative treatment in order to improve her cardiac and renal function, and to control her blood sugar levels, so as to improve her tolerance to surgery. Ureteroscopy detected a papillary neoplasm with a pedicle in the upper calyx of the left kidney. Subsequently, the patient underwent LPN with segmental renal artery clamping. After entering the retroperitoneal space and dissociating the renal artery and renal vein, the target artery was clamped beyond the final bifurcation before entering the parenchyma. Access and clamping strategies for target arteries were preoperatively determined on the basis of the 3D models by the radiologist and surgeon. After incision of the left renal parenchyma and exposure of the upper calyceal neck, the tumor was found confined to the upper calyx. Later, the renal calyx and parenchyma were sutured successively after complete resection of the neoplasm. During

the operation, a double J tube was placed for drainage of urine and for postoperative infusion therapy. The tumor was found to be confined to the upper calyx of the left kidney. Histopathological examination of the surgical specimens confirmed a diagnosis of papillary Grade I carcinoma of the renal pelvis, with massive hemorrhage, with the tumor measuring 18 mm × 10 mm × 7 mm and confined to the mucosal layer (Fig. 3). All surgical margins were negative.

The patient received postoperative intravesical instillation of pharmorubicin fortnightly for 3 months. Subsequently, the double J tube was removed. A cystoscopy was performed every 3 months for the first 3 years. CT was performed to check for the recurrence or metastasis of the tumor every 6 months for the first 3 years, and annually thereafter. There was no evidence of recurrence during the follow-up period for more than 43 months after surgery till the time of writing this report. The most recent SCr level and eGFR of the patient were 82.9 μmol/L and 69.78 mL/min/1.73 m^2, respectively.

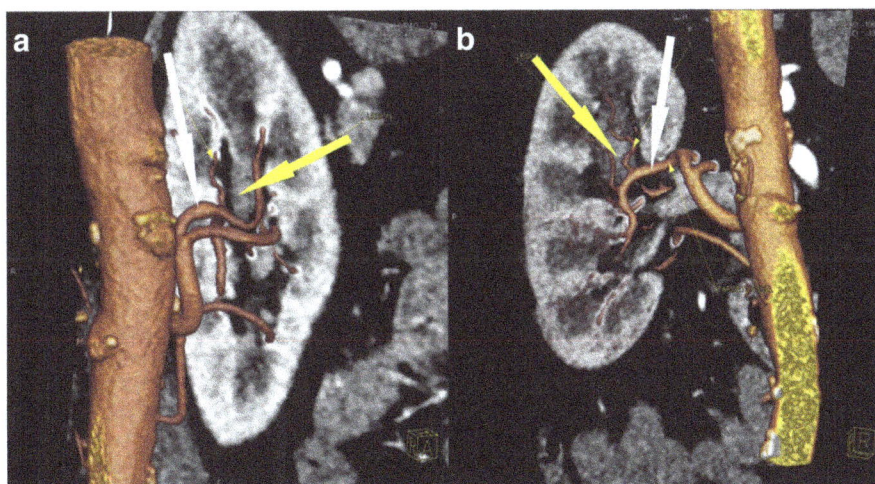

Fig. 2 Computed tomography angiography showing the blood supply vessels (*white arrow*) of tumor region (*yellow arrow*) (**a**) Anterior view (**b**) Right view

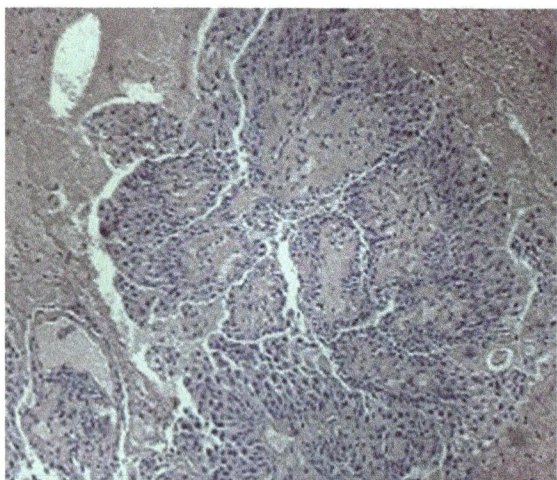

Fig. 3 Histopathologic examination of the surgical specimens revealing grade I papillary carcinoma of the renal pelvis

Discussion

Urothelial carcinomas (UCs) are the fourth most common tumors after prostate (or breast), lung, and colorectal cancer [1]. Bladder tumors are the most common malignancy of the urinary tract and account for 90%–95% of the UCs [2]. In contrast, UTUCs are uncommon and account for only 5%–10% of the UCs [3]. Renal pelvic carcinoma accounts for the vast majority of UTUCs. In more than 95% of the cases, renal pelvic carcinoma is derived from the urothelium [4]. The WHO classification of bladder cancer in 1973 that distinguished it into three grades (G1, G2, and G3) is the most widely used method of tumor classification. The most common symptom of pyelo-carcinoma is gross or microscopic hematuria, observed in 70%–80% of the cases [5], followed by flank pain and a lumbar mass. UTUCs that invade the muscle wall usually have a very poor prognosis. The 5-year specific survival is less than 50% for pT2/pT3 tumors and less than 10% for pT4 tumors [6].

Radical nephroureterectomy with excision of the bladder cuff is the gold standard treatment for renal pelvis carcinoma [7]. However, for the superficial isolated tumor localized to one particular calyx, the advantage of LPN with segmental renal artery clamping is more obvious in patients with renal insufficiency or in those with high risk factors. Compared with radical nephrectomy, our novel segmental clamping techniques block the feeding arteries to the tumor, thus avoiding whole renal ischemia and protecting residual renal function. Compared with endoscopic management, this technique has the advantages of more thorough excision and low tumor recurrence rate.

The indication for this operation is superficial low-grade cancer of the renal pelvis that is localized to one particular calyx.

This technique (retroperitoneal laparoscopic partial nephrectomy with segmental renal artery clamping) was pioneered by our team and has been routinely carried out in our department [8]. After long-term promotion and verification, this technology has been proved to be safe and effective.

The key points of this operation were as follows. Firstly, the target artery was determined preoperatively by building a CTA model [8]. Secondly, the renal artery was blocked selectively to protect renal function. Thirdly, after clamping the target artery, the renal parenchyma was incised to expose the upper calyceal neck. A wedge resection was performed to ensure that the neoplasm had been resected in extenso. Lastly, a double J tube was placed during the operation to reduce the risk of postoperative leakage of urine and to facilitate postoperative perfusion treatment.

There do exist risk of tumor spillage and seeding. In this case, to prevent cancer spillage or seeding, we suggest guaranteeing the resection range be sufficient and avoiding touching and squeezing the tumor. When the tumor is cut off, immediately put it into a specimen bag and then suture the wound. At last, we could flush the surgical area with sterile water.

Until the time of writing this report, there was no evidence of recurrence during the follow-up period for more than 43 months after surgery, and the kidney function of the patient afforded her a normal daily life.

Conclusions

In a word, for patients having superficial low-grade renal pelvic cancer localized to one particular calyx, retroperitoneal LPN with segmental renal artery clamping provides a new feasible strategy to ensure complete resection of the tumor, while simultaneously preserving normal renal function.

Abbreviations

CT: Computed tomography; CTA: Computed tomography angiography; eGFR: estimated glomerular filtration rate; LPN: Laparoscopic partial nephrectomy; SCr: Serum creatinine; UCs: Urothelial carcinomas; UTUCs: Upper tract urothelial carcinomas

Acknowledgments

The authors thank the patient for allowing us to publish this case report.

Funding

This work was supported by a grant from the National Natural Science Foundation of China (No.81201998).

Authors' contributions

ZW participated in the design of this study, MB performed the statistical analysis. PS carried out the study. CL collected important background information. YY drafted the manuscript. PS conceived of this study, and participated in the design and helped to draft the manuscript. All authors have read and approved the final manuscript.

Competing interests
The authors' declare that they have no competing interests.

Author details
[1]Department of Urology, The First Affiliated Hospital of Nanjing Medical University, Nanjing 210029, China. [2]Department of Pathology, The First Affiliated Hospital of Nanjing Medical University, Nanjing 210029, China.

References
1. Munoz JJ, Ellison LM. Upper tract urothelial neoplasms: incidence and survival during the last 2 decades. J Urol. 2000;164:1523–5.
2. Ploeg M, Aben KK, Kiemeney LA. The present and future burden of urinary bladder cancer in the world. World J Urol. 2009;27:289–93.
3. Siegel R, Naishadham D, Jemal A. Cancer statistics, 2012. CA Cancer J Clin. 2012;62:10–29.
4. Olgac S, Mazumdar M, Dalbagni G, et al. Urothelial carcinoma of the renal pelvis: a clinicopathologic study of 130 cases. Am J Surg Pathol. 2004;28:1545–52.
5. Raman JD, Shariat SF, Karakiewicz PI, et al. Does preoperative symptom classification impact prognosis in patients with clinically localized upper-tract urothelial carcinoma managed by radical nephroureterectomy? Urol Oncol. 2011;29:716–23.
6. Jeldres C, Sun M, Isbarn H, et al. A population-based assessment of perioperative mortality after nephroureterectomy for upper-tract urothelial carcinoma. Urology. 2010;75:315–20.
7. Rouprêt M, Babjuk M, Comperat E, et al. European guidelines on upper tract urothelial carcinomas: 2013 update. Eur Urol. 2013;63:1059–71.
8. Shao P, Qin C, Yin C, et al. Laparoscopic partial nephrectomy with segmental renal artery clamping: technique and clinical outcomes. Eur Urol. 2011;59:849–55.

The "Guidewire-Coil"-Technique to prevent retrograde stone migration of ureteric calculi during intracorporeal lithothripsy

Nici Markus Dreger[1*], Friedrich Carl von Rundstedt[2,3], Stephan Roth[1], Alexander Sascha Brandt[1] and Stephan Degener[1]

Abstract

Background: Stone retropulsion represents a challenge for intracorporeal lithotripsy of ureteral calculi. The consequences are an increased duration and cost of surgery as well as decreased stone-free rates. The use of additional tools to prevent proximal stone migration entails further costs and risks for ureteral injuries. We present the simple technique of using a coil of the routinely used guidewire to prevent stone retropulsion.

Methods: We retrospectively evaluated all patients with mid-to-proximal ureteral stones in 2014, which were treated by ureteroscopic lithotripsy (Ho: YAG and/or pneumatic lithotripsy). The preoperative stone burden was routinely assessed using low dose CT scan (if available) and/or intravenous pyelogram.

Results: The study population consisted of 55 patients with 61 mid-to-proximal calculi. Twentyseven patients underwent semirigid ureterorenoscopy using the "Guidewire-Coil-Technique", the second group ($n = 28$) served as control group using the guidewire as usual. There has been a statistically significant reduction of accidental stone retropulsion (2/27 vs. 8/28, $p < 0.05$) as well as a decreased use of auxiliary procedures ($p < 0.05$) compared to the control group. No difference was observed in operative time. One ureteral injury in the control group required a prolonged ureteral stenting.

Conclusion: The "Guidewire-Coil-Technique" is a simple and safe procedure that may help to prevent proximal calculus migration and therefore may increase stone-free rates without causing additional costs.

Keywords: Stone migration, Stone retropulsion, Intracorporeal lithotripsy, Ureterorenoscopy, Ureteric calculi

Background

During the past two decades, there have been many improvements regarding the endoscopic treatment of urolithiasis. Ureterorenoscopy (URS) with and without lithotripsy is a standard method to treat ureteral calculi depending on different factors including location, stone size, individual patient factors as well as equipping [1, 2]. A particular challenge limiting the success of ureteroscopic lithotripsy is stone retropulsion due to insertion of the ureteroscope, pressure by the irrigation fluid and/or the lithotripsy itself [2]. Stone migration occurs in 28–60% of proximal calculi [3–6]. Hereby an increase in operative time, a decrease in stone-free rates and the need for further auxiliary procedures (i.e. shockwave lithotripsy (SWL), flexible ureterorenoscopy (fURS)) with affiliated morbidities and health-care costs have been reported [2, 7, 8]. Novel stone retrieval devices have been introduced to address the problem of accidental stone migration: Stone baskets [9, 10], suction devices [11], balloon catheters [12, 13] guidewire [14–16] and gel-based devices [17, 18] significantly reduced the incidence of stone retropulsion. On the contrary, these devices are associated with additional costs and some of them with a higher risk for ureteral injuries [2].

Because of this predicament, we assessed a new technique only using the usually recommended guidewire to

---
* Correspondence: nici-markus.dreger@helios-kliniken.de
[1]Department of Urology, Helios Medical Center Wuppertal, Helios University Hospital Wuppertal, University of Witten/Herdecke, Heusnerstraße 40, Wuppertal 42283, Germany
Full list of author information is available at the end of the article

prevent proximal stone migration. We here describe our experience and the efficacy of this method.

Methods

From January 2014 to December 2014, 55 patients with upper ureteral calculi ($n = 61$) were treated in our institution by primary intracorporeal lithotripsy according to the current guidelines [19]. Preoperative stone location and size were confirmed by abdomen and pelvis computed tomography (CT) scan or in rare cases by intravenous pyelography (IVP), if CT scan was not available. All patients underwent semirigid ureterorenoscopy and intracorporeal lithotripsy has been performed using holmium-YAG laser (Ho:YAG) and/or pneumatic lithotriptor. The "Guidewire-Coil-Technique" in this study was performed by a single faculty urologist (S.R.) with more than 2000 ureterorenoscopies. IRB approval was obtained (no. 43/2016, Witten/Herdecke University).

All 55 patients were analyzed retrospectively: Of these patients 27 were treated using the "Guidewire-Coil-Technique" and 28 patients served as control group using the guidewire in regular fashion. Plain film radiographs of the kidneys, ureters, and bladder (KUB) and sonography were obtained to verify stone-free rate and migration rate.

Patients were stratified by the kind of use of the guidewire. The primary endpoint was the stone-free rate. The incidence of stone retropulsion, need for further auxiliary procedures, operative time and complication rate were defined as secondary endpoints. Statistical assessment was performed using Fisher's exact test for categorical variables and Mann–Whitney U test for continuous variables respectively. P values < 0.05 were considered significant. Statistical analysis was performed using SPSS 21® for Mac® (SPSS Inc., Chicago, IL, USA).

The "Guidewire-Coil-Technique"

In all patients a hydrophilic guidewire with nitinol core and angled tip (outer diameter 0.89 mm (0.035"), length 150 cm, flexible length 30 mm) was used. In our case series, we used a 9.8 F (8 F tip, 9.8 F base) semirigid ureteroscope (Karl Storz, Germany) with a 5 F working channel. After careful retrograde pyelography (RPG, Figs. 1a-b, 2a-b), the guidewire is advanced beyond the stone. After reaching the renal pelvis, the angled tip was placed in the upper calix and then pushed until a loop of the guidewire was achieved. The loop in the upper calix facilitates a direct turn back into the ureter (and prevents a coiling in renal pelvis without turn back in the ureter). By rotating the guidewire manually or with a Halstead clamp (can be helpful with clammy gloves), the angled tip can be used to navigate the guidewire in the desired direction. Additionally, we don't recommend a guidewire with a straight distal curve because it's stiffness makes a precise loop in the upper calix much more difficult. The reverted guidewire was placed consecutively directly proximal to the stone (Fig. 1c). At this position, the reverted guidewire acts as a counterfort, which will help to prevent retrograde stone migration during intracorporeal lithotripsy (Figs. 2c and 3).

Results

The two groups were comparable with regard to gender, age, size or location (Table 1). Upward stone or fragment retropulsion to the kidney occurred in two patients (7.4%) in the treatment and eight patients (28.6%) in the control group, a statistically significant difference ($p < 0.05$, Table 2). In the treatment group a guidewire coiling could be achieved in every patient after 1–8 attempts (median 3 attempts). There was no relevant difference concerning the mean operative

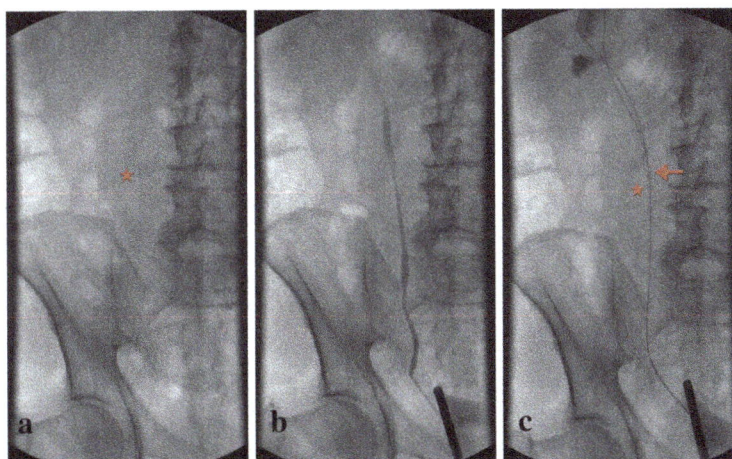

Fig. 1 Step-by-step description of the "Guidewire-Coil-Technique" based on the example of a mid ureteric stone. **a**: Plain x-ray; **b**: Retrograde pyelography; **c**: Correctly placed coil of the guidewire. *Asterisk = Ureteral calculus, arrow = Reverted guidewire acting as a counterfort*

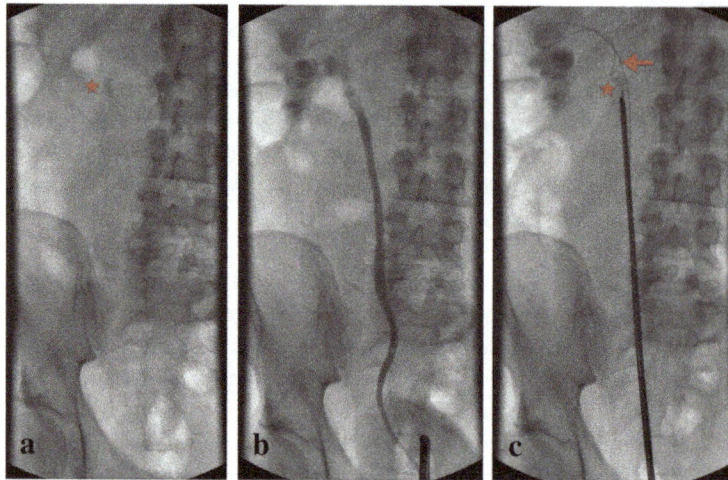

Fig. 2 Step-by-step description of the "Guidewire-Coil-Technique" based on the example of a proximal stone. **a**: Plain x-ray; **b**: Retrograde pyelography; **c**: Correctly placed coil of the guidewire. *Asterisk = Ureteral calculus, arrow = Reverted guidewire acting as a counterfort*

time (67.6 versus 70.3 minutes, $p = 0.901$) and the type of lithotripsy used for fragmentation of the stones (Ho:YAG versus pneumatic lithotripsy, $p = 0.500$). Auxiliary procedures such as flexible ureterorenoscopy were necessary in three patients (11%) in the treatment group compared to ten patients (35.7%) in the control group ($p < 0.05$). Postoperatively, patients were followed up with KUB and sonography as described before. The stone-free rates were 92.6% in the treatment and 75% in the control group, respectively. The difference between the two groups was statistically borderline significant ($p = 0.079$). Only one notable ($\geq$ III, classified according to the Clavien system) complication was observed: one patient (3.6%) in the control group had a ureteral wall injury, which resulted in a prolonged ureteral stenting.

Discussion

Stones larger than 5 mm in diameter require intracorporeal fragmentation before extraction through the ureteroscope [20]. A wide variety of endoscopic lithotriptors have become available for stone fragmentation including laser, electrohydraulic and the pneumatic lithotriptor. The ballistic nature of the energy occasionally displaces calculi towards the kidney. Stone migration into the collecting system makes stone retrieval substantially more challenging especially into a lower pole or anterior calyx, which necessitates additional procedures such as adjuvant extracorporeal SWL [8, 21].

Novel stone retrieval devices have been recommended for the prevention of retrograde stone displacement including ureteral stone baskets, balloon catheters, stone cone, etc. (Table 3). However, all of these add to the costs and some increase the risk for ureteral injuries [2].

The stone-free rate in the current work was different between the 2 groups (92.6% for the treatment group and 75% for the control group). The control group consequently had a higher rate of ancillary procedures as reflected by the significantly different efficiency quotient. This was partly due to stone retropulsion requiring an auxiliary procedure. In comparison to the before mentioned (expensive) stone retrieval devices and their associated stone-free rates (Table 3), our technique was not inferior.

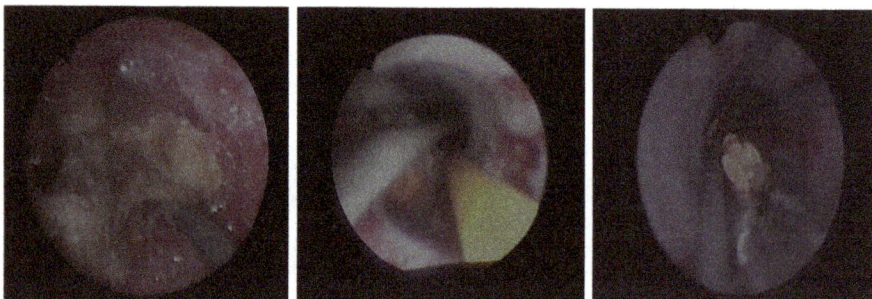

Fig. 3 Examples of the endoscopic point of view while using the "Guidewire-Coil-Technique"

Table 1 Preoperative characteristics of both groups

	Guidewire-Coil n = 27		Control n = 28		P value
		±SD		±SD	
Gender					0.527[†]
Male	22		22		
Female	5		6		
Age [a]					
Mean	58.0	16.0	55.0	15.5	0.622*
Median	54.0		56.5		
Number of stones	28		33		
Size [mm]					
Mean	9.8	3.4	10.0	3.5	0.953*
Median	8.6		9.2		
Calculus location					
Proximal ureter	13		15		0.571[†]
Mid ureter	15		18		

SD = standard deviation
*Significant at p value < 0.05 by Mann–Whitney test
[†]Significant at p value < 0.05 by Fisher's-exact test

Table 2 Postoperative comparison of both groups

	Guidewire-Coil n = 27		Control n = 28		P value
		±SD		±SD	
Operative time [min]					
Mean	67.6	29.8	70.3	34.0	0.901*
Median	61.0		58.5		
Stone migration					0.044[†]
Yes	2 [7.4%]		8 [28.6%]		
No	25		20		
Auxiliary procedures					0.032[†]
Yes	3 [11%]		10 [35.7%]		
Flexible URS	2		5		
SWL	0		4		
Secondary URS	0		1		
No	24		18		
Stone-free rate					0.079[†]
Yes	25 [92.6%]		21 [75%]		
No	2		7		
Lithotripsy					0.500[†]
Ho:YAG	20		19		
Pneumatic	8		9		

Operative time was determined using the anesthesia protocols
SD = standard deviation; URS = ureterorenoscopy; Ho:YAG = Holmium-YAG laser lithotripter
*Significant at p value < 0.05 by Mann–Whitney test
[†]Significant at p value < 0.05 by Fisher's-exact test

Table 3 Overview of different devices and techniques to prevent accidental stone migration

Author	Year	Device/Technique	n	Stone migration [%]	SFR [%]
Kesler et al. [10]	2008	Stone basket (Escape®)	23	n.a.	87
Eisner et al. [22]	2009	Guidewire (Stone Cone®)	133	1.5	98.5
Sen et al. [23]	2014	Guidewire (Stone Cone®)	25	4.5	95.5
Sen et al. [23]	2014	Guidewire (PercSys®)	25	8.7	91.3
Wang et al. [24]	2011	Guidewire (NTrap®)	56	0.0	100
Sen et al. [23]	2014	Gel-based (Lidocaine jelly)	25	21.7	82.6
Mohseni et al. [18]	2006	Gel-based (Lidocaine jelly)	16	12.4	93.7
Rane et al. [25]	2010	Thermosensitive polymer (BackStop®)	34	8.8	87.8
Dretler et al. [13]	2000	Balloon catheter (Passport®)	29	10.3	89.7

In two patients in the group managed with the guidewire-coil-technique we were not able to prevent stone migration towards the kidney. While we did not observe any proximal stone migration during the placement of the wire there may be an association with the diameter of the dilated ureter (similar to balloon catheters) [2, 13]. Although possible in every patient in the treatment group, it took 1–8 (median 3) attempts to coil the guidewire in the renal pelvis and get a loop back into the ureter. To our experience the most important step is a direct loop in the upper calix to achieve a quick and direct turn back into the ureter. We do acknowledge that there there is a learning curve to the procedure but the steps are easily learned by the residents in our programme. Furthermore there might be anatomical conditions that make this step of the procedure challenging (e.g. a duplex collecting system).

Contrary to our expectations, we did not observe significant differences in operative time between the two groups (67.6 versus 70.3 min, P = 0.901). While multiple attempts of directing the guidewire back in the ureter can be time consuming it has been our experience that the actual procedure can be performed more efficiently and possibly faster because of a higher flow of irrigation fluid. This can result in improved vision without an increased risk of stone retropulsion.

This was not a prospective study. Patients were not randomized. By that, the retrospective character and the small number of patients are limitations of this study. Nevertheless, we were able to show the feasibility of this technique and its potential utility in the prevention of stone migration during ureteroscopy and lithotripsy.

Conclusion

Coiling the routinely used guidewire just proximal to the stone in the ureter prior to lithotripsy during ureteroscopy may be a simple and inexpensive option to significantly reduce inadvertent stone migration and achieve higher stone-free rates.

Abbreviations

CT: Computerized tomography; fURS: Flexible ureterorenoscopy; Ho:YAG: Holmium:YAG laser; IRB: Institutional review board; IVP: Intravenous pyelography; KUB: Plain film radiographs of the kidneys, ureters, and bladder; SWL: Shock wave lithotripsy; URS: Ureterorenoscopy

Acknowledgements

None.

Authors' contribution

NMD and SD have made substantial contributions to conception and design, acquisition of data as well as analysis and interpretation of data; have been involved in drafting the manuscript and have given final approval of the version to be published. FCvonR, SR and ASB made substantial contributions to conception and design as well as interpretation of data; have been involved in revising the manuscript critically for important intellectual content; have given final approval of the version to be published. Each author has participated sufficiently in the work to take public responsibility for appropriate portions of the content and agreed to be accountable for all aspects of the work in ensuring that questions related to the accuracy or integrity of any part of the work are appropriately investigated and resolved.

Competing interests

The authors declare that they have no competing interests.

Author details

[1]Department of Urology, Helios Medical Center Wuppertal, Helios University Hospital Wuppertal, University of Witten/Herdecke, Heusnerstraße 40, Wuppertal 42283, Germany. [2]Scott Department of Urology, Baylor College of Medicine Medical Center, 7200 Cambridge, Houston, TX, USA. [3]Department of Urology, Jena Medical Center, Friedrich-Schiller University, Bachstraße 18, Jena 07743, Germany.

References

1. Ahmed M, Pedro RN, Kieley S, Akornor JW, Durfee WK, Monga M. Systematic evaluation of ureteral occlusion devices: insertion, deployment, stone migration, and extraction. Urology. 2009;73(5):976–80.
2. Elashry OM, Tawfik AM. Preventing stone retropulsion during intracorporeal lithotripsy. Nat Rev Urol. 2012;9(12):691–8.
3. Chow GK, Patterson DE, Blute ML, Segura JW. Ureteroscopy: effect of technology and technique on clinical practice. J Urol. 2003;170(1):99–102.
4. Knispel HH, Klan R, Heicappell R, Miller K. Pneumatic lithotripsy applied through deflected working channel of miniureteroscope: results in 143 patients. J endourol Soc. 1998;12(6):513–5.
5. Osorio L, Lima E, Soares J, Autorino R, Versos R, Lhamas A, Marcelo F. Emergency ureteroscopic management of ureteral stones: why not? Urology. 2007;69(1):27–31. discussion 31–23.
6. Tunc L, Kupeli B, Senocak C, Alkibay T, Sozen S, Karaoglan U, Bozkirli I. Pneumatic lithotripsy for large ureteral stones: is it the first line treatment? Int Urol Nephrol. 2007;39(3):759–64.

7. Dretler SP. The stone cone: a new generation of basketry. J Urol. 2001; 165(5):1593–6.
8. Lee H, Ryan RT, Teichman JM, Kim J, Choi B, Arakeri NV, Welch AJ. Stone retropulsion during holmium:YAG lithotripsy. J Urol. 2003;169(3):881–5.
9. El-Gabry EA, Bagley DH. Retrieval capabilities of different stone basket designs in vitro. J Endourol Soc. 1999;13(4):305–7.
10. Kesler SS, Pierre SA, Brison DI, Preminger GM, Munver R. Use of the Escape nitinol stone retrieval basket facilitates fragmentation and extraction of ureteral and renal calculi: a pilot study. J Endourol Soc. 2008;22(6):1213–7.
11. Delvecchio FC, Kuo RL, Preminger GM. Clinical efficacy of combined lithoclast and lithovac stone removal during ureteroscopy. J Urol. 2000; 164(1):40–2.
12. Dellabella M, Milanese G, d'Anzeo G, Muzzonigro G. Rapid, economical treatment of large impacted calculi in the proximal ureter with ballistic ureteral lithotripsy and occlusive, percutaneous balloon catheter: the high pressure irrigation technique. J Urol. 2007;178(3 Pt 1):929–33. discussion 933–924.
13. Dretler SP. Ureteroscopy for proximal ureteral calculi: prevention of stone migration. J Endourol Soc. 2000;14(7):565–7.
14. Ding H, Wang Z, Du W, Zhang H. NTrap in prevention of stone migration during ureteroscopic lithotripsy for proximal ureteral stones: a meta-analysis. J Endourol Soc. 2012;26(2):130–4.
15. Maislos SD, Volpe M, Albert PS, Raboy A. Efficacy of the Stone Cone for treatment of proximal ureteral stones. J Endourol Soc. 2004;18(9):862–4.
16. Pagnani CJ, El Akkad M, Bagley DH. Prevention of stone migration with the accordion during endoscopic ureteral lithotripsy. J Endourol Soc. 2012;26(5):484–8.
17. Ali AA, Ali ZA, Halstead JC, Yousaf MW, Ewah P. A novel method to prevent retrograde displacement of ureteric calculi during intracorporeal lithotripsy. BJU Int. 2004;94(3):441–2.
18. Mohseni MG, Arasteh S, Alizadeh F. Preventing retrograde stone displacement during pneumatic lithotripsy for ureteral calculi using lidocaine jelly. Urology. 2006;68(3):505–7.
19. Preminger GM, Tiselius HG, Assimos DG, Alken P, Buck C, Gallucci M, Knoll T, Lingeman JE, Nakada SY, Pearle MS, et al. 2007 guideline for the management of ureteral calculi. J Urol. 2007;178(6):2418–34.
20. Leveillee RJ, Lobik L. Intracorporeal lithotripsy: which modality is best? Curr Opin Urol. 2003;13(3):249–53.
21. Aghamir SK, Mohseni MG, Ardestani A. Treatment of ureteral calculi with ballistic lithotripsy. J Endourol Soc. 2003;17(10):887–90.
22. Eisner BH, Dretler SP. Use of the stone cone for prevention of calculus retropulsion during holmium:YAG laser lithotripsy: case series and review of the literature. Urol Int. 2009;82(3):356–60.
23. Sen H, Bayrak O, Erturhan S, Urgun G, Kul S, Erbagci A, Seckiner I. Comparing of different methods for prevention stone migration during ureteroscopic lithotripsy. Urol Int. 2014;92(3):334–8.
24. Wang CJ, Huang SW, Chang CH. Randomized trial of NTrap for proximal ureteral stones. Urology. 2011;77(3):553–7.
25. Rane A, Bradoo A, Rao P, Shivde S, Elhilali M, Anidjar M, Pace K, JR DAH. The use of a novel reverse thermosensitive polymer to prevent ureteral stone retropulsion during intracorporeal lithotripsy: a randomized, controlled trial. J Urol. 2010;183(4):1417–21.

Supra-costal tubeless percutaneous nephrolithotomy is not associated with increased complication rate: a prospective study of safety and efficacy of supra-costal versus sub-costal access

Meng-Yi Yan[1], Jesun Lin[1], Heng-Chieh Chiang[1,3], Yao-Li Chen[2,3] and Pao-Hwa Chen[1*]

Abstract

Background: To assess the morbidities of tubeless percutaneous nephrolithotomy (PCNL) using supra-costal access and re-evaluate traditional concept of increased complications with supra-costal access.

Methods: From January 2010 to December 2014, a single surgeon performed 118 consecutive one-stage fluoroscopic guided PCNL's for complex renal and upper ureteral stone. Our definition for complex renal stone is defined as partial or complete staghorn stone, multiple renal stones in more than 2 calyxes, obstructive uretero-pelvic stone > 2 cm, and a renal stone in single functional kidney. Inclusion criteria include: staghorn stones, renal calculi > 2 cm in diameter, upper ureteral stone > 1.5 cm in diameter. Exclusion criteria for tubeless PCNL include: significant bleeding or perforation of the collecting system, large residue stone, multiple PCNL tract and obstructive renal anatomy. Morbidity, operation time, analgesia requirement, length of hospital stay, stone- free rate, were analyzed.

Results: Of the 118 consecutive PCNL, eighty-six patients underwent tubeless PCNL (56 supra-costal and 30 sub-costal) and included in our prospective follow-up period. The mean age, operation side, stone locations were similar. The male to female ratio is higher in supra-costal than sub-costal. Large renal stones and staghorn stones makes up for most patients (supra-costal: 75%, sub-costal: 80%). The stone–free rate of supra-costal group was 59% (33/56) and in sub-costal group was 50% (15/30). The operative times, length of stay, post-op analgesic use, hematocrit change was similar in both groups. The overall complication rate is 6% [supra-costal (1/56), sub-costal (4/30)] with the majority being infectious complications.

Conclusions: Supra-costal access above 12th rib during tubeless PCNL is safe and effective procedure and is not associated with higher incidence of post-op complications in experience hands.

Keywords: Tubeless PCNL, Surgical complications, Supra-costal, Nephrolithotomy

* Correspondence: 149690@gmail.com
[1]From the Division of Urology, Department of Surgery, Changhua Christian
Hospital, 135, Nanxiao St., Changhua City, Changhua County 500, Taiwan
Full list of author information is available at the end of the article

Background

Since Fernstrom and Johansson performed the first percutaneous nephrolithotomy (PCNL) was performed in 1976, endourological approach has taken an increase role in management of complex urinary calculi [1, 2]. In the recent periods, minimally invasive surgical procedures using advanced instruments and techniques have gradually replaced open surgery for treating large, complex renal and upper ureteral stones. According to the American Urological Association (AUA) guidelines and European Association of Urology (EAU) guideline on urolithiasis, percutaneous nephrolithotripsy (PCNL) is the first-line treatment for renal staghorn stones and renal stones larger than 2 cm. During standard PCNL, the placement of a nephrostomy tube after the operation is a common practice which provides hemostasis, adequate drainage and retaining access for future endoscopic procedures. In selected cases with minimal bleeding and those not needing subsequent percutaneous access, tubeless PCNL has been found to be a safe and effective practice. In previous studies, tubeless PCNL has been showed to reduce hospital stay and post-operative pain compared to conventional nephrostomy tube placement [3–10].

According to results of Hopper & Yakes' study, intercostal percutaneous approach between the 11th and 12th rib into the collecting system would result in lung injury in 14% on the left and 29% in right side. [11] If the puncture is in the 10th–11th rib intercostal space, lung injury is expected in 86% on the left and 93% right side. The key factor in a successful PCNL surgery is selecting the appropriate calyx to gain access to the collecting system. In certain situation such as large or complicated renal stone, an upper pole access will ensure better stone free rate. In most cases, supra-costal approach (intercostal space between 11th and 12th rib) will provide the easiest and the most direct access of the upper calyx in the collecting system. Therefore for large complicated stones, an supra-costal approach is necessary to obtain the best stone free rate [12]. On the other hand, the increased risk of injury to the surrounding organs (pleura, lung, spleen or liver) reported in previous literatures of supra-costal approach is strongly discouraged [13, 14].

In recent studies, tubeless PCNL offers the potential advantages of decreased post-operative pain leading to decrease analgesic use and hospital stay without increasing the complications [4, 5, 8–10, 15, 16]. Since there is a very limited literatures discussing tubeless PCNL using supra-costal approach, the questions of increased complication and morbidities associated with supra-costal approach when compared to sub-costal (below 12th rib) approach is still debatable [4, 15]. Therefore, we set out to prospectively analyze the morbidity associated with supra-costal and sub-costal approach using tubeless percutaneous nephrolithotomy.

Methods

After obtaining Institutional review board (IRB number: 140315), the data from patients underwent PCNL at Changhua Christian Hospital were collected analyzed. Percutaneous nephrolithotomy was first introduced at Changhua Christian Hospital in 1987. Since 2009, the Urology department averaged around 150 PCNL per year has 8 board certified urologist and performed the procedure. From January 2010 to December 2014, a single urologist (MYY) performed one-stage fluoroscopic-guide percutaneous nephrolithotomy for complex renal and upper ureteral stone on 118 consecutive patients. We define complex renal stone as partial or complete staghorn stone, multiple renal stones in more than 2 calyxes, obstructive uretero-pelvic stone > 2 cm, and a renal stone in single functional kidney. Surgical indications were renal staghorn stones, large renal calculi (larger diameter > 2 cm), large upper ureteral stone (transverse diameter > 1.5 cm) or mixed. The decision on either supra-costal or sub-costal approach will be decided after intra-operative injection of contrast through retrograde ureter catheter. We usually choose puncture site that would result in maximum stone clearance and ease of double-J insertion in mind. If the desired entry point into the collecting system is feasible in subcostal, then subcostal approach is chosen and vice versa. All the patient received double-J ureteral stent. The decision to use nephrostomy was made at the end of the procedure. Exclusion criteria for tubeless procedure included: significant postoperative bleeding, significant perforation of the collecting system, much residue stone burden, multiple percutaneous tracts and obstructive renal anatomy. Patients were informed about the decision making prior to agreeing on undertaking the procedure. Of the 118 patients, eighty-six patients underwent tubeless percutaneous nephrolithotomy during the study period. Of the 86 tubeless cases, fifty-six patients underwent supra-costal approach and 30 patients underwent standard sub-costal approach. If the patients experience intrathoracic complication during the procedure, a pigtail drain would be inserted at the end of the procedure and would not defer from tubeless procedure. Fortunately, none of the patients experienced intrathoracic complications during the study period. Stone-free is defined as no visible stone at end of procedure taken with intraoperative fluoroscopy or stone ≤2 mm at follow-up KUB imaging. If large residual stone ≥20 mm which require staged operation, a nephrostomy tube would also be placed. If there is residual symptomatic (ie. hydronephrosis, renal colic pain, hematuria, etc) stone ≥5 mm, adjuvant treatment with ureteroscopic lithotripsy or extracorporeal shockwave were used.

Pre-operative survey, operative method, and post-operative care

Preoperative evaluation of patients includes urine analysis, urine culture, serum creatinine, a kidneys ureter and bladder (KUB) X-ray, renal ultrasonography and intravenous pyelogram. Prophylactic antibiotics (1000 mg of cefazolin) was administered 30 min prior to the start of the operation, unless the patient is allergic to cephalosporine then alternative antibiotics would be used. All the procedure is performed under general anesthesia. With the patient in the lithotomy position, a 5.0 Fr. ureteral catheter was placed in the ipsilateral renal pelvis and secured on to the Foley's catheter. The patient was then changed to the prone position, with all the pressure points protected with padding. Contrast medium was used to opacify the calyceal system via the ureteral catheter or a Chiba needle under ultrasonic guidance puncture. The "eye-of-the-needle" technique, as described by Dr. Arthur Smith, was used in establishing percutaneous access [17]. Most of the time, upper or middle post calyx is chosen for puncture under fluoroscopic guidance. After selecting the suitable calyx for puncture, a small 0.5 cm incision was made at the skin to help facilitate the insertion of the puncture needle. Once the puncture needle enters the collecting system and confirmed with fluoroscopy, a 0.038 in. guide wire is then passed into the collecting system and whenever possible into the renal pelvis or into the ureter. The skin incision is then extended to 1 cm and the nephrostomy tract is then dilated using Amplatz fascia dilator (Microvasive, Natick, MA, USA) until 26 Fr. diameter. A 26 Fr. access sheath is then placed in the collecting system and a 24 Fr. nephroscope (Richard Wolf GmbH, Knittlingen, Germany) coupled with ultrasonic lithotripter was used for stone fragmentation. The stone fragments were then removed using a 3-clawed forceps or suction. After all the visible stone is removed, a 6 Fr. double-J stent is placed in antegrade fashion for all the patients. In order to check for feasibility of tubeless cases, a guidewire in the collecting system then the access sheath is slowly removed while the nephroscope inspect the nephrostomy tract for any pulsating bleeders. After completely removing the access sheath, we further observe for pulsating or excessive bleeding from the nephrostomy tract. If there is pulsating or excessive bleeding, the access sheath is inserted into the collecting system with help of guidewire and a nephrostomy tube is inserted, otherwise the wound is closed with 2–0 nylon suture with a pressure dressing. Patients will start oral intake as soon as possible with the use of diclofenac 25 mg 3 times daily as oral analgesia if eGFR > 60. For patients with eGFR < 60, we will prescribe acetaminophen 500 mg 4 times daily. If the pain persists, intravenous pethidine 50 mg every 6 h pro re nata will be used for further pain control and the amount of intravenous analgesia would be recorded and analyzed. Cefazolin would be used up to 3 days as post-operative antibiotics. The Foley's catheter is removed on post-operative day 1 and patients were on the average discharged on post-operative day 4 depending on their conditions. All patients were assessed with renal ultrasonography, KUB and CXR before discharge to confirm stone-free status and exclude the presence of urinoma or perirenal hematoma and hemothorax or pneumothorax before discharge. Double-J stents were removed 2 weeks after the operation. KUB and renal sonography will be arranged 1 month after the operation during clinic hours.

Statistical analysis

Morbidity, operation time, analgesics requirement, length of hospital stay, stone- free rate, were analyzed. Statistical analysis was done using 1-way ANOVA, Pool t test and Chi-Square test, with $p < 0.05$ considered statistically significant. Calculations were performed using commercial software (JMP 6).

Results

Thirty-two cases did not receive tubeless treatment and were excluded from our study. Eighteen cases had large residual stone burden, 10 had excessive nephrostomy tract bleeding, 1 underwent multiple percutaneous tracts, 2 underwent bilateral PCNL on the same day and 1 experienced pelvis perforation. A total of 86 tubeless cases (56 in supra-costal group and 30 in sub-costal group) were included in this study. The mean age, operation side, stone locations were similar in both groups. The male to female ratio is higher in supra-costal group (39/17) than in sub-costal group (13/17) ($p = 0.0174$). Large renal stones and staghorn stones occupied most of the stone cases (supra-costal group 75%, sub-costal group 80%) (Table 1). The mean operation time is 100 min in supra-costal group and 110 min in sub-costal group (Table 2). Stone location is related to the operative time with upper ureter stone being the shortest and staghorn stone being the longest (Table 3). Upper and middle calyx were the main entry sites in both groups. The initial stone-free rate is higher in the supra-costal group 59% (33/56) when compared to sub-costal group was 50% (15/30) ($p = 0.4274$) with the overall stone-free rate was 56%. All non-stone free patients will undertake post-operative ancillary procedures (extracorporeal shockwave lithotripsy or ureteroscopic lithotripsy) 3 months later, the total stone-free rate increased to 90% (Table 2). Upper ureteral stone group had the highest initial stone-free rate (10 out of 11 patients) and the staghorn stone group being the lowest (3 out of 25 patients, 1 in supra-costal and 2 in sub-costal) ($p < 0.0001$) (Table 4). Mean length of stay is similar in both group (4 days). There was no statistically significant difference in use of post-operative intravenous analgesia requirements (supra-costal 25.76 mg, sub-costal 33.92 mg) and hematocrit change (supra-costal 3.5%, sub-costal 3.3%) (Table 2). The overall complication rate is 6% including 1 patient supra-costal group (2%) and 4 patients in

Table 1 Patients Demographics profile

	Supra-costal(n = 56) No. (%)	Subcostal(n = 30) No. (%)	Total(n = 86) No. (%)	P value
Sex				
F	17 (30)	17 (57)	34 (40)	0.0174
M	39 (70)	13 (43)	52 (60)	
Age(years)[a]	52.33 ± 11.75	55.43 ± 12.59		
Side				
Left	26 (46)	12 (40)	38 (44)	0.5672
Right	30 (54)	18 (60)	48 (56)	
Stone location				
Renal+upper ureter	8 (14)	1 (3)	9 (10)	0.4159
Renal	26 (46)	15 (50)	41 (48)	
Staghorn	16 (29)	9 (30)	25 (29)	
Upper ureter	6 (11)	5 (17)	11 (13)	
Stone Burden				
Length (mm)	42.59 ± 19.76	33.41 ± 18.00	38.73 ± 19.42	0.077
Width (mm)	27.03 ± 12.28	24.38 ± 13.98	25.92 ± 12.97	0.577
Dimension (L x W)	1346.51 ± 1111.07	999.46 ± 1166.55	1200.38 ± 1137.63	0.259

1. Chi-square test
2. [a]Pool t-test

Table 2 Operation Outcomes

	Supra-costal(n = 56) No. (%)	Subcostal(n = 30) No. (%)	Total(n = 86) No. (%)	P value
Puncture calyx				
Lower	1 (2)	3 (10)	4 (5)	0.2195
Middle	31 (55)	16 (53)	47 (55)	
Upper	24 (43)	11 (37)	35 (41)	
Op time(mins)[a]	100.71 ± 23.46	110 ± 27.38		
LOS (days)[a]	4.03 ± 2.33	4 ± 0.94		
Pethidine(mg) required[a]	25.76 ± 42.02	33.92 ± 56.60		
HCT change (%)[a]	3.53 ± 2.36	3.36 ± 2.40		
Stone-free (post op)				
No	23 (41)	15 (50)	38 (44)	0.4274
Yes	33 (59)	15 (50)	48 (56)	
Stone-free (3 months)				
No	6 (11)	3 (10)	9 (10)	0.9179
Yes	50 (89)	27 (90)	77 (90)	
Ancillary procedures	23 (41)	15 (50)		
Complications				
No	55 (98)	26 (87)	81 (94)	0.0292
Yes	1 (2)	4 (13)	5 (6)	

1. Chi-square test
2. [a]Pool t-test

Table 3 Stone Location and Operation Time(minutes)

Level	Number	Mean	Std Dev	Std Err Mean	Lower 95%	Upper 95%
Renal+upper ureter	9	90	17.5	5.83	76.55	103.45
Renal	41	98.29	20.26	3.16	91.9	104.69
Stghorn	25	121.6	27.90	5.58	110.08	133.12
Upper ureter	11	96.36	21.57	6.50	81.87	110.86

1. Chi-square test, $p < 0.0001$

sub-costal group (13%) ($p = 0.0292$, Table 2). One patient in the supra-costal group was transferred to intensive care unit due to sepsis with respiratory failure. The complications in the sub-costal group includes three patients with acute pyelonephritis and one patient needing blood transfusion. All patients with complications recovered uneventfully (Table 5). Post-operative renal ultrasonography did not show evidence of perirenal hematoma or fluid accumulation.

Discussion

Percutaneous renal surgery is a useful tool for urologists in treating conditions in the upper urinary tract. For complex renal stone, PCNL is as effective as open operation but with less post-operative discomfort and a shorter hospital stay. An optimal and atraumatic access to the desired calyx is the first step in a successful PCNL. In most cases, sub-costal puncture is preferred access; however, an upper pole access (via supra-costal area) is favored in cases of complex proximal. The advantage of upper pole over lower pole access is direct access to all calyces and the upper ureter but at a cost of increase risk of intrathoracic complications. In a study by Hopper & Yakes, percutaneous nephrostomy puncture in the intercostal space between the 11th–12th rib result in a lung injury in 14 to 29% of the patients while a 10th–11th rib intercostal space puncture result in lung injury in 86 to 93% of patients. After careful inspection of pleura anatomy, we noticed that the lowest point of the costo-diaphragmatic recess is at the medial half of the 12th rib, therefore an intercostal puncture on the lateral half 12th rib will less likely result in a punctured pleura. In cases of large complex renal stone, upper posterior calyx is the preferred access point to obtain maximum stone clearance [12, 18]. Due to the anatomical restrictions, supra-costal puncture is necessary for an

Table 4 Stone Location and Results Analysis

	Renal + upper ureter No. (%)	Renal No.(%)	Staghorn No. (%)	Upper ureter No. (%)	Total ($n = 86$) No. (%)	P value
Sex						
F	1 (11)	14 (34)	16 (64)	3 (27)	34 (40)	0.0148
M	8 (89)	27 (66)	9 (36)	8 (73)	52 (60)	
Side						
Left	4 (44)	18 (44)	12 (48)	4 (36)	38 (44)	0.9357
Right	5 (56)	23 (56)	13 (52)	7 (64)	48 (56)	
Puncture calyx						
Lower	0 (0)	2 (5)	2 (8)	0 (0)	4 (5)	0.3119
Middle	3 (33)	20 (49)	17 (68)	7 (64)	47 (55)	
Upper	6 (67)	19 (46)	6 (24)	4 (36)	35 (41)	
Operation-access						
Supra-costal	8 (89)	26 (63)	16 (64)	6 (55)	56 (65)	0.4159
Subcostal	1 (11)	15 (37)	9 (36)	5 (45)	30 (35)	
Stone-free						
No	1 (11)	14 (34)	22 (88)	1 (9)	38 (44)	< 0.0001
Yes	8 (89)	27 (66)	3 (12)	10 (91)	48 (56)	
Complication						
No	8 (89)	39 (95)	23 (92)	11 (100)	81 (94)	0.6999
Yes	1 (11)	2 (5)	2 (8)	0 (0)	5 (6)	

1. Chi-square test

Table 5 Comorbidities

Supra-costal (n = 1)		
Clavien-Dindo Classifications	number	
Grade 4	1	ICU admission due to sepsis with respiratory failure
Sub-costal (n = 4)		
Clavien-Dindo Classifications	number	
Grade 2	4	Pyelonephritis [3], blood transfusion [1]

adequate access into the upper posterior calyx. The stone–free rate in our series for supra-costal group was 59% (33/56) compared to 50% (15/30) in the sub-costal group ($p = 0.4274$). Since our series comprised of mostly large renal stone and staghorn stone, our overall stone-free rate of 56.9% is similar to CROES data for staghorn patients [19]. The reasons for initial low stone-free rate in our series compared to other tubeless studies include higher percentage of staghorn stone (77%), single nephrostomy tract, and use of rigid nephoscopy [10, 16, 19]. However, the use of post ancillary procedures improved the stone-free rate at 3 months to 90%. Sub-analysis showed that patients with proximal ureter stone is more prone to be stone-free due to smaller size. Length of stay and analgesic requirement did not have statistically significant difference between our supra-costal and sub-costal group, but the average amount of analgesia is less in supra-costal group (25 mg vs. 34 mg).

In the late 1980's to early 2000, several studies report contradictory results about "tubeless" PCNL. Placement of nephrostomy tube at the end of PCNL procedure is routine for most urologist to assist renal healing, avoid urine extravasation, aid hemostasis and future access in staged procedures [20]. However, nephrostomy tube is associated post-operative pain and discomfort, analgesic use, and urine leak from nephrostomy tract [9, 21]. In 1997 Bellman et al. started using the term "tubeless" PCNL, the study included fifty patients underwent PCNL procedures with only internal double-J stent. In their series, tubeless PCNL resulted in lower length of stay (LOS) and less analgesic use with faster return to normal activity when compared to the standard PCNL [3]. In subsequent studies comparing to standard PCNL, the safety and efficacy of tubeless PCNL is confirmed with similar morbidities, while offering shorter LOS and less analgesic use [3–10, 15, 22, 23].

Fever and bleeding are the most common complications associated with percutaneous renal surgery. The overall complication rate in our study is 6% (5 of 86 patients), with infection being the most common (Table 5). The combination of pre-operative urine culture and prophylactic antibiotics helped manage post-operative infection without resulting in any mortality during our study period. Post-PCNL bleeding can arise from a variety of sources such as the collecting system, renal parenchyma, arteriovenous fistula, pseudo-aneurysm, or the intercostal or subcutaneous vessels. The most frequent source of bleeding after PCNL seems to be from the renal parenchyma-collecting system junction. In our opinion, a careful calyx selection and puncture angle is very essential in minimizing post-PCNL bleeding. Since most of our puncture site are either middle or upper calyx, supra-costal approach into the posterior calyx will ensure a more direct angle into the desired calyx through the avascular plane of Brodel that is parallel with the minor calyx. A punctured tract parallel with minor calyx will minimize injury to interlobar vessels. In contrast for sub-costal puncture to reach middle or upper calyx, the puncture angle would be wider and not as parallel as the supra-costal puncture which results in higher chance of injuring interlobular vessels. Only one patient (sub-costal puncture) in our current series experienced severe bleeding which required blood transfusion.

In order to minimize post-PCNL bleeding, several studies investigate different hemostatic methods and agents. Noller et al. reported the use of fibrin sealant in renal parenchyma defect which resulted in average 2% decrease of hematocrit and no patients needing blood transfusion [24]. Hemostatic agents such as gelatin, Surgicel (oxidized cellulose), and Tisseel sealants were also investigated and showed contradictory results [15, 22]. Jou et al. investigated the use of electrocauterization to stop bleeder in the PCNL tracts in 249 patients, which results in 84 patients (34%) not needing a nephrostomy tube [25]. In our series, no additional hemostatic agents or electrocauterization over nephrostomy tracts were used. Instead, we gauge the amount of bleeding in the nephrostomy tract while retracting the nephroscope to determine the necessity of nephrostomy tube. In our series, the average hematocrit decrease was 3.53% ± 2.36% (supra-costal) and 3.36% ± 2.40% (sub-costal). Our study shows the initial puncture selection is more crucial in developing post-PCNL bleeding than the use of other adjuvant hemostatic agents or electrocautery.

In Munver's series of 300 percutaneous renal surgery, the overall complication rate was 8.3% (16.3% for supra-costal and 4.5% for sub-costal access) with supra-costal access having the most intrathoracic complications [13]. In our study, we did not experience any intrathoracic complications in the supra-costal (11th -12th intercostal) access group. Low incidence of intrathoracic injury can be attributed to careful review of anatomy and puncture selection. A careful anatomy puncture on the lateral half of 12th rib is a key in preventing intrathoracic injury. Limitations of our study include small study population and non-randomizing between the study groups.

Conclusions

Traditionally, a supra-costal access is associated with significantly higher intrathoracic complication rates compared to sub-costal access in standard PCNL. From the low complication rate in our current study, tubeless PCNL is a safe and effective procedure in selected patients. With careful anatomical position and an experienced operator, tubeless PCNL with supra-costal puncture within the 11th and 12th intercostal space is not associated with increase intrathoracic complication or morbidity.

Abbreviations

CROES: Clinical Research Office of the Endourological Society; DM: Diabetes mellitus; ESWL: Extracorporeal shockwave lithotripsy; IRB: Institutional review board; KUB: Kidney, Ureter, Bladder X-ray; PCNL: Percutaneous nephrolithotomy; WBC: White blood cells

Acknowledgements

Not applicable

Funding

Not applicable

Authors' contributions

All listed authors' contributions are in line with ICMJE guidelines. All authors read and approved the final manuscript.

Competing interests

The authors declare that they have no competing interests.

Author details

[1]From the Division of Urology, Department of Surgery, Changhua Christian Hospital, 135, Nanxiao St., Changhua City, Changhua County 500, Taiwan. [2]From the Transplant Medicine and Surgery Research Center, Changhua Christian Hospital, Changhua, Taiwan. [3]School of Medicine, Kaohsiung Medical University, Kaohsiung, Taiwan.

References

1. Preminger GM, Clayman RV, Hardeman SW, Franklin J, Curry T, Peters PC. Percutaneous nephrostolithotomy vs open surgery for renal calculi. A comparative study. JAMA. 1985;254(8):1054–8.
2. Segura JW, Patterson DE, LeRoy AJ, Williams HJ Jr, Barrett DM, Benson RC Jr, et al. Percutaneous removal of kidney stones: review of 1,000 cases. J Urol. 1985;134(6):1077–81.
3. Bellman GC, Davidoff R, Candela J, Gerspach J, Kurtz S, Stout L. Tubeless percutaneous renal surgery. J Urol. 1997;157(5):1578–82.
4. Shah HN, Kausik VB, Hegde SS, Shah JN, Bansal MB. Tubeless percutaneous nephrolithotomy: a prospective feasibility study and review of previous reports. BJU Int. 2005;96(6):879–83.
5. Karami H, Jabbari M, Arbab AH. Tubeless percutaneous nephrolithotomy: 5 years of experience in 201 patients. J Endourol. 2007;21(12):1411–3.
6. Mouracade P, Spie R, Lang H, Jacqmin D, Saussine C. "Tubeless" percutaneous nephrolithotomy: a series of 37 cases. Prog Urol. 2007;17(7):1351–4.
7. Shaikh AH, El Khalid S, Nabi N. Safety and efficacy of tubeless percutaneous nephrostolithotomy. J Pak Med Assoc. 2007;57(12):584–6.
8. Tefekli A, Altunrende F, Tepeler K, Tas A, Aydin S, Muslumanoglu AY. Tubeless percutaneous nephrolithotomy in selected patients: a prospective randomized comparison. Int Urol Nephrol. 2007;39(1):57–63.
9. Gupta NP, Mishra S, Suryawanshi M, Seth A, Kumar R. Comparison of standard with tubeless percutaneous nephrolithotomy. J Endourol. 2008; 22(7):1441–6.
10. Malcolm JB, Derweesh IH, Brightbill EK, Mehrazin R, DiBlasio CJ, Wake RW. Tubeless percutaneous nephrolithotomy for complex renal stone disease: single center experience. Can J Urol. 2008;15(3):4072–6.
11. Hopper KDYW. The posterior intercostal approach for percutaneous renal procedures: risk of puncturing the lung, spleen, and liver as determined by CT. Am J Roentgenol. 1990;154(1):115–7.
12. Lojanapiwat B, Prasopsuk S. Upper-pole access for PCNL - comparison of supracostal and infracostal approaches. J Endourol. 2006;20(7):491–4.
13. Munver R, Delvecchio FC, Newman GE, Preminger GM. Critical analysis of supracostal access for percutaneous renal surgery. J Urol. 2001;166(4):1242–6.
14. Radecka E, Brehmer M, Holmgren K, Magnusson A. Complications associated with percutaneous nephrolithotripsy: supra- versus subcostal access. A retrospective study. Acta Radiol. 2003;44(4):447–51.
15. Shah HN, Hegde SS, Shah JN, Bansal MB. Safety and efficacy of supracostal access in tubeless PCNL. J Endourol. 2006;20(12):1016–21.
16. Falahatkar S, Khosropanah I, Roshani A, Neiroomand H, Nikpour S, Nadjafi-Semnani M, et al. Tubeless percutaneous nephrolithotomy for staghorn stones. J Endourol. 2008;22(7):1447–51.
17. Marcovich RSA. Percutaneous renal access: tips and tricks. BJU Int. 2005; 95(syupplement 2):78–84.
18. Raza A, Moussa S, Smith G, Tolley DA. Upper-pole puncture in percutaneous nephrolithotomy: a retrospective review of treatment safety and efficacy. BJU Int. 2008;101(5):599–602.
19. Desai M, De Lisa A, Turna B, Rioja J, Walfridsson H, D'Addessi A, et al. The clinical research office of the endourological society percutaneous nephrolithotomy global study: staghorn versus nonstaghorn stones. J Endourol. 2011;25(8):1263–8.
20. Winfield HN, Weyman P, Clayman RV. Percutaneous nephrostolithotomy: complications of premature nephrostomy tube removal. J Urol. 1986;136(1):77–9.
21. Agrawal MS, Agrawal M, Gupta A, Bansal S, Yadav A, Goyal J. A randomized comparison of tubeless and standard percutaneous nephrolithotomy. J Endourol. 2008;22(3):439–42.
22. Shah HN, Kausik V, Hedge S, Shah JN, Bansal MB. Initial experience with hemostatic fibrin glue as adjuvant during tubeless PCNL. J Endourol. 2006;20(3):194–8.
23. Cormio L, Ibarlucea G, Tolley D, et al. Exit strategies following percutaneous nephrolithotomy (PCNL): a comparison of surgical outcomes in the clinical research Office of the Endourological Society (CROES) PCNL global study. World J Urol. 2013;31(5):1239–44.
24. Noller MW, Baughman SM, Morey AF, Auge BK. Fibrin sealant enables tubeless percutaneous stone surgery. J Urol. 2004;172(1):166–9.
25. Jou YC, Cheng MC, Sheen JH, Lin CT, Chen PC. Electrocauterization of bleeding points for percutaneous nephrolithotomy. Urology. 2004;64(3):443–6 discussion 6-7.

27

Robot-assisted laparoscopic reconstructed management of multiple aneurysms in renal artery primary bifurcations

Hai-bin Wei[1†], Xiao-long Qi[1†], Feng Liu[1*], Jie Wang[2], Xiao-feng Ni[3], Qi Zhang[1], En-hui Li[1], Xuan-yu Chen[1] and Da-hong Zhang[1*]

Abstract

Background: Renal artery aneurysm (RAA) is rare and its incidence in the general population remains elusive. There have been few reports on the repair of multiple aneurysms conducted with the Da Vinci robot-assisted surgical platform (Intuitive Surgical Inc., Sunnyvale, CA, USA), especially for those located in renal artery primary bifurcations.

Case presentation: We report our experience in the surgical management of two expanding right-sided RAAs in a 64-year-old man using a robot-assisted laparoscopic approach. Two aneurysms were located in renal artery primary bifurcations, whose diameter was 1.8 and 1.2 cm. The aneurysms were resected and the renal artery branch reconstructed by in situ arteriorrhaphy. The operation lasted for 2 h and 35 min with a warm ischemia time of 26 min and estimated blood loss of 150 ml. The hospital stay was 6 days. The computed tomography (CT) scan performed 2 months after the surgery showed resolution of the aneurysms. Additionally, split renal function indicated the preservation of right renal function in the follow-up period.

Conclusions: The robot-assisted laparoscopic procedure is a safe and effective surgical technique, which may be considered as an alternative to open surgery for complex multiple RAAs in the future.

Keywords: Renal artery aneurysms, Robotic surgery, Reconstruction, Renovascular disease, Case report

Background

Renal artery aneurysm (RAA) is an uncommon clinical condition, whose actual annual incidence rate in the general population remains unclear. The incidence rate of RAAs is estimated to range from 0.03% to 0.09%, according to previous autopsy series reports [1, 2]. There is an increasing detection of RAAs along with the widespread use of ultrasonography and computed tomography (CT) as tools for medical examination and diagnostic purposes.

A later research report found an incidence of 0.3% to 2.5% according to some angiographic and CT studies [3]. However, the incidence of multiple RAAs is still uncommon.

The Da Vinci robot-assisted surgical platform (Intuitive Surgical Inc., Sunnyvale, CA, USA) was introduced to our hospital in 2014 and has been used in a variety of minimally invasive urological surgery. It provides possibilities and alternatives for various complicated and delicate surgeries, and has only shown great superiority compared with conventional laparoscopic surgery. Until now, there has been no report on the treatment of multiple RAAs with the Da Vinci robot-assisted surgery. To determine the feasibility of using this approach, we performed a robot-assisted laparoscopic reconstruction of multiple aneurysms at major bifurcations of the renal artery in a 64-year-old man and evaluated the safety and efficiency of the Da Vinci robot-assisted surgery.

* Correspondence: liufeng2408@sina.com; zhangdahong88@yeah.net
†Equal contributors
[1]Department of Urology, Zhejiang Provincial People's Hospital, No. 158, Shangtang Road, Xiacheng District, Hangzhou, Zhejiang 310014, China
Full list of author information is available at the end of the article

Case presentation

A 64-year-old man was admitted to our department due to incidentally discovered RAAs. A previous enhanced CT scan of the local hospital showed two saccular RAAs in the right renal artery. The two aneurysms were located at primary bifurcations of renal artery, with a diameter of 1.8 cm and 1.2 cm, respectively, as shown in Fig. 1. The smaller one was located at the first bifurcation of the first segmental artery of the renal artery, while the other one is at the second bifurcation of the another segmental artery of the renal artery. The patient had no history of comorbidities other than a hepatitis B infection and partial hepatectomy, cholecystectomy and splenectomy due to hepatic carcinoma in 2002. Also, there were no typical clinical symptoms, such as flank pain, hematuria, or a sense of abdominal distension. His blood pressure was 106/56 mmHg at admission and the usual hypertension was absent.

Split renal function was evaluated through glomerular filtration rate (GFR) before surgery and then 2 months after surgery. We obtained the GFR using the camera-based Gate's method to measure the renal uptake of ^{99m}Technetium (^{99m}Tc) diethylenetriaminepentaacetic acid (DTPA). The preoperatively estimated GFRs were 30.16 ml/min/1.69 m^2 (right renal) and 36.09 ml/min/1.69 m^2 (left renal). The class 2 classification was deemed according to the American Society of Anesthesiologists (ASA).

The patient was secured in the left lateral position. A Veress needle was used to establish a carbon dioxide (CO_2) pneumoperitoneum of 12 mmHg lateral to the right rectus muscle at the level of the umbilicus, and then a 12-mm laparoscopic camera port was placed at the same position. A 30° lens was introduced to position the other ports under direct vision. A 12-mm port was placed 3 cm below the umbilicus position. Then, two ports of 8-mm were placed at 10 cm below the xiphoid at the ventral midline and below the 12th rib costochondral margin at the mid-clavicle. The 5-mm assistant port was inserted at 2 cm below the xiphoid at the ventral midline.

The renal hilum was completely dissected anteriorly and posteriorly, and the right renal artery and segmental arteries were isolated at the level of the renal hilum. The two RAAs were fully exposed and turned out to be saccular in accordance with the preoperative CT scan. The vascular bulldog clamp was used to clamp the inflow of renal artery. Then, the RAAs were resected from the proximal inflow to the distal outflow by cold monopolar shears, preserving the vascular back wall intact for the ensuing repair process. The bifurcations were then reconstructed with continuous suture using 5–0 Prolene (Ethicon US, LLC., Somerville, NJ, USA). Before the last suture, the vascular bulldog clamp was removed and then blood filled the entire renal artery to exclude intravascular air. Subsequently, intraoperative ultrasound was adopted for arterial perfusion and hemodynamic evaluation. The surgical procedure is depicted in Fig. 2. Finally, the Da Vinci device was undocked after removal of the resected RAAs by the Endocatch bag.

The warm ischemia time was 26 min. The total operative duration and estimated blood loss was 155 min and 150 ml, respectively. There was no perioperative complication. The serum creatinine and blood urea nitrogen was stable within the reference range. On postoperative day 6 the patient was discharged home. The CT scan performed 2 months later, shown in Fig. 3, demonstrated resolution of the aneurysms without any recurrence or artery stenosis; the estimated GFR were 29.76 ml/min/1.69 m^2 (right renal) and 34.03 ml/min/1.69 m^2 (left renal).

Discussion and conclusions

RAA is a rare disorder, and multiple RAAs, which occur in about 18% of the RAA cases, are even more rare in the general population [4]. It is difficult to reach a consensus on the appropriate indications for intervention in RAAs, due to the numerous aspects involved, such as the clinical symptoms (hematuria, refractory hypertension, persistent back pain and renal infarction), the anatomical and morphological characteristics of RAAs (size, location, wall calcification and enlarging lesion), and general clinical features (life expectancy, comorbidities and planned pregnancy) [5]. Currently, widely accepted indications for RAA include more than 2 cm in size, women in reproductive age planning for pregnancy and positive clinical manifestation, such as pain, hematuria and refractory hypertension attributable to the RAA. In our opinion, the

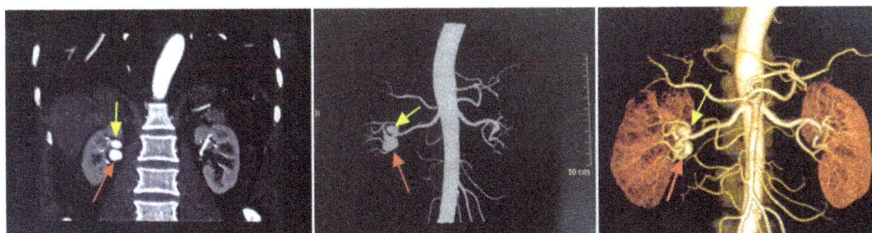

Fig. 1 CT angiogram and reconstruction preoperative. Red asterisk indicates the RAA of 1.8 cm. Yellow asterisk represents the RAA of 1.2 cm

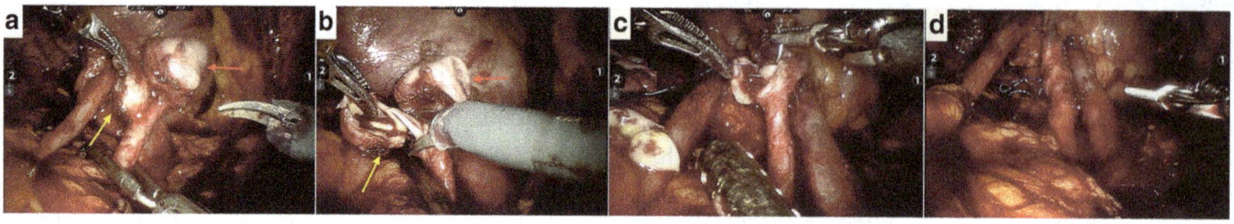

Fig. 2 The surgical procedure of reconstruction. **a**, RAA dissected and renal hilar control. **b**, resection of RAA. **c**, reconstruction of RAA. **d**, completed reconstruction of renal artery main trunk. Red asterisk indicates the RAA of 1.8 cm. Yellow asterisk represents the RAA of 1.2 cm

coexistence of two RAAs in the renal artery added to the risk of rupture and progression, which also required active intervention.

RAAs can be managed by surgical or percutaneous interventional radiological treatments. Due to lower invasiveness and reduced morbidity, percutaneous interventional radiological techniques surpass traditional surgical techniques and have become increasingly popular [5]. However, endovascular techniques are not preferred for all conditions, such as aneurysms located at the artery bifurcations or distal branches. As the gold standard for RAAs, open surgery results in the most considerable blood loss, prolonged recovery, and the heaviest patient burden [6, 7]. Since a report on laparoscopic repair of RAAs by Gill et al., in 2001, more and more successful laparoscopic repairs have been reported [8].

The laparoscopic technique has not been widely accepted because laparoscopic surgical reconstruction of RAA is still a challenging and time-consuming task under the constraint of the warm ischemia time (WIT), especially for those involving multiple aneurysms. First, intracorporeal suturing for angioplasty remains technically difficult, especially for aneurysms located at artery bifurcations, as well as those located at distal branches. Second, intracorporeal angioplasty is a time-consuming step after the renal artery is clamped with the bulldog clamp. It is generally considered that optimal ischemia time should not exceed 35 min [9]. In addition, there are considerable perioperative complications, such as unplanned nephrectomy and artery reintervention resulting from anastomotic stenosis or thrombosis [6]. The Da

Vinci surgical platform can provide precise suturing thanks to the perfect features of the "wristed" manipulators and 3-D stereo imaging. Accordingly, robot-assisted laparoscopic surgery may overcome some of the challenges of suturing and angioplasty, and offers an alternative surgical approach for the treatment of RAAs.

One of the key limiting factors for surgery is the WIT. Every minute of WIT matters when the renal artery is clamped, since an additional minute of WIT is associated with a 6% increase in the risk of new-onset stage IV chronic kidney disease during the follow-up [10]. Two artery aneurysms were resected and reconstructed with a WIT of 26 min, which was in a controllable range. There are several main reasons for a shorter WIT. First, the flexible "wristed" instruments and 3-D optical imaging of the Da Vinci surgical platform make it easier to cut and suture for reconstruction. Second, arteriorrhaphy greatly reduced the difficulty of angioplasty and avoided more artery suturing due to vascular anastomosis and aneurysmectomy with bypass. Third, the vascular bulldog clap was removed before the last suture. Such early withdrawal of the bulldog clap further reduced the WIT and intravascular air was excluded by the filling blood. Also, since the two aneurysms were close in the renal artery, the reconstruction of the two aneurysms was completed after only one clamping of the renal artery, which avoided acute kidney injury caused by repeatedly occluding the renal artery. Due to a WIT of less than 30 min, the cooled (4 °C) renal perfusion supplemented with mannitol or prostaglandin E was avoided. Thus, despite having performed two reconstructions in the renal artery, the split renal function

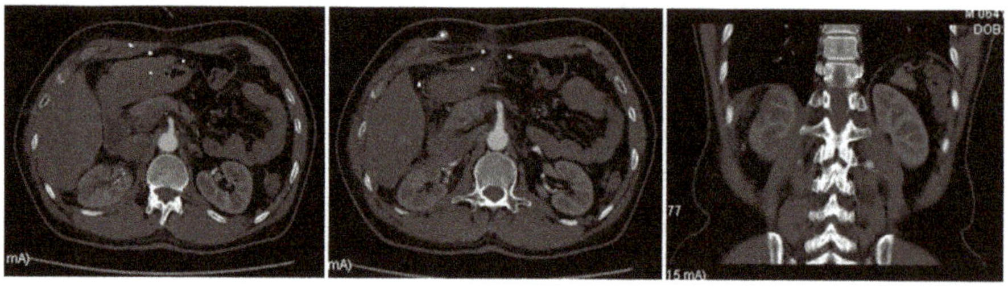

Fig. 3 CT angiogram postoperative

Table 1 Summary of case series of robot-assisted laparoscopic RAA reconstruction

	Our study-2015	Luke-2006	Giulianotti-2010	Samarasekera-2014
Patient number	1	1	5	1
Robot	DaVinci Si	DaVinci	DaVinci	DaVinci Si
Size (cm)	1.8 and 1.2	2.5	1.94 (range, 9–28)	1.6
Suture type	Arteriorrhaphy	End-to-end anastomosis	1 end-to-end anastomosis and 4 graft angioplasty	Arteriorrhaphy
Perioperative characteristic				
WIT (min)	26	59	10 and 38.5 (range, 20–60)	44
Operative time (min)	155	360	288 (range, 170–360)	240
Blood loss (ml)	150	650	100 (range, 50–300)	260
Hospital stay (d)	6	3	5.6 (range, 3–7).	-
Follow-up (months)	10	-	28 (range, 6–48)	2
Complications				
Perirenal hematoma	0	0	0	0
Haemorrhage	0	0	0	0
Renal dysfunction	0	0	1	0
Unimproved hypertension	0	0	3	0
Stenosis	0	0	1 patient treat with percutaneous angioplasty	0

RAA renal artery aneurysm, *WIT* warm ischemia time

was not affected, as shown on the ^{99m}Tc-DTPA renogram performed 2 months later.

We systematically searched the Medline electronic database, and summarized the case series on robot-assisted laparoscopic RAA reconstruction. To the best of our knowledge, there are only a few reports on the Da Vinci robot-assisted reconstruction of RAA [7, 11, 12], as listed in Table 1. Like our study, the study by Luke as well as that by Samarasekera, are all single case reports, and there were no severe complications requiring acute reintervention [7, 11]. In the study by Giulianotti, one out of 5 patients had elevated postoperative serum creatinine level, which spontaneously returned to normal range by postoperative day three [12]. In addition, another patient experienced stenosis in the reconstructed branch 6 months after the repair, and responded well to percutaneous angioplasty [12]. Although we performed arteriorrhaphy for two RAAs at the same time, the complications did not increase compared with the other three studies. In general, the Da Vinci robot-assisted reconstruction of RAA is a safe technique associated with a low complication rate, despite the adoption of different angioplasty ways to reconstruct.

In summary, the results of our study demonstrate the safety and efficiency of the robot-assisted laparoscopic technique to treat complex multiple RAAs. Although more technical refinements and longer follow-up period is necessary, the robot-assisted laparoscopic technique represents a valid alternative to open surgery for complex multiple RAAs in the future.

Abbreviations
ASA: American Society of Anesthesiologists; CO_2: Carbon dioxide; CT: Computed tomography; GFR: Glomerular filtration rate; RAA: Renal artery aneurysm; WIT: Warm ischemia time

Acknowledgements
We would like to thank the Department of Urology, Zhejiang Provincial People's Hospital for the population and optimization of Robot-assisted laparoscopic techniques in order to benefit patients. In addition, we would like to thank the patient for giving us the permission to use the medical information for this publication.

Funding
No funding from any source for this study.

Authors' contributions
DHZ made substantial contributions to conception and design and acquisition of data. HBW has been involved in drafting the manuscript. HBW, XLQ and FL made substantial contributions to conception and design. JW, XFN and QZ made substantial contributions to analysis and interpretation of data. EHL and XYC revised it critically for important intellectual content. All authors have read and given final approval of the version to be published.

Competing interests
The authors declare that they have no competing interests.

Author details
[1]Department of Urology, Zhejiang Provincial People's Hospital, No. 158, Shangtang Road, Xiacheng District, Hangzhou, Zhejiang 310014, China.

[2]Department of Nephrology, Sir Run Run Shaw Hospital, No. 3, East Qingchun Road, Jianggan District, Hangzhou, Zhejiang 310076, China.
[3]Department of general surgery, Central Hospital of Huzhou, No. 198, Hongqi Road, Wuxing District, Huzhou, Zhejiang 313003, China.

References

1. Orion KC, Abularrage CJ. Renal artery aneurysms: movement toward endovascular repair. Semin Vasc Surg. 2013;26(4):226–32.
2. Stanley JC, Rhodes EL, Gewertz BL, et al. Renal artery aneurysms: significance of macroaneurysms exclusive of dissections and fibrodysplastic mural dilations. Arch Surg. 1975;110(11):1327–33.
3. Coleman DM, Stanley JC. Renal artery aneurysms. J Vasc Surg. 2015;62(3):779–85.
4. Wayne EJ, Edwards MS, Stafford JM, et al. Anatomic characteristics and natural history of renal artery aneurysms during longitudinal imaging surveillance. J Vasc Surg. 2014;60(2):448–52.
5. Rossi M, Varano GM, Orgera G, et al. Wide-neck renal artery aneurysm: parenchymal sparing endovascular treatment with a new device. BMC Urol. 2013;14(1):1–5.
6. Henke PK, Cardneau JD, Jr UG, et al. Renal artery aneurysms: a 35-year clinical experience with 252 aneurysms in 168 patients. Ann Surg. 2001; 234(234):454–63.
7. Dinesh S, Riccardo A, Ali K, et al. Robot-assisted laparoscopic renal artery aneurysm repair with selective arterial clamping. Int J Urol. 2014;21(1):114–6.
8. Gill IS, Murphy DP, Hsu THS, et al. Laparoscopic repair of renal artery aneurysm. J Urol. 2001;166(1):202–5.
9. Frank B, Hein VP, Hakenberg OW, et al. Assessing the impact of ischaemia time during partial nephrectomy. Eur Urol. 2009;56(4):625–35.
10. Thompson RH, Lane BR, Lohse CM, et al. Every minute counts when the renal Hilum is clamped during partial Nephrectomy. Eur Urol. 2010;58(3):340–5.
11. Patrick L, Knudsen BE, Nguan CY, et al. Robot-assisted laparoscopic renal artery aneurysm reconstruction. J Vasc Surg. 2006;44(3):651–3.
12. Pier Cristoforo G, Francesco Maria B, Pietro A, et al. Robot-assisted laparoscopic repair of renal artery aneurysms. J Vasc Surg. 2010;51(4):1062.

28

Aortic calcification burden predicts deterioration of renal function after radical nephrectomy

Ken Fukushi[1], Shingo Hatakeyama[1*] (iD), Hayato Yamamoto[1], Yuki Tobisawa[1], Tohru Yoneyama[2], Osamu Soma[1], Teppei Matsumoto[1], Itsuto Hamano[1], Takuma Narita[1], Atsushi Imai[1], Takahiro Yoneyama[1], Yasuhiro Hashimoto[2], Takuya Koie[1], Yuriko Terayama[3], Tomihisa Funyu[3] and Chikara Ohyama[1,2]

Abstract

Background: Radical nephrectomy for renal cell carcinoma (RCC) is a risk factor for the development of chronic kidney disease (CKD), and the possibility of postoperative deterioration of renal function must be considered before surgery. We investigated the contribution of the aortic calcification index (ACI) to the prediction of deterioration of renal function in patients undergoing radical nephrectomy.

Methods: Between January 1995 and December 2012, we performed 511 consecutive radical nephrectomies for patients with RCC. We retrospectively studied data from 109 patients who had regular postoperative follow-up of renal function for at least five years. The patients were divided into non-CKD and pre-CKD based on a preoperative estimated glomerular filtration rate (eGFR) of ≥60 mL/min/1.73 m^2 or <60 mL/min/1.73 m^2, respectively. The ACI was quantitatively measured by abdominal computed tomography before surgery. The patients in each group were stratified between low and high ACIs. Variables such as age, sex, comorbidities, and pre- and postoperative renal function were compared between patients with a low or high ACI in each group. Renal function deterioration-free interval rates were evaluated by Kaplan-Meier analysis. Factors independently associated with deterioration of renal function were determined using multivariate analysis.

Results: The median age, preoperative eGFR, and ACI in this cohort were 65 years, 68 mL/min/1.73 m^2, and 8.3%, respectively. Higher ACI (≥8.3%) was significantly associated with eGFR decline in both non-CKD and pre-CKD groups. Renal function deterioration-free interval rates were significantly lower in the ACI-high than ACI-low strata in both of the non-CKD and pre-CKD groups. Multivariate analysis showed that higher ACI was an independent risk factor for deterioration of renal function at 5 years after radical nephrectomy.

Conclusions: Aortic calcification burden is a potential predictor of deterioration of renal function after radical nephrectomy.

Keywords: Aortic calcification, Chronic kidney disease, Radical nephrectomy, Renal cell carcinoma, Renal function

* Correspondence: shingoh@hirosaki-u.ac.jp
[1]Department of Urology, Hirosaki University Graduate School of Medicine, 5 Zaifu-chou, Hirosaki 036-8562, Japan
Full list of author information is available at the end of the article

Background

Various studies have shown that radical nephrectomy for renal cell carcinoma (RCC) is an independent risk factor for the development of chronic kidney disease (CKD) [1, 2]. A radical nephrectomy remains the standard treatment for patients, depending on factors such as tumor size, tumor location, and comorbidities, nevertheless CKD increases the risk of cardiovascular events and overall mortality [3]. Although it is suggested that CKD as a consequence of surgery (such as nephrectomy) may be associated with a relatively lower risk of progression and mortality than CKD attributed to medical disorders (such as hypertension, type 2 diabetes, and/or cardiovascular disease) [4, 5], any CKD is associated with an increased risk of cardiovascular events and all-cause mortality in large, population based studies [6–8]. Therefore, when discussing the therapeutic option of radical nephrectomy, it is essential to estimate the risk of postoperative deterioration of renal function. Potential factors associated with severe postoperative renal impairment have been reported, such as old age, preexisting stage 3 CKD, hypertension, type 2 diabetes, and cardiovascular disease [1–3].

Aortic calcification is one of the sequelae of aortic degeneration and has recently been considered a major complication and independent risk factor for coronary artery disease, heart failure, and stroke [9, 10]. Several studies have addressed the clinical importance of arterial calcification in patients at high risk for cardiovascular disease; however, only a few studies have demonstrated the impact of arterial calcification on renal function [11–13]. In addition, the clinical relevance of the aortic calcification index (ACI) with regard to postoperative renal function outcome in patients undergoing radical nephrectomy has not been well studied. Therefore, we hypothesized that preexisting aortic calcification may play a crucial role in the deterioration of renal function after radical nephrectomy and investigated the contribution of the ACI in predicting postoperative renal function in such patients. This study was registered as a clinical trial: UMIN000023577 (http://rctportal.niph.go.jp/en/detail?trial_id=UMIN000023577).

Methods

Patient selection and variables evaluated

Between January 1995 and December 2012, we performed 511 consecutive radical nephrectomies in patients with RCC. Of those, we excluded 95 patients who deceased within five years, 165 patients without baseline abdominal computed tomography (CT) prior to radical nephrectomy, and 142 patients without postoperative regular assessment of renal function for five years after the surgery. The remaining 109 patients were included in the present study. Blood tests including renal function were routinely performed at least once a year after radical nephrectomy. The estimated glomerular filtration rate (eGFR) was calculated using the Modification of Diet in Renal Disease equation for Japanese patients [14].

The patients were divided in two groups depending on the preoperative eGFR, a non-CKD group with an eGFR of ≥ 60 mL/min/1.73 m^2 and a pre-CKD group with an eGFR <60 mL/min/1.73 m^2.

Using abdominal CT images (TSX-301B, Toshiba Medical Systems Corp., Ohtawara, Japan, or CT750HD, GE Healthcare Japan, Tokyo, Japan), the ACI was quantitatively measured by scanning 10 slices of the aorta at 5-mm intervals above the bifurcation of the common iliac arteries as previously described [15]. Intimal calcification was scored in each of 12 radial sectors of each slice and reported as a percentage. For example, if 5 of 12 sectors were calcified in section 1, it was scored as 5/12 = 41.7% (Fig. 1). The ACI (%) was calculated as the average intimal calcification values of sections 1–10. ACI measurement was performed by an investigator who was blind to patients' clinical parameters.

The patients in each group were stratified depending on whether their ACIs were higher or lower than 8.3%, based on the median value of ACI in this cohort. Variables including age; sex; history of hypertension, type 2 diabetes, or cardiovascular disease; clinicopathologic data on the renal cancer; and renal function before and

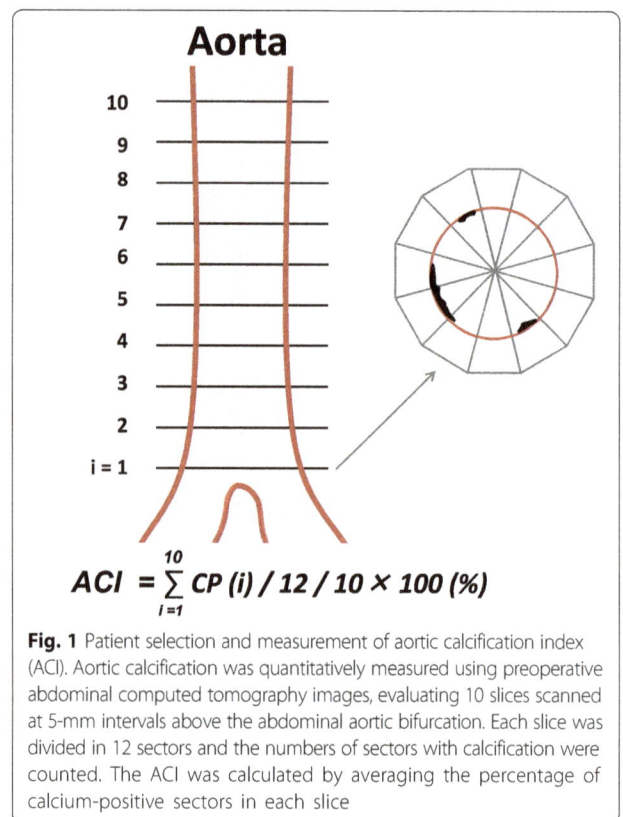

$$ACI = \sum_{i=1}^{10} CP\,(i)\,/\,12\,/\,10 \times 100\ (\%)$$

Fig. 1 Patient selection and measurement of aortic calcification index (ACI). Aortic calcification was quantitatively measured using preoperative abdominal computed tomography images, evaluating 10 slices scanned at 5-mm intervals above the abdominal aortic bifurcation. Each slice was divided in 12 sectors and the numbers of sectors with calcification were counted. The ACI was calculated by averaging the percentage of calcium-positive sectors in each slice

for 5 years after surgery were compared between patients with low and high ACI in each group. Hypertension was defined as taking any antihypertensive medications or preoperative systolic and diastolic blood pressure measurements of >140 and >90 mmHg. Diabetes was defined a history of type 2 diabetes or meeting the relevant diagnostic criteria and requiring glycemic control. Cardiovascular disease was defined as a positive history of cardiac surgery, angina, myocardial infarction, or stroke or taking any cardiotonic agents or coronary vasodilators.

The interval until the progression of CKD was measured from 3 months after surgery until the eGFR decreased in the non-CKD group to <60 ml/min/1.73 m^2 (defined as CKD3-free interval) or in the pre-CKD group to <45 ml/min/1.73 m^2 (defined as CKD3B-free interval).

Statistical analysis

Statistical analysis was performed using SPSS v. 22.0 (IBM Corporation, Armonk, NY, USA) and GraphPad Prism v. 5.03 (GraphPad Software, San Diego, CA, USA). Categorical variables were reported as percentages and compared using Fisher's exact test. Quantitative data were expressed as medians with quartiles 1 and 3 (Q1, Q3). Differences between the groups were compared using a t test for normally distributed data or Mann—Whitney U test for data with a non-normal distribution. Probability (P) values of <0.05 were considered statistically significant. Renal function deterioration-free intervals were evaluated

by Kaplan-Meier analysis. Independent factors associated with the renal function deterioration-free interval were identified by multivariate analysis using a Cox regression model. Hazard ratios (HR) with 95% confidence intervals (95% CI) were calculated after adjusting for potential confounders. Multivariate logistic regression analysis was performed to identify significant risk factors for eGFR loss >30% after radical nephrectomy at 5 years. Odds ratios (OR) with 95% CI were calculated after adjusting for potential confounders. Liner regression analysis was performed to develop a 5-year eGFR prediction formula, and correlation was analyzed using Spearman's correlation coefficient.

Results

Table 1 summarizes patients' characteristics. The median age, preoperative eGFR, and ACI in this cohort were 65 years, 68 mL/min/1.73 m^2, and 8.3%, respectively. The median ACI value of 8.3% was used as a cut-off between low and high ACI. Although there were statistically significant differences in ages between the low and high ACI strata in the non-CKD and pre-CKD groups, sex, renal function, comorbidities, and tumor stage did not differ significantly (Table 1). In the non-CKD group, longitudinal evaluation of eGFR revealed that the postoperative median eGFR at 5 years in patients with low and high ACI were 58 and 50 ml/min/1.73 m^2, respectively ($P = 0.0061$). It also showed significantly poorer renal function in patients with a high than a low ACI in

Table 1 Comparison of clinical and pathological patient's characteristics between low (<8.3%) and high (≥8.3%) ACI

	non-CKD			pre-CKD		
	low ACI	high ACI	P value	low ACI	high ACI	P value
n	40	36		13	20	
Age, years	57 (44–63)	67 (62–75)	<0.001	62 (53–71)	76 (74–79)	<0.001
Sex (Male)	26 (65%)	26 (72%)	0.499	9 (69%)	13 (65%)	1.000
Comorbidities						
Hypertension	9 (23%)	11 (31%)	0.426	1 (8%)	9 (45%)	0.050
Diabetes	3 (8%)	7 (19%)	0.177	1 (8%)	3 (15%)	1.000
Cardiovascular disease	2 (5%)	2 (6%)	1.000	0 (0%)	1 (5%)	1.000
Preoperative eGFR	77 (68–87)	74 (67–84)	0.202	50 (42–54)	42 (33–55)	0.152
ACI (%)	0.8 (0.0–5.8)	18 (14–27)	<0.001	0.8 (0.0–3.3)	18 (16–44)	<0.001
Tumor stage						
T1/2/3/4	25/6/7/2	23/3/10/0	0.394	7/4/2/0	13/3/3/1	0.810
Pathological subtype			0.277			1.000
Clear cell	35 (88%)	35 (97%)		12 (92%)	18 (90%)	
Papillary	1 (2.5%)	1 (3%)		1 (8%)	1 (5%)	
Chromophobe	1 (2.5%)	0 (0%)		0 (0%)	1 (5%)	
Others	3 (7.5%)	0 (0%)		0 (0%)	0 (0%)	
Distant metastasis	6 (15%)	3 (8%)	0.494	2 (15%)	3 (15%)	1.000
Tumor recurrence	9 (23%)	5 (14%)	0.334	2 (15%)	2 (10%)	1.000

Median and interquartile range (Q1, Q3) was used for consecutive variables. *ACI* aortic calcification index, *eGFR* estimated glomerular filtration rate

the non-CKD group (Fig. 2a). The decline ratio at 5 years after radical nephrectomy was higher in patients with a high (36%) than a low ACI (28%) (Fig. 2b). Similarly, the postoperative median eGFR at five years in the pre-CKD group was significantly poorer in those with a high rather than a low ACI (32 ml/min/1.73 m^2 vs. 42 ml/min/1.73 m^2, respectively, $P = 0.0058$) (Fig. 2c). In the pre-CKD group, the eGFR showed 28% reduction at 1 year after radical nephrectomy in patients with a high ACI, whereas it was 13% in low ACI (Fig. 2d).

In terms of the rates of decline in eGFR, significant differences were observed in both groups between patients with low and high ACI (Fig. 3a, b). The median rate of decline at 5 years was significantly higher in patients with a high (32%) versus low ACI (28%) in the non-CKD group ($P = 0.0430$) (Fig. 3a). Similarly, patients with high ACI in the pre-CKD group exhibited remarkably higher rates of decline (27%) than did those with low ACI (6%) at 5 years after radical nephrectomy ($P = 0.0446$) (Fig. 3b).

In the non-CKD group, CKD stage 3-free interval was significantly shorter in patients with high ACI than in those with low ACI ($P = 0.0025$) (Fig. 4a). Five-year CKD stage 3-free rates were 19.4% and 42.5% in patients with high and low ACI, respectively. Similarly, in the pre-CKD group, the CKD stage 3B-free intervals were significantly shorter in patients with high than with low ACI ($P = 0.0037$) (Fig. 4b) Five-year CKD stage 3-free rates were 0% and 15.4% in patients with a high or low ACI, respectively.

Multivariate Cox regression analysis revealed that age, preoperative eGFR, and ACI were independent risk factors for CKD progression (Table 2). Multivariate logistic regression analysis revealed that age, preoperative eGFR, and ACI were independent risk factors for eGFR loss >30% at five years after radical nephrectomy (Table 3). Based on the significant variables, we developed a formula by linear regression analysis to predict eGFR at five years after radical nephrectomy: Y (estimated 5-year eGFR) = (0.351 x preoperative eGFR) + (−0.232 x age) + (−0.208 x ACI) + 41.758. The correlation between actual eGFR and predicted values were significant ($P < 0.001$, $r^2 = 0.4623$) (Fig. 5). The minimal data set of the present study is available in Additional file 1: Dataset S1.

Discussion

In the present study, we demonstrated that a higher burden of aortic calcification was an independent risk factor for deterioration of renal function in patients after radical nephrectomy. In addition, the postoperative decline in renal function was significantly worse in patients with a high ACI regardless of their preoperative eGFR. Multivariate analysis revealed that the association of ACI with deterioration of renal function was statistically significant. Our findings suggest that a patient's ACI may be useful in predicting renal function after unilateral nephrectomy.

Because aortic calcification is one of the results of aortic degeneration, we hypothesized that it might predict deterioration of renal function after unilateral nephrectomy. Indeed, our previous study suggested that the burden of aortic calcification has impact on poor postoperative renal function in renal transplant patients [12], as well as with persistent hypertension after unilateral adrenalectomy in patients with aldosterone-producing

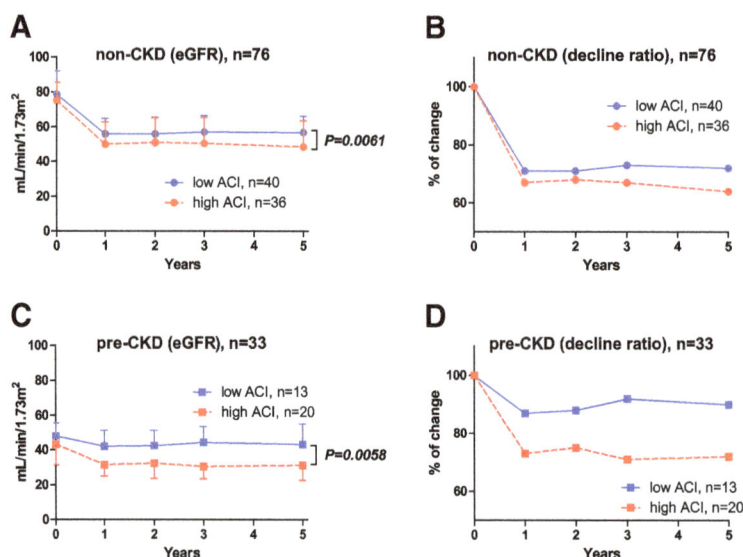

Fig. 2 Renal function compared in patients with low and high ACI in non-CKD and pre-CKD groups. Longitudinal evaluation of eGFR reveals significantly poorer renal function in patients with a high than a low ACI in the non-CKD group (**a**) and in the pre-CKD group (**c**). The decline ratios are higher in patients with high rather than low ACI in the non-CKD group (**b**) and in the pre-CKD group (**d**)

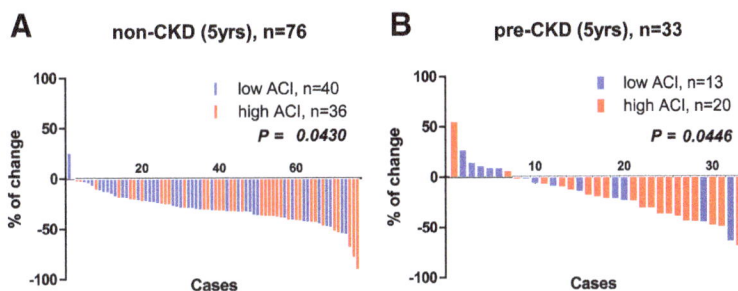

Fig. 3 Rate of decline of eGFR over 5 years in non-CKD and pre-CKD groups. Waterfall plots show significant differences between patients with a high or low ACI in the non-CKD group (**a**) and pre-CKD group (**b**). In the pre-CKD group, patients with a high ACI had greater rates of decline (27%) than those with a low ACI (6%) at 5 years after radical nephrectomy

adenomas [16]. Although the mechanisms by which aortic calcification might influence glomerular microcapillary degeneration remain unclear, it is not hard to anticipate that vascular damage occurs first and more severely in small vessels such as afferent arterioles and glomeruli.

Risk factors for aortic calcification include older age, higher systolic blood pressure, smoking, increased oxidative stress, dyslipidemia, the presence of diabetes and/or cardiovascular disease, and CKD [17, 18]. However, as all these factors are correlated with each other, the association is confusing, similar to asking whether the chicken or the egg comes first. The element that is common to all such risk factors is chronic, low grade, systemic inflammation, which has been defined as a metabolic syndrome [19]. A recent large study revealed that aortic valve calcification involves inflammatory, lipid, and mineral metabolism pathways [20]. In addition, inflammation and oxidative stress have been linked to vascular calcification in patients with CKD [18]. Therefore, chronic, low grade, systemic inflammation may accelerate arterial degeneration, resulting in arterial calcification and reduced renal reserve. Further studies are necessary to address the detailed association

between aortic calcification, inflammation, oxidative stress, and CKD.

Aortic calcification was once believed to be a simple passive process of aging. However, it is now recognized as a complex and highly regulated systemic process that involves the activation of cellular signaling pathways, genetic factors, and hormones. It had been assumed to be irreversible, and no agents were available to prevent it. However, a recent study reported that policosanol has the potential to inhibit vascular calcification [21]. Elseweidy et al. reported that treating diabetic hyperlipidemic rats with policosanol, omega-3 fatty acids, and atorvastatin for eight weeks significantly increased high-density lipoprotein cholesterol (HDL-C) and vitamin D, decreased the number of aortic vacuoles, and inhibited the calcification process. Of the agents used, policosanol induced more remarkable reduction in the density and number of foam cells and improved intimal lesions of the aorta more than atorvastatin. The key effects of policosanol are inhibition of inflammation, oxidative stress, and calcium deposition, all of which are essential pathways in aortic calcification.

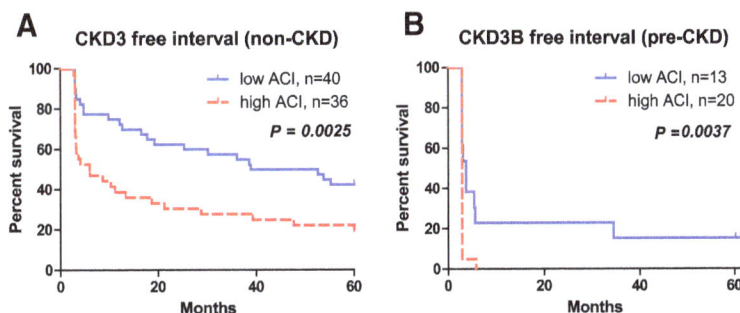

Fig. 4 CKD stage progression-free interval after radical nephrectomy. The CKD stage progression-free interval rates are significantly lower in the patients with high ACI after radical nephrectomy in the non-CKD group (**a**) and in the pre-CKD group (**b**). CKD stage progression is defined as CKD stage 0–2 progressing to stage 3 in the non-CKD group and CKD stage 3A progressing to 3B in the pre-CKD group

Table 2 Multivariate Cox regression analysis for risk factors for stage 3 CKD (eGFR < 60 mL/min/1.73 m^2) in non-CKD group, or stage 3B CKD (eGFR < 45 mL/min/1.73 m^2) in pre-CKD group

Cox regression analyses	Risk factor	P value	HR	95% CI
Age, years	Continuous	0.224	1.01	0.99–1.04
Sex	Male	0.520	0.85	0.53–1.38
Diabetes	Positive	0.936	0.97	0.51–1.86
Cardiovascular disease	Positive	0.542	1.35	0.52–3.51
ACI (%)	Continuous	0.044	1.02	1.00–1.03
Metastatic disease	Positive	0.053	0.47	0.22–1.01
Preoperative eGFR (ml/min/1.73 m^2)	Continuous	<0.001	0.97	0.96–0.99

ACI aortic calcification index, *CKD* Chronic kidney disease, *eGFR* estimated glomerular filtration rate

In the present study, we found that patients in the pre-CKD group who had a higher ACI had a marked decrease in renal function (Fig. 2d). Because older patients were included in this group, the result might reflect selection bias. However, multivariate analysis showed that preoperative eGFR and ACI were independent predictors' deterioration of renal function after controlling for other patient variables. Therefore, our findings suggest that patients with RCC who have both preoperative CKD and a high ACI are at significant risk for severe deterioration in renal function after unilateral nephrectomy. Although our observation needs further investigation, aortic calcification appears to be a potential surrogate marker for diminished renal reserve after unilateral nephrectomy.

Several limitations need to be acknowledged. First, selection of RCC patients with renal function for 5 years is a main limitation of our study. The small sample size and single-institution retrospective design prevent definitive conclusions on the influence of aortic calcification on postoperative renal function. The fact that only one observer calculated the ACI parameter could be another limitation. Significant differences in ages between the low and high ACI stratified groups in the non-CKD and pre-CKD groups are a strong limitation that restricts the value of the findings. We could not exclude the multiple collinearity among variables including age, eGFR, Hypertension,

and ACI. Definition of hypertension is not suitable for detection postoperative renal impairment. Whether our findings are generalizable to non-Asian populations is also unclear. In addition, we were unable to include in the analysis certain other established risk factors for renal dysfunction, such as cigarette smoking, dyslipidemia, proteinuria, blood pressure control, and medications.

Second, our study did not assess the influence of aortic calcification on cardiovascular events or overall survival after radical nephrectomy in patients with RCC. Because CKD resulting from surgery may not increase mortality as much as CKD that is secondary to medical conditions, [5] the association between a decline in renal function after radical nephrectomy and mortality is under debate. Recent research suggests that survival is better with CKD occurring after surgery rather than with other diseases, particularly if the postoperative eGFR is greater than 45 ml/min/1.73 m^2, whereas patients with preexisting CKD are at risk of a significant decline in renal function after surgery [8]. Therefore, further large-scale, long-term studies are required to resolve these issues.

Despite these limitations, the strength of this study is its novel finding of the association between aortic calcification and deterioration renal function after radical nephrectomy. Using a non-invasive modality of measuring ACI, we were able to demonstrate an independent association between aortic calcification and postoperative renal

Table 3 Multivariate logistic regression analyses for risk factors for loss of renal function greater than 30% at 5 years after nephrectomy

Logistic regression analysis	Risk factor	P value	OR	95% CI
Age, years	Continuous	0.137	1.03	0.99–1.08
Sex	Male	0.714	1.20	0.46–3.14
Diabetes	Positive	0.202	0.40	0.10–1.63
Cardiovascular disease	Positive	0.735	1.36	0.23–8.19
ACI (%)	Continuous	0.016	1.05	1.01–1.09
Metastatic disease	Positive	0.763	0.81	0.21–3.18
Preoperative eGFR (ml/min/1.73 m^2)	Continuous	<0.001	1.07	1.03–1.10

ACI aortic calcification index, *CKD* Chronic kidney disease, *eGFR* estimated glomerular filtration rate

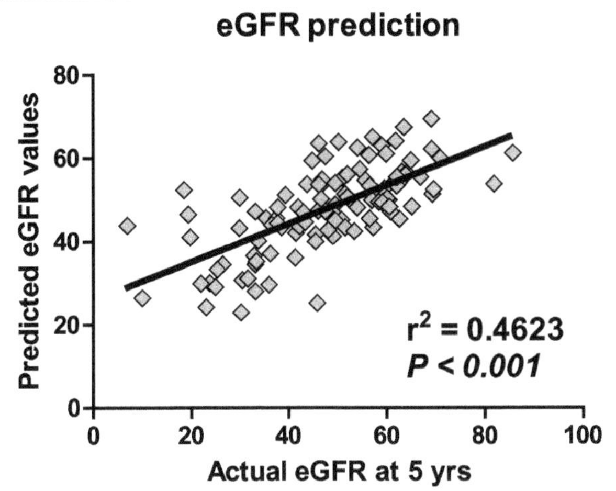

Fig. 5 The 5-year eGFR prediction model after radical nephrectomy. The formula to predict 5-year eGFR was developed by linear regression analysis including three key factors (age, preoperative eGFR, and ACI). The formula is: Y (estimated 5 years eGFR) = (0.351 x preoperative eGFR) + (−0.232 x age) + (−0.208 x ACI) + 41.758. The predicted 5-year eGFR is significantly correlated with actual eGFR at 5 years after radical nephrectomy

impairment. Our findings may assist in recognizing patients who are at high risk of CKD after radical nephrectomy, which will help to inform the preoperative discussion of therapeutic options.

Conclusions

In conclusion, the aortic calcification burden is a potential predictor for postoperative renal impairment. It may be useful to identify patients who are at high risk for renal impairment after radical nephrectomy.

Additional file

Additional file 1: Dataset-S1, Simple data set. Simple data set is available in supplemental file (Dataset S1, MS Excel). Mean (± standard deviation) and median (interquartile range) age were 63 ± 13 and 65 (55–73) years old, respectively. Median height (cm) and body weight (kg) were 161 (155–167) and 63 (54–72), respectively.

Abbreviations

ACI: Aortic calcification; CKD: Chronic kidney disease; CT: Computed tomography; eGFR: Estimated glomerular filtration rate; HDL-C: High-density lipoprotein cholesterol; HR: Hazard ratio; OR: Odds ratio; Q1: First quartile; Q3: Third quartile; RCC: Renal cell carcinoma

Acknowledgements

We thank Yuriko Tanabe, Yuki Fujita and Mihoko Osanai for their invaluable help with the data collection.

Authors' contributions

All authors read and approved the final manuscript, and author contributions are in line with the ICMJE guidelines. Conceived and designed the experiments: SH, CO, TK, TF. Performed the experiments: KF, HY, OS, TM, AI, TaY, YH, IH, NT. Analyzed the data: YTe, SH. Contributed reagents/materials/analysis tools: YTo, ToY. Wrote the manuscript: KF, SH.

Authors' information

KF: postgraduate student, SH: assistant professor, HY: assistant professor, YT (Yuki Tobisawa): assistant professor, TY (Tohru Yoneyama): assistant professor, OS: postgraduate student, TM: postgraduate student, IT: postgraduate student, NT: postgraduate student, AI: assistant professor, YT (Takahiro Yoneyama): assistant professor, YH: associate professor, TK: associate professor, YT (Yuriko Terayama): academic researcher, TF: administrative director, CO: professor and chairman.

Competing interests

The authors declare that they have no competing interests, and no financial conflict of interest.

Financial disclosure

This work was supported by a Grant-in-Aid for Scientific Research (No. 23791737, 24659708, 22390301, 15H02563, and 15 K15579) from the Japan Society for the Promotion of Science. The funders had no role in study design, data collection and analysis, decision to publish, or preparation of the manuscript.

Author details

^{1}Department of Urology, Hirosaki University Graduate School of Medicine, 5 Zaifu-chou, Hirosaki 036-8562, Japan. ^{2}Department of Advanced Transplant and Regenerative Medicine, Hirosaki University Graduate School of Medicine, Hirosaki, Japan. ^{3}Department of Urology, Oyokyo Kidney Research Institute, Hirosaki, Japan.

References

1. Yokoyama M, Fujii Y, Takeshita H, Kawamura N, Nakayama T, Iimura Y, et al. Renal function after radical nephrectomy: development and validation of predictive models in Japanese patients. Int J Urol. 2014;21:238–42.
2. Kawamura N, Yokoyama M, Fujii Y, Ishioka J, Numao N, Matsuoka Y, et al. Recovery of renal function after radical nephrectomy and risk factors for postoperative severe renal impairment: a Japanese multicenter longitudinal study. Int J Urol. 2016;23:219–23.
3. Takeshita H, Yokoyama M, Fujii Y, Chiba K, Ishioka J, Noro A, et al. Impact of renal function on cardiovascular events in patients undergoing radical nephrectomy for renal cancer. J Urol. 2012;19:722–8.
4. Lane BR, Campbell SC, Demirjian S, Fergany AF. Surgically induced chronic kidney disease may be associated with a lower risk of progression and mortality than medical chronic kidney disease. J Urol. 2013;189:1649–55.
5. Demirjian S, Lane BR, Derweesh IH, Takagi T, Fergany A, Campbell SC. Chronic kidney disease due to surgical removal of nephrons: relative rates of progression and survival. J Urol. 2014;192:1057–62.
6. Go AS, Chertow GM, Fan D, McCulloch CE, Hsu CY. Chronic kidney disease and the risks of death, cardiovascular events, and hospitalization. N Engl J Med. 2004;351:1296–305.
7. Levey AS, Coresh J. Chronic kidney disease. Lancet. 2012;379:165–80.
8. Lane BR, Demirjian S, Derweesh IH, Takagi T, Zhang Z, Velet L, et al. Survival and functional stability in chronic kidney disease due to surgical removal of nephrons: Importance of the new baseline glomerular filtration rate. Eur Urol. 2015;68:996–1003.
9. Walsh CR, Cupples LA, Levy D, Kiel DP, Hannan M, Wilson PW, et al. Abdominal aortic calcific deposits are associated with increased risk for congestive heart failure: the framingham heart study. Am Heart J. 2002;144:733–9.
10. Nakagami H, Osako MK, Morishita R. New concept of vascular calcification and metabolism. Curr Vasc Pharmacol. 2011;9:124–7.

11. Thomas IC, Ratigan AR, Rifkin DE, Ix JH, Criqui MH, Budoff MJ, et al. The association of renal artery calcification with hypertension in community-living individuals: the multiethnic study of atherosclerosis. J Am Soc Hypertens. 2015;10:167–74.

12. Imanishi K, Hatakeyama S, Yamamoto H, Okamoto A, Imai A, Yoneyama T, et al. Post-transplant renal function and cardiovascular events are closely associated with the aortic calcification index in renal transplant recipients. Transplant Proc. 2014;46:484–8.

13. Li LC, Lee YT, Lee YW, Chou CA, Lee CT. Aortic arch calcification predicts the renal function progression in patients with stage 3 to 5 chronic kidney disease. Biomed Res Int. 2015; doi:10.1155/2015/131263

14. Imai E, Horio M, Iseki K, Yamagata K, Watanabe T, Hara S, et al. Prevalence of chronic kidney disease (CKD) in the Japanese general population predicted by the MDRD equation modified by a Japanese coefficient. Clin Exp Nephrol. 2007;11:156–63.

15. Tsushima M, Terayama Y, Momose A, Funyu T, Ohyama C, Hada R. Carotid intima media thickness and aortic calcification index closely relate to cerebro- and cardiovascular disorders in hemodialysis patients. Int J Urol. 2008;15:48–51.

16. Fujita N, Hatakeyama S, Yamamoto H, Tobisawa Y, Yoneyama T, Yoneyama T, et al. Implication of aortic calcification on persistent hypertension after laparoscopic adrenalectomy in patients with primary aldosteronism. Int J Urol. 2016;23:412–7.

17. Canepa M, Ameri P, AlGhatrif M, Pestelli G, Milaneschi Y, Strait JB, et al. Role of bone mineral density in the inverse relationship between body size and aortic calcification: results from the baltimore longitudinal study of aging. Atherosclerosis. 2014;235:169–75.

18. Byon CH, Chen Y. Molecular mechanisms of vascular calcification in chronic kidney disease: the link between bone and the vasculature. Curr Osteoporos Rep. 2015;13:206–15.

19. Nishimura S, Manabe I, Nagasaki M, Eto K, Yamashita H, Ohsugi M, et al. CD8+ effector T cells contribute to macrophage recruitment and adipose tissue inflammation in obesity. Nat Med. 2009;15:914–20.

20. Bortnick AE, Bartz TM, Ix JH, Chonchol M, Reiner A, Cushman M, et al. Association of inflammatory, lipid and mineral markers with cardiac calcification in older adults. Heart. 2016; doi:10.1136/heartjnl-2016-309404.

21. Elseweidy MM, Zein N, Aldhamy SE, Elsawy MM, Saeid SA. Policosanol as a new inhibitor candidate for vascular calcification in diabetic hyperlipidemic rats. Exp Biol Med. 2016;241:1943–9.

29

Multiparametric ultrasound: evaluation of greyscale, shear wave elastography and contrast-enhanced ultrasound for prostate cancer detection and localization in correlation to radical prostatectomy specimens

Christophe K. Mannaerts[1][*] ⓘ, Rogier R. Wildeboer[2], Arnoud W. Postema[1], Johanna Hagemann[3], Lars Budäus[3], Derya Tilki[3], Massimo Mischi[2], Hessel Wijkstra[1,2] and Georg Salomon[3]

Abstract

Background: The diagnostic pathway for prostate cancer (PCa) is advancing towards an imaging-driven approach. Multiparametric magnetic resonance imaging, although increasingly used, has not shown sufficient accuracy to replace biopsy for now. The introduction of new ultrasound (US) modalities, such as quantitative contrast-enhanced US (CEUS) and shear wave elastography (SWE), shows promise but is not evidenced by sufficient high quality studies, especially for the combination of different US modalities. The primary objective of this study is to determine the individual and complementary diagnostic performance of greyscale US (GS), SWE, CEUS and their combination, multiparametric ultrasound (mpUS), for the detection and localization of PCa by comparison with corresponding histopathology.

Methods/design: In this prospective clinical trial, US imaging consisting of GS, SWE and CEUS with quantitative mapping on 3 prostate imaging planes (base, mid and apex) will be performed in 50 patients with biopsy-proven PCa before planned radical prostatectomy using a clinical ultrasound scanner. All US imaging will be evaluated by US readers, scoring the four quadrants of each imaging plane for the likelihood of significant PCa based on a 1 to 5 Likert Scale. Following resection, PCa tumour foci will be identified, graded and attributed to the imaging-derived quadrants in each prostate plane for all prostatectomy specimens. Primary outcome measure will be the sensitivity, specificity, negative predictive value and positive predictive value of each US modality and mpUS to detect and localize significant PCa evaluated for different Likert Scale thresholds using receiver operating characteristics curve analyses.

Discussion: In the evaluation of new PCa imaging modalities, a structured comparison with gold standard radical prostatectomy specimens is essential as first step. This trial is the first to combine the most promising ultrasound

(Continued on next page)

* Correspondence: c.k.mannaerts@amc.uva.nl
[1]Department of Urology, Amsterdam University Medical Centers, University of Amsterdam, Amsterdam, The Netherlands
Full list of author information is available at the end of the article

(Continued from previous page)

modalities into mpUS. It complies with the IDEAL stage 2b recommendations and will be an important step towards the evaluation of mpUS as a possible option for accurate detection and localization of PCa.

Keywords: Prostate cancer, Imaging, Ultrasound, Multiparametric, Radical prostatectomy, Detection, Accuracy

Background

To date, patients with a clinical suspicion of prostate cancer (PCa) based on elevated serum prostate specific antigen (PSA) and/or a suspicious digital rectal examination (DRE) should undergo a transrectal ultrasound (TRUS)-guided systematic biopsy as next step in assessing presence of PCa [1]. This combination of tests results in a considerable rate of benign biopsy results, overdiagnosis of clinically insignificant PCa and underdiagnosis and undergrading of clinically significant PCa [2, 3]. Moreover, systematic transrectal biopsy carries significant morbidity [4]. As a consequence, the diagnostic pathway for PCa has begun to lean towards an imaging-driven targeted biopsy approach. Multiparametric magnetic resonance imaging (mpMRI) of the prostate and targeted biopsies of suspicious mpMRI lesions has evolved into an increasingly appealing tool in the PCa diagnostic arsenal and is currently recommended in men with a sustained suspicion of PCa after a negative initial biopsy [1]. The exact role for mpMRI in PCa diagnosis remains unclear, however; improved clinically significant PCa detection compared with systematic biopsy is controversial in biopsy-naïve patients and mpMRI as a triage test before biopsy seems to miss significant PCa [5, 6]. Moreover, universal implementation of an mpMRI pathway seems unlikely for now, given the relatively high cost, low specificity with high rates of false positives, moderate inter-reader reproducibility and radiology training burden, limiting its broad use outside expert centres [7–9].

Ultrasound modalities as well as their combination in a multiparametric approach are gaining increasing interest [10, 11]. Although conventional greyscale (GS) TRUS as imaging modality has a limited role in PCa diagnosis with sensitivity and positive predictive value (PPV) generally reported to be around 11–35% and 27–57%, respectively, ultrasound-based imaging offers many advantages [12, 13]. Ultrasound imaging is widely available, portable, less expensive in machine purchase and usage than MRI with the additional possibility of real-time imaging and biopsy needle monitoring. These advantages have motivated towards the development of various new ultrasound modalities striving to increase PCa detection including contrast-enhanced ultrasound (CEUS), computerized TRUS and (shear wave) elastography. Particularly, CEUS with quantitative parametric imaging and shear wave elastography (SWE) have produced encouraging results in recent studies [14, 15].

In CEUS, a suspension of gas-filled microbubbles, i.e. ultrasound contrast agents (UCAs) is used for visualization of microvascular flow patterns. Contrast-specific imaging is achieved by differentiating the non-linear scattering produced by the microbubbles from the linear tissue reflections. In PCa, abnormal blood flow patterns can be observed with CEUS and adding CEUS-targeted cores to the systematic biopsy procedure resulted in improved per-patient PCa detection rates [16, 17]. However, angiogenic microvascular cancer patterns can be ambiguous as higher blood flow by shunt formation and a higher microvascular density are counteracted by an increase in interstitial pressure and tortuosity [18]. To overcome this ambiguous effect of angiogenesis on blood flow limiting visual interpretation and perfusion-based quantification of CEUS, dispersion quantification techniques have been developed for a more detailed assessment of the UCA kinetics in the prostate. Several promising dispersion parameters have been extracted from recorded time-intensity-curves (TICs) and converted into parametric maps of the prostate with encouraging results in clinical prediction of PCa presence [14, 19].

SWE estimates tissue elasticity and can discriminate PCa, as malignancy typically shows increased stiffness, because of higher cellular density and collagen depositions [20]. In an SWE examination, an acoustic radiation force push pulse, induces a shear wave whose propagation is captured with an ultrafast ultrasonic imaging protocol. The speed of the shear wave is linked to the stiffness properties of the medium through which it propagates. SWE provides a dynamic quantitative map of soft-tissue elastic properties in near real time and is parametrically presented as a colour-coded overlay on the greyscale images [12, 21]. In two prostate biopsy studies, suspicious findings on SWE were at high risk of harboring clinically significant PCa while SWE targeted biopsy demonstrated equal per-core detection rates compared to systematic biopsy [22, 23]. Moreover, one study demonstrated that SWE allowed the identification of resection pathology proven PCa foci based on SWE density thresholds, potentially allowing for reader independent localization of prostate cancer foci [15].

Combining CEUS and SWE in a multiparametric ultrasound (mpUS) approach, in a similar fashion as mpMRI, could potentially reduce the risk of missing tumours that are not visible to one of the modalities and discriminate benign prostatic diseases like prostatitis that sometimes mimic malignant characteristics. Brock. et al. demonstrated in their mpUS study of 86 patients, with radical prostatectomy specimens as reference standard, that the addition of CEUS for lesions detected on strain elastography significantly decreased false-positive results (34.9% to 10.3%) and improved PPV from 65.1 to 89.7% [10]. With the known learning curve to perform strain elastography, the use of quantification software, inherent in SWE and as adjunct to CEUS, can not only improve diagnostic accuracy but also decrease user-dependency and training time while improving clinical applicability.

In this study protocol paper we will describe our present study evaluating the diagnostic accuracy of GS, SWE and CEUS with parametric mapping and its combination mpUS for the detection and localization of (clinically significant) PCa with radical prostatectomy specimens as reference standard. Additionally, this study will contribute to the development of a classifier algorithm, fully exploiting and integrating the complementary information of the different ultrasound modalities into a single parametric map.

Methods/design
Study objectives
Primary objectives
To determine the diagnostic performance i.e. sensitivity, specificity, PPV and negative predictive value (NPV) of GS, SWE, CEUS with quantitative mapping and their combination, mpUS, for the localization of clinically significant PCa foci.

Clinically significant PCa for the purpose of the primary objectives will be defined as the presence of a histopathologically confirmed Gleason $\geq 3 + 4 = 7$ tumour focus with a tumour volume > 0.5 cm^3.

Secondary objective(s)
To determine the diagnostic performance i.e. sensitivity, specificity, PPV and NPV of GS, SWE, CEUS with quantitative mapping and their combination mpUS for the detection and localization of PCa foci:

- for different thresholds of clinical significance; namely presence of a Gleason $\geq 4 + 3 = 7$ tumour focus and presence of a Gleason $\geq 3 + 4 = 7$ tumour focus, independent of volume, respectively
- in relation to the specific region of the prostate (peripheral zone versus transition zone)

To assess the technical feasibility, image quality and procedure related adverse events

To assess the interobserver agreement between US readers with difference levels of experience

To develop a classifier algorithm combining complementary information in the different ultrasound modalities into one single multiparametric map.

Expected outcomes
It is expected that mpUS has the potential to improve PCa diagnosis and clinical decision making compared to currently applied diagnostic tests, as combining modalities has the potential to detect more tumours while being more specific as more different characteristics of suspicious lesions are evaluated. There is however limited data on the performance of combinations of ultrasound modalities [12]. Nelson et al. compared GS, Colour Doppler ultrasound and (strain) elastography targeted biopsies with sextant systematic biopsies as reference standard in 137 patients [24]. GS, Colour Doppler and elastography were positive in 16%, 29% and 25% of the 106 biopsy sites, respectively while the combination was positive in 46%, showing that the three modalities detect different tumours. Previously mentioned, Brock et al. demonstrated in their study that the addition of CEUS for lesions detected on real-time elastography decreased false-positive results and improved PPV [10]. None of these studies have included the quantitative techniques of our current study. Recently, Wildeboer et al. demonstrated in their study with 45 CEUS recordings, in 19 patients referred for radical prostatectomy, that the combination of CEUS parameters extracted from TICs performed better in detecting PCa than a single CEUS parameter with an accuracy of 81% for the combination compared to 73% for the best performing single parameter. Moreover the NPV increased to 83% from 70% [19]. Based on the available data, we expect that our mpUS will demonstrate higher diagnostic performance than the ultrasound techniques as stand alone.

Study design
This study is a prospective, single center, single group, in-vivo study in humans in which we will perform ultrasound imaging in patients with biopsy-proven PCa scheduled for radical prostatectomy. These patients will undergo ultrasound imaging using a clinical ultrasound scanner (Aixplorer®, Supersonic Imagine, Aix-en-Provence, France) with an endfire endorectal probe (Super Endocavity™ SE12–3, Supersonic Imagine, Aix-en-Provence, France). The ultrasound scanner and probe are illustrated in Fig. 1. CEUS imaging requires the administration of a UCA bolus. SonoVue® (Bracco, Geneva, Switzerland), a well-tolerated and commonly used UCA, will be used through an intravenous cannula for the purpose of this study. After written informed consent, patients will undergo mpUS imaging the day prior to surgery. The prostate is examined in 3 planes (base, mid and apex of the prostate) using the 3 principal scanning

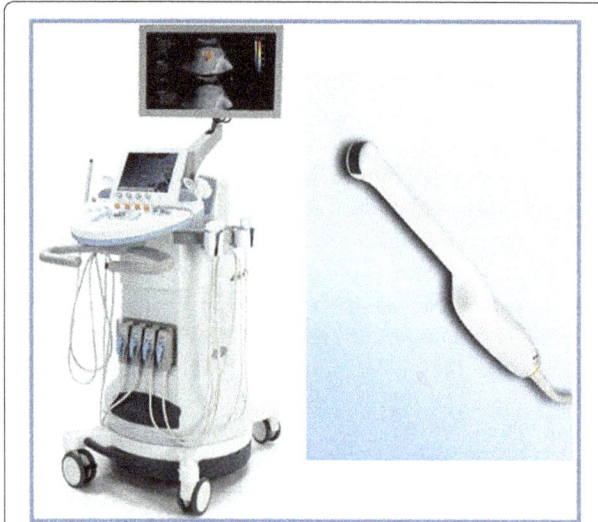

Fig. 1 The ultrasound system and endorectal probe. Legend: Ultrasound scanner (Aixplorer®, Supersonic Imagine, Aix-en-Provence, France) and endorectal probe (SuperEndocavity™ SE12–3 with number of elements: 192 and bandwith: 3–12 MHz, Supersonic Imagine, Aix-en-Provence, France) used for the purpose of this study

modalities (GS, SWE and CEUS) sequentially. Usage of Colour Doppler and Power Doppler are left to the discretion of the ultrasound performer to avoid excessive scanning times. All scans will be recorded and exported as DICOM files with quantitative analysis of the CEUS recordings carried out remotely after the scan. At a later stage, recorded images will be evaluated independently by blinded readers, scoring the four quadrants of each imaging plane for the likelihood of clinically significant PCa based on a 1 to 5 Likert-scale for the different ultrasound modalities alone and for mpUS. Following resection, histopathologic analysis is performed according to institution standards with PCa tumour foci identified, graded and attributed to the imaging-derived quadrants in each prostate plane for all the prostatectomy specimens. Accurate registration of imaging and histopathology is reached using a standardized histopathology correlation protocol consisting of three-dimensional (3D) histopathological and imaging modelling, a registration procedure and a correlation step [25, 26]. This explorative study is in agreement with the IDEAL stage 2b recommendations [27].

Population
Study population
The study population consists of the men with biopsy-proven prostate cancer that are scheduled for a radical prostatectomy. All patients will be recruited in the Martini Clinic, Prostate Cancer Center (Hamburg, Germany) and all study procedures will be performed in this institution. Patients will be informed about the study in oral and written form. Patient inclusion is confirmed

by signing written informed consent. A total of 50 consecutive patients will be included in the study.

Inclusion and exclusion criteria
All inclusion and exclusion criteria are presented in Table 1. Exclusion criteria are based on contra-indications for ultrasound contrast agent usage and selected to allow a complete and reliable histopathological specimen analysis (no previous PCa therapy or hormonal therapy) and to maintain SWE image quality (upper prostate volume threshold of 80 mL). To better reflect the clinical practice where mpUS will be applied in the future if proven valuable, high risk patients with highly elevated PSA levels above 20 ng/mL and/or a clinical T3 digital rectal examination, will be excluded, as diagnostic imaging is less relevant in these patients.

Study procedures
Multiparametric ultrasound
After placement of an intravenous access, transrectal ultrasound imaging will be performed in the left-lateral decubitus position by one ultrasound performer. A total scanning time of 30 min is anticipated.

Greyscale
After standard prostate volumetry and evaluation of the prostate capsule and seminal vesicles, transversal and sagittal sweeps of the entire prostate are slowly captured using GS ultrasound. Abnormal echogenicity patterns (calcifications, cysts and hypo-echoic lesions) are documented while the operator visually determines and stores pictures of the base, mid and apical transverse plane of

Table 1 Inclusion and exclusion criteria

Inclusion Criteria

1. Patients ≥18 years old

2. Biopsy proven prostate cancer

3. Treatment by radical prostatectomy (open or robot-assisted)

4. Signed informed consent

Exclusion Criteria

1. PSA > 20 ng/mL and or clinical T3 rectal examination

2. Prostate volume above 80 mL measured on TRUS

3. Radiation therapy, focal therapy and/or chemotherapy for prostate cancer

4. Inability to undergo TRUS

5. Any form of hormonal therapy or androgen deprivation therapy within 6 months prior to procedure

6. Any contraindication for the ultrasound contrast agent including cardiac right to left shunt, pulmonary hypertension, uncontrolled hypertension, instable coronary disease

7. Has any medical condition or circumstance which would significantly decrease the chances of obtaining reliable data, achieving study objectives, or completing the study

interest taking into account the anatomical shape of the prostate. If areas of the prostate are considered more suspicious outside the anatomically chosen imaging planes, these are also brought into view and stored.

Shear wave elastography

Before SWE imaging, SWE specific settings (maximized penetration and appropriate elasticity scale) are checked and if necessary optimized while SWE examinations will be performed with minimal preload (pre-compressions). Each pre-defined transverse plane will be scanned with the SWE box in unilateral (left/right only) and bilateral (entire plane; maximum prostate plane coverage) fashion. For each scan, the transducer is maintained in a steady position for 5 s to make sure the signal is stable. Pictures and cine loops are stored for determination of elasticity values at a later stage. If areas of the prostate are considered more suspicious on SWE outside the predetermined imaging planes, these are also brought into view. An example of SWE is provided in Fig. 2.

Contrast-enhanced ultrasound and quantification

CEUS settings (dynamic range, focus zone and mechanical index) are checked and optimized per patient. A total of 3 CEUS recordings will be made: One for each of the pre-defined planes. Each of the 2-min recordings will be started following the administration of a 2.4-mL bolus of UCA. After each recording a pause of 3 min is observed to allow the inflow of the next UCA bolus after sufficient UCA breakdown. A 4th bolus can be used if imaging quality due to e.g. patient movement is determined to be insufficient for quantitative analysis or for an area outside the imaging planes that is considered more suspicious on greyscale and/or SWE.

CEUS recordings will be stored and transferred for quantitative analysis. In this study, we will use the Contrast Ultrasound Dispersion Imaging (CUDI) analysis of the Eindhoven University of Technology with computer-aided quantification and parametric mapping [28, 29]. In short, this method quantifies the dispersive effects in the contrast concentration kinetics on a pixel basis by spatiotemporal analysis of the UCA in- and outflow during the CEUS recording. Several dispersion parameters have been derived that show promising results in prediction of PCa presence using radical prostatectomy specimens as the reference standard with a receiver-operating-characteristic (ROC) area under the curve (AUC) ranging from 0.84–0.89 [28, 30–32]. The resulting colour-coded parametric maps can be used to assess PCa presence. An example of CEUS and CUDI is provided in Fig. 3.

Radical prostatectomy and histopathology

The radical prostatectomy (open or robot-assisted laparoscopic) will be performed in accordance to institution standards. In the majority of patients (> 90%) an intraoperative neurovascular structure-adjacent frozen section examination technique will therefore be performed. In this procedure, frozen sections are taken from one or both lateral side(s) of the prostate to enable the sparing of nerves while decreasing positive surgical margins [33]. These frozen sections are processed separately from the resected specimen in the pathology lab. Following the radical prostatectomy, the whole specimen and frozen sections will be macroscopically photographed. The resection specimen is fixated and dissected in 4-mm thick transversal slices and quadrant sections with the location and orientation of all coupes recorded. Pathologic analysis will be performed by dedicated genitourinary pathologists, unaware of imaging results, who will evaluate the entire specimen for presence of tumour (marking each lesion's Gleason score), extracapsular invasion and seminal vesicle invasion. Individual foci of tumour will be outlined.

Histopathologic correlation of imaging

All US imaging, each sequence separate and combined, will be evaluated by US readers in blinded fashion. The four quadrants (left and right peripheral zone and left and right transition zone, respectively) of each imaging plane (base, mid and apex) will be evaluated for the likelihood of clinically significant PCa based on a five-point Likert Scale (1: highly unlikely; 2: unlikely; 3: equivocal; 4: likely; and 5: highly likely), resulting in a total of 12 regions of interest (ROIs) per prostate. Examiners are blinded for clinical and pathological data but aware that patients are scheduled for radical prostatectomy.

Matching of US imaging with histopathology is a challenge; not only do the deformations of the prostate after resection have to be taken into account, but also the mismatch in orientation between imaging planes and pathology slices and deformation due to transrectal probe usage. To provide for an accurate histopathologic correlation a three-step process combing reconstruction, registration and correlation is used in line with our previous published work [25, 26, 34]. First, a 3D histopathological reconstruction with adequate interpolation of tumour delineations into tumour volumes is performed based on the pathology slices. Hereafter, a 3D US model of the in-vivo prostate is reconstructed from the 2D greyscale sweeps [25, 26]. Thirdly, a 3D, surface-based elastic registration method is used to fuse the in-vivo 3D US model with the 3D histopathological model. This method avoids the need of landmarks or a high level of detail, often lacking in greyscale US, while no manual intervention is required during the registration [26]. Lastly, the registered 3D models are correlated to the actual images with superposition of histopathology onto the ultrasound imaging with its 12 ROIs per prostate. Figure 4 provides a schematic overview of a full registration procedure.

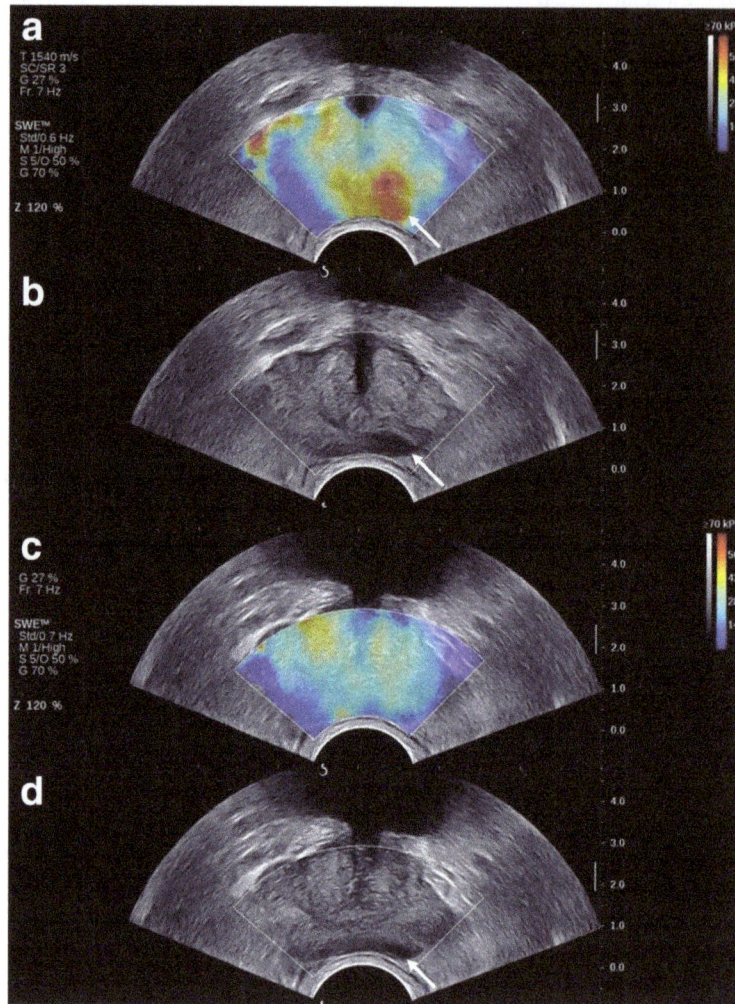

Fig. 2 Shearwave elastography imaging of the prostate. Legend: An area with decreased tissue elasticity is visible in the left side of the prostate in the mid plane on SWE (white arrow) (**a**). This area is also visible as hypo-echogenious lesion on the corresponding greyscale image (white arrow) (**b**). A normal SWE pattern is visible in the base plane with the peripheral zone homogeneous coded in blue and the transition zone slightly heterogeneous in yellow (**c**). There is still some hypoechogenicity visible on the corresponding greyscale image (white arrow) (**d**). Radical prostatectomy revealed a Gleason 3 + 4 = 7 PCa with its primary focus in the left mid and apex of the prostate while the left base of the prostate was free of PCa tumour

Statistical analysis and sample size

Demographic and disease specific characteristics of the study population will be descriptively reported. For localization of PCa, a logistic generalized estimating equation (GEE) model, accounting for the fact that 12 ROIs will be analysed in the same patient, will be used to estimate the sensitivity, specificity, PPV and NPV for the three different US modalities and any combination of those, both for different Likert scale thresholds (Likert ≥3 and Likert ≥4) as for the predefined criteria of clinically significant PCa. In principle, the model will contain US modality, reader and their interaction. Sensitivity is defined as the probability of correctly identifying a tumour focus in a given ROI. Specificity is defined as the probability of correctly identifying ROIs negative for tumour. The effect of histopathological variables (Gleason score, lesion size and

pT-stage) will be tested for the sensitivity of each US modality. For detection, readers with Likert scores ≥4 for any clinically significant PCa-containing ROI are considered to have detected PCa in that particular patient. The interobserver agreement will be evaluated using the intraclass correlation coefficient.

No formal sample size calculation was performed. In line with the IDEAL recommendations for explorative studies and published (mpMRI) studies with a similar design a total of 50 patients will be included in the study [35–37].

Quality and patient safety

Quality of data and patient safety will be continuously monitored by the investigators. Periodical reporting of study progression and patient safety will be performed to the reviewing Institutional Review Board (IRB). The

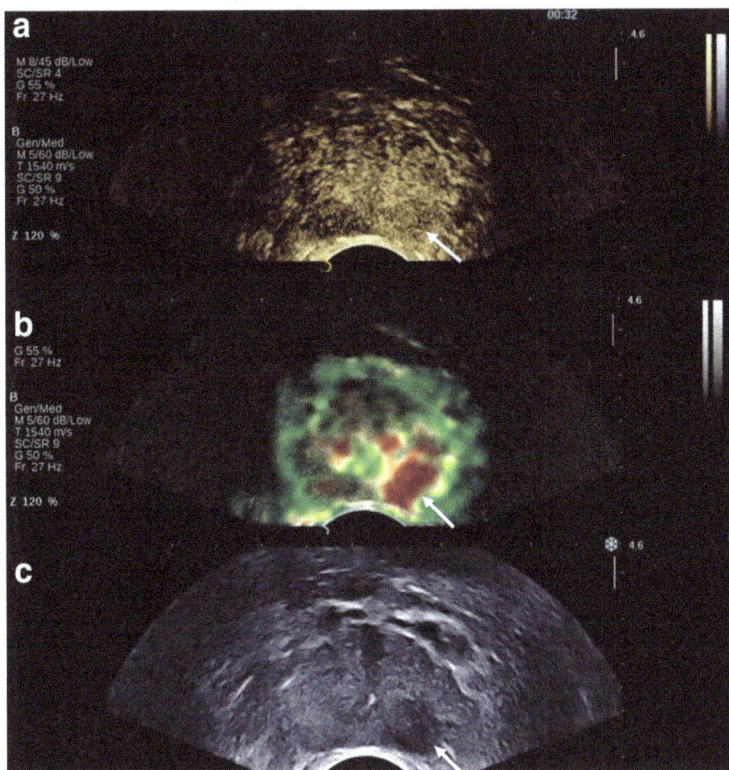

Fig. 3 Contrast-enhanced ultrasound and contrast dispersion ultrasound imaging of the prostate. Legend: An area of early contrast enhancement is visible in the left peripheral zone of the prostate in the apical plane (white arrow) (**a**). Quantitative analysis with the Péclet CUDI parameter demonstrates a suspicious red lesion on the parametric image (white arrow) (**b**). The suspicious area is also visible as hypo-echogenious lesion on the corresponding greyscale image (white arrow) (**c**). Radical prostatectomy revealed a pT3a, Gleason 3 + 4 = 7 with tertiary pattern 5 PCa on the left apical side of the prostate

investigator will inform the subjects and the reviewing IRB if anything occurs of which the disadvantages of participation may be significantly greater than was foreseen in the research proposal. The investigators will notify the IRB without undue delay of a temporary halt including reason for such an action. The investigators will take care that all subjects are kept informed.

Risks and benefits

TRUS imaging of the prostate is safe and well tolerated. There is a small anticipated risk in this study because of the UCA usage. After its use in thousands of patients, adverse events related to UCAs appear to be mild, rare and transient [38–40]. Sensations of warmth, facial or general flushes and itching (at injection site) are the

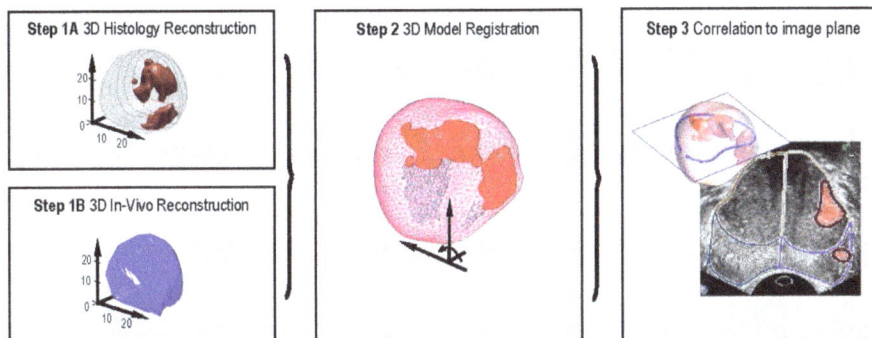

Fig. 4 Schematic overview of a full registration framework for the correlation of the ultrasound image with histopathology. Legend: A 3D reconstruction of the ex-vivo radical prostatectomy specimen and in-vivo gland (Step 1A and 1B); registration between the in-vivo and ex-vivo model (Step 2); Correlation of the pathology data and ultrasound image (Step 3); Pixel-wise superposition of the histopathological data onto the ultrasound image

most frequently reported minor side effects. Serious adverse reactions, which consists of hypersensitivity allergic reactions are rare (< 0.01%), but comprehensive rescue measures are prepared and available for all the patients in the study. There is no direct benefit for patients included in this study. Results of this study, however, can be important for future patients in the diagnostic work-up for PCa. Patients will be informed of the risks and absence of benefit, and both will be described in the study information

Discussion

New ultrasound modalities with quantitative techniques, such as SWE and CEUS with parametric mapping, are gaining interest. The exploration of these techniques in a multiparametric fashion is essential for the development of an ultrasound-based imaging approach with the potential of real-time PCa imaging and targeted biopsy. This study, including a ground truth reference standard, will give insight into different US features of PCa and into its combined diagnostic value. Furthermore this study will provide information on the question whether mpUS could potentially be used as a triage test to exclude significant PCa or should be used to target specific regions suspicious for significant PCa or both. With accurate registration and fusion gaining attention for reliable image-targeted biopsies and (focal) treatment, we believe that our study also contributes to the introduction of suitable registration/fusion options.

Its design with radical prostatectomy specimens as reference standard, however also comes with some disadvantages. First, the population is different from the primary diagnostic setting since men must have PCa and choose to have surgery (spectrum bias). Second, the reader examining the images is aware that there must be PCa, potentially biasing readers towards higher sensitivity readings (observer bias). However, studies using a more appropriate population with prostate biopsy specimens as reference standard, fail to detect all clinically significant lesions found after radical prostatectomy, even in a template-guided transperineal saturation setting [1, 41]. Despite this important limitation of prostate biopsy as reference standard, a biopsy study can be foreseen as next step in the clinical assessment of mpUS imaging for PCa diagnosis. After all, the clinical utility of a targeted biopsy approach for mpUS suspicious lesions cannot be accurately assessed in this study as a targeted biopsy procedure is not only dependent on the scoring of lesions on mpUS but also dependent on other factors such as targeting accuracy, biopsy operator experience and patient movement.

Another limitation of this study is that the prostate is evaluated in 2D US imaging planes. There is a risk of missing tumours outside the predefined imaging planes while the UCA transport kinetics have to be modelled

with strong assumptions in its directionality [31]. Although a 3D approach can overcome these limitations and reduce the number of UCA bolus injections, no clinical US device is currently available with both 3D SWE and 3D CEUS imaging.

We have chosen for a stringent 12 region based template per prostate for our analysis. Although, in comparison with the prostate imaging reporting and data system version 2 (PI-RADSv2), this is a limited number of regions, we assume that this approach is the best approximation for US and pathology matching as more ROIs per template would increase the risk of registration errors. Besides the well-known errors in the registration procedure of ultrasound imaging and pathology caused by gland deformation, fixation-related shrinkage and a mismatch in US imaging and pathology orientation, the intraoperative frozen section examination have to be taken into account in our study [42, 43]. To assess the influence of the registration between imaging and histopathology on the final results, separate analyses including and excluding ROIs with small tumors (with respect to the ROIs) and inconsistencies across multiple ROIs are foreseen. Besides, studies with PI-RADSv2 or more ROIs per template often also simplify their template for analysis or use more tolerant approaches for misalignment with inclusion of neighboring regions [44–46].

Lastly, further research regarding improvements to the standardization and reproducibility of these ultrasound modalities as stand-alone tools and in a multiparametric fashion is still required. Various ultrasound manufacturers have introduced SWE into their ultrasound scanners and computer-aided quantification and parametric mapping of CEUS recording with CUDI is not limited to a specific ultrasound scanner. Therefore, there is an increasing need to define quality criteria for these new techniques, provided that results of our study are positive, in order to improve clinical application and generalizability of these techniques in other centres with their own local expertise and resources [47, 48].

Despite these limitations, we expect that the results of this study will contribute to the assessment of the role of mpUS imaging for the diagnosis of PCa in clinical practice. In light of current limitations of prostate biopsy and mpMRI, mpUS holds the potential for an accessible imaging-based PCa approach.

Abbreviations

(PI-RADSv2): Prostate imaging reporting and data system version 2; AUC: Area under the curve; CEUS: Contrast - enhanced ultrasound; CUDI: Contrast ultrasound dispersion imaging; DRE: Digital rectal examination; EAU: European Association of Urology; GS: Gleason score; IRB: Institutional Review Board; mpMRI: Multiparametric magnetic resonance imaging; mpUS: Multiparametric ultrasound; NPV: Negative predictive value; PCa: Prostate cancer; PPV: Positive predictive value; PSA: Prostate specific antigen; SWE: Shear wave elastography; TIC: Time-intensity-curve; TRUS: Transrectal ultrasound; UCA: Ultrasound contrast agent

Acknowledgements
We acknowledge Supersonic Imagine (Aix-en-Provence, France) for providing the Aixplorer® Ultrasound Platform and technical support.

Funding
This trial is funded by the Dutch Cancer Society (grant number: UVA 2013–5941). The funding body had no role in the design of the study and collection, analysis, and interpretation of data and in writing the manuscript.

Authors' contributions
CKM, AWP, HW and GS conceived the trial concept and designed the protocol for IRB approval. CKM, RRW, JH and GS organized the trial logistics. RRW and MM facilitate quantitative CEUS analysis. CKM, RRW oversee the interpretation for this study. CKM and RRW drafted the manuscript. All authors (CKM, RRW, AWP, JH, LB, DT, MM, HW and GS) reviewed and approved the final manuscript. CKM, RRW, GS and HW had full access to the final trial dataset.

Ethics approval and consent to participate
This trial will be conducted in accordance to the Good Clinical Practice standards, with the ethical principles that have their origins in the Declaration of Helsinki (Fortealiza, Brazil, October 2013). The trial protocol has been reviewed and approved by the IRB of the University Hospital Hamburg-Eppendorf (Ethik-Kommission der Ärztekammer Hamburg), Germany under study ID: PV5439 on February 13, 2017 and prospectively registered on the clinicaltrials.gov database (NCT03091231) on March 14, 2017. Any amendments to the trial protocol will be submitted for review by the IRB. Trial registrations will be updated and participants will be informed about the risks and benefits of participation both verbally by one of the investigators and in writing in the form of an extensive patient information brochure. Participants will only be included after written informed consent has been obtained by the medical doctor performing the multiparametric ultrasound imaging. Patients can leave the study at any time for any reason if they wish to do so without any consequences. The investigator can decide to withdraw a subject from the study for urgent (medical) reasons. Patient data will be anonymized and stored in a secure database.

Consent for publication
Not applicable

Competing interests
All authors of this manuscript declare no relationships with any companies, products or services related to the matter of the study.

Author details
[1]Department of Urology, Amsterdam University Medical Centers, University of Amsterdam, Amsterdam, The Netherlands. [2]Department of Electrical Engineering, Eindhoven University of Technology, Eindhoven, The Netherlands. [3]Martini Clinic, Prostate Cancer Center, University Hospital Hamburg-Eppendorf, Hamburg, Germany.

References
1. Mottet N, Bellmunt J, Bolla M, Briers E, Cumberbatch MG, De Santis M, et al. EAU-ESTRO-SIOG Guidelines on Prostate Cancer. Part 1: Screening, Diagnosis, and Local Treatment with Curative Intent. Eur Urol. 2016;1–12. https://doi.org/10.1016/j.eururo.2016.08.003.
2. Bjurlin MA, Carter HB, Schellhammer P, Cookson MS, Gomella LG, Troyer D, et al. Optimization of initial prostate biopsy in clinical practice: sampling, labeling and specimen processing. J Urol. 2013;189:2039–46.
3. Abraham NE, Mendhiratta N, Taneja SS. Patterns of repeat prostate biopsy in contemporary clinical practice. J Urol. 2015;193:1178–84. https://doi.org/10.1016/j.juro.2014.10.084.
4. Loeb S, Vellekoop A, Ahmed HU, Catto J, Emberton M, Nam R, et al. Systematic review of complications of prostate biopsy. Eur Urol. 2013;64: 876–92. https://doi.org/10.1016/j.eururo.2013.05.049.
5. Schoots IG, Roobol MJ, Nieboer D, Bangma CH, Steyerberg EW, Hunink MGM. Magnetic resonance imaging-targeted biopsy may enhance the diagnostic accuracy of significant prostate Cancer detection compared to standard Transrectal ultrasound-guided biopsy: a systematic review and meta-analysis. Eur Urol. 2015;68:438–50.
6. Moldovan PC, Van den Broeck T, Sylvester R, Marconi L, Bellmunt J, van den Bergh RCN, et al. What is the negative predictive value of multiparametric magnetic resonance imaging in excluding prostate Cancer at biopsy? A Systematic Review and Meta-analysis from the European Association of Urology Prostate Cancer Guidelines Panel. Eur Urol. 2017;72:250–66.
7. Mertan FV, Greer MD, Shih JH, George AK, Kongnyuy M, Muthigi A, et al. Prospective evaluation of the prostate imaging reporting and data system version 2 for prostate Cancer detection. J Urol. 2016;196:690–6. https://doi.org/10.1016/j.juro.2016.04.057.
8. Muller BG, Shih JH, Sankineni S, Marko J, Rais-Bahrami S, George A, et al. Prostate Cancer: Interobserver Agreement and Accuracy with the Revised Prostate Imaging Reporting and Data System at Multiparametric MR Imaging. Radiology. 2015;277 May 2016:142818.
9. Zhao C, Gao G, Fang D, Li F, Yang X, Wang H, et al. The efficiency of multiparametric magnetic resonance imaging (mpMRI) using PI-RADS version 2 in the diagnosis of clinically significant prostate cancer. Clin Imaging. 2016;40:885–8. https://doi.org/10.1016/j.clinimag.2016.04.010.
10. Brock M, Eggert T, Palisaar RJ, Roghmann F, Braun K, Löppenberg B, et al. Multiparametric ultrasound of the prostate: adding contrast enhanced ultrasound to real-time elastography to detect histopathologically confirmed cancer. J Urol. 2013;189:93–8. https://doi.org/10.1016/j.juro.2012.08.183.
11. Grey A, Scott R, Charman S, Der J Van, Frinking P, Acher P, et al. The CADMUS trial – Multi-parametric ultrasound targeted biopsies compared to multi-parametric MRI targeted biopsies in the diagnosis of clinically significant prostate cancer. Contemp Clin Trials. 2017. https://doi.org/10.1016/J.CCT.2017.10.011.
12. Postema A, Mischi M, de la Rosette J, Wijkstra H. Multiparametric ultrasound in the detection of prostate cancer: a systematic review. World J Urol. 2015; 33:1651–9. https://doi.org/10.1007/s00345-015-1523-6.
13. Smeenge M, de la Rosette JJMCH, Wijkstra H. Current status of transrectal ultrasound techniques in prostate cancer. Curr Opin Urol. 2012;22:297–302. https://doi.org/10.1097/MOU.0b013e3283548154.
14. Postema AW, Frinking PJA, Smeenge M, De Reijke TM, De La Rosette JJMCH, Tranquart F, et al. Dynamic contrast-enhanced ultrasound parametric imaging for the detection of prostate cancer. BJU Int. 2016;117:598–603.
15. Boehm K, Salomon G, Beyer B, Schiffmann J, Simonis K, Graefen M, et al. Shear wave elastography for localization of prostate cancer lesions and assessment of elasticity thresholds: implications for targeted biopsies and active surveillance protocols. J Urol. 2015;193:794–800. https://doi.org/10.1016/j.juro.2014.09.100.
16. Russo G, Mischi M, Scheepens W, De La Rosette JJ, Wijkstra H. Angiogenesis in prostate cancer: Onset, progression and imaging. BJU Int. 2012;110 11 C:794–808.
17. Van Hove A, Henri P, Maurin C, Brunelle S, Gravis G, Salem N, et al. Comparison of image - guided targeted biopsies versus systematic randomized biopsies in the detection of prostate cancer: a systematic literature review of well - designed studies. World J Urol. 2014;32:847–58.
18. Carmeliet P, Jain RK. Angiogenesis in cancer and other diseases. Nature. 2000;407:249–57.
19. Wildeboer RR, Postema AW, Demi L, Kuenen MPJ, Wijkstra H, Mischi M. Multiparametric dynamic contrast-enhanced ultrasound imaging of prostate cancer. Eur Radiol. 2017;27:3226–34. https://doi.org/10.1007/s00330-016-4693-8.
20. Good DW, Stewart GD, Hammer S, Scanlan P, Shu W, Phipps S, et al. Elasticity as a biomarker for prostate cancer: a systematic review. BJU Int. 2014;113:523–34.
21. Cosgrove D, Barr R, Bojunga J, Cantisani V, Chammas MC, Dighe M, et al. WFUMB guidelines and recommendations on the clinical use of ultrasound Elastography: part 4. Thyroid. Ultrasound Med Biol. 2017;43:4–26. https://doi.org/10.1016/j.ultrasmedbio.2016.06.022.
22. Boehm K, Budeaus L, Tennstedt P, Beyer B, Schiffmann J, Larcher A, et al. Prediction of significant prostate Cancer at prostate biopsy and per Core detection rate of targeted and systematic biopsies using real-time shear wave Elastography. Urol Int. 2015;95:189–96.

23. Barr RG, Memo R, Schaub CR. Shear wave ultrasound Elastography of the prostate. Ultrasound Q. 2012;28:13–20. https://doi.org/10.1097/RUQ.0b013e318249f594.
24. Nelson ED, Slotoroff CB, Gomella LG, Halpern EJ. Targeted biopsy of the prostate: the impact of color Doppler imaging and Elastography on prostate Cancer detection and Gleason score. Urology. 2007;70:1136–40.
25. Wildeboer RR, Schalk SG, Demi L, Wijkstra H, Mischi M. Three-dimensional histopathological reconstruction as a reliable ground truth for prostate cancer studies. Biomed Phys Eng Express. 2017;3.
26. Schalk SG, Postema A, Saidov TA, Demi L, Smeenge M, De JJMCH, et al. 3D surface-based registration of ultrasound and histology in prostate cancer imaging. Comput Med Imaging Graph. 2016;47:29–39. https://doi.org/10.1016/j.compmedimag.2015.11.001.
27. McCulloch P, Altman DG, Campbell WB, Flum DR, Glasziou P, Marshall JC, et al. No surgical innovation without evaluation: the IDEAL recommendations. Lancet. 2009;374:1105–12.
28. Kuenen MPJ, Saidov TA, Wijkstra H, Mischi M. Contrast-ultrasound dispersion imaging for prostate cancer localization by improved spatiotemporal similarity analysis. Ultrasound Med Biol. 2013;39:1631–41.
29. Kuenen MP, Mischi M, Wijkstra H. Contrast-ultrasound diffusion imaging for localization of prostate cancer. IEEE Trans Med Imaging. 2011;30:1493–502.
30. Kuenen MP, Saidov TA, Wijkstra H, de la Rosette JJ, Mischi M. Spatiotemporal correlation of ultrasound contrast agent dilution curves for angiogenesis localization by dispersion imaging. IEEE Trans Ultrason Ferroelectr Freq Control. 2013;60:2665–9.
31. van Sloun RJ, Demi L, Postema AW, de la Rosette JJ, Wijkstra H, Mischi M. Ultrasound-contrast-agent dispersion and velocity imaging for prostate cancer localization. Med Image Anal. 2017;35:610–9.
32. Van Sloun RJ, Demi L, Postema AW, Jmch De La Rosette J, Wijkstra H, Mischi M. Entropy of Ultrasound-Contrast-Agent Velocity Fields for Angiogenesis Imaging in Prostate Cancer. IEEE Trans Med Imaging. 2017;36:826–37.
33. Schlomm T, Tennstedt P, Huxhold C, Steuber T, Salomon G, Michl U, et al. Neurovascular structure-adjacent frozen-section examination (NeuroSAFE) increases nerve-sparing frequency and reduces positive surgical margins in open and robot-assisted laparoscopic radical prostatectomy: experience after 11 069 consecutive patients. Eur Urol. 2012;62:333–40.
34. Schalk S, Demi L, Bouhouch N, Kuenen M, Postema A, de la Rosette J, et al. Contrast-enhanced ultrasound angiogenesis imaging by mutual information analysis for prostate Cancer localization. IEEE Trans Biomed Eng. 2016;9294(c):1–1.
35. Turkbey B, Mani H, Shah V, Rastinehad AR, Bernardo M, Pohida T, et al. Multiparametric 3T prostate magnetic resonance imaging to detect cancer: histopathological correlation using prostatectomy specimens processed in customized magnetic resonance imaging based molds. J Urol. 2011;186:1818–24.
36. Hoeks CCM A, Barentsz JJO, Hambrock T, Yakar D, Somford DM, Heijmink SWTPJ, et al. Prostate cancer: multiparametric MR imaging for detection, localization, and staging. Radiology 2011;261:46–66. https://doi.org/10.1148/radiol.11091822.
37. Isebaert S, Van Den Bergh L, Haustermans K, Joniau S, Lerut E, De Wever L, et al. Multiparametric MRI for prostate cancer localization in correlation to whole-mount histopathology. J Magn Reson Imaging. 2013;37:1392–401.
38. Bokor D, Chambers JB, Rees PJ, Mant TG, Luzzani F, Spinazzi A. Clinical safety of SonoVue™, a new contrast agent for ultrasound imaging, in healthy volunteers and in patients with chronic obstructive pulmonary disease. Investig Radiol. 2001;36:104–9.
39. Tang C, Fang K, Guo Y, Li R, Fan X, Chen P, et al. Safety of sulfur hexafluoride microbubbles in sonography of abdominal and superficial organs: retrospective analysis of 30,222 cases. J Ultrasound Med. 2017;36:531–8. https://doi.org/10.7863/ultra.15.11075.
40. Piscaglia F, Bolondi L, Aiani L, Luigi Angeli M, Arienti V, Barozzi L, et al. The safety of Sonovue® in abdominal applications: retrospective analysis of 23188 investigations. Ultrasound Med Biol. 2006;32:1369–75.
41. Mai Z, Xiao Y, Yan W, Zhou Y, Zhou Z, Liang Z, et al. Comparison of lesions detected and undetected by template-guided transperineal saturation prostate biopsy. BJU Int. 2017. https://doi.org/10.1111/bju.13977.
42. Weinreb JC, Barentsz JO, Choyke PL, Cornud F, Haider MA, Macura KJ, et al. Pi-Rads v2. Am Coll Radiol. 2015.
43. Wildeboer RR, van Sloun RJG, Postema AW, Mannaerts CK, Gayet M, Beerlage HP, et al. Accurate validation of ultrasound imaging of prostate cancer: a review of challenges in registration of imaging and histopathology. J Ultrasound. 2018;21:197–207. https://doi.org/10.1007/s40477-018-0311-8.
44. Isebaert S, Bergh L Van Den, Haustermans K, Joniau S, Lerut E, Wever L De, et al. Multiparametric MRI for Prostate Cancer Localization in Correlation to Whole-Mount Histopathology 2012;0:1–10.
45. Turkbey B, Pinto PA, Mani H, Bernardo M, Pang Y, McKinney YL, et al. Prostate cancer: value of multiparametric MR imaging at 3 T for detection--histopathologic correlation. Radiology. 2010;255:89–99. https://doi.org/10.1148/radiol.09090475.
46. Greer MD, Brown AM, Shih JH, Summers RM, Marko J, Law YM, et al. Accuracy and agreement of PIRADSv2 for prostate cancer mpMRI: a multireader study. J Magn Reson Imaging. 2017;45:579–85.
47. Mulazzani L, Salvatore V, Ravaioli F, Allegretti G, Matassoni F, Granata R, et al. Point shear wave ultrasound elastography with Esaote compared to real-time 2D shear wave elastography with supersonic imagine for the quantification of liver stiffness. J Ultrasound. 2017;21(20):213–25.
48. Postema AW, Scheltema MJV, Mannaerts CK, Van Sloun RJG, Idzenga T, Mischi M, et al. The prostate cancer detection rates of CEUS-targeted versus MRI-targeted versus systematic TRUS-guided biopsies in biopsy-naïve men: a prospective, comparative clinical trial using the same patients. BMC Urol. 2017;17(1):27. https://doi.org/10.1186/s12894-017-0213-7.

30

Performance characteristics of prostate-specific antigen density and biopsy core details to predict oncological outcome in patients with intermediate to high-risk prostate cancer underwent robot-assisted radical prostatectomy

Masahiro Yashi[1*], Akinori Nukui[1], Yuumi Tokura[1], Kohei Takei[1], Issei Suzuki[1], Kazumasa Sakamoto[1], Hideo Yuki[1], Tsunehito Kambara[1], Hironori Betsunoh[1], Hideyuki Abe[1], Yoshitatsu Fukabori[1], Yoshimasa Nakazato[2], Yasushi Kaji[3] and Takao Kamai[1]

Abstract

Background: Many urologic surgeons refer to biopsy core details for decision making in cases of localized prostate cancer (PCa) to determine whether an extended resection and/or lymph node dissection should be performed. Furthermore, recent reports emphasize the predictive value of prostate-specific antigen density (PSAD) for further risk stratification, not only for low-risk PCa, but also for intermediate- and high-risk PCa. This study focused on these parameters and compared respective predictive impact on oncologic outcomes in Japanese PCa patients.

Methods: Two-hundred and fifty patients with intermediate- and high-risk PCa according to the National Comprehensive Cancer Network (NCCN) classification, that underwent robot-assisted radical prostatectomy at a single institution, and with observation periods of longer than 6 months were enrolled. None of the patients received hormonal treatments including antiandrogens, luteinizing hormone-releasing hormone analogues, or 5-alpha reductase inhibitors preoperatively. PSAD and biopsy core details, including the percentage of positive cores and the maximum percentage of cancer extent in each positive core, were analyzed in association with unfavorable pathologic results of prostatectomy specimens, and further with biochemical recurrence. The cut-off values of potential predictive factors were set through receiver-operating characteristic curve analyses.

Results: In the entire cohort, a higher PSAD, the percentage of positive cores, and maximum percentage of cancer extent in each positive core were independently associated with advanced tumor stage $\geq$ pT3 and an increased index tumor volume > 0.718 ml. NCCN classification showed an association with a tumor stage $\geq$ pT3 and a Gleason score $\geq$8, and the attribution of biochemical recurrence was also sustained. In each NCCN risk group, these preoperative factors showed various associations with unfavorable pathological results. In the intermediate-risk group, the percentage of positive cores showed an independent predictive value for biochemical recurrence. In the high-risk group, PSAD showed an independent predictive value.

(Continued on next page)

* Correspondence: yashima@dokkyomed.ac.jp
[1]Department of Urology, Dokkyo Medical University, 880 Kitakobayashi, Mibu, Shimotsuga, Tochigi 321-0293, Japan
Full list of author information is available at the end of the article

(Continued from previous page)

Conclusions: PSAD and biopsy core details have different performance characteristics for the prediction of oncologic outcomes in each NCCN risk group. Despite the need for further confirmation of the results with a larger cohort and longer observation, these factors are important as preoperative predictors in addition to the NCCN classification for a urologic surgeon to choose a surgical strategy.

Keyword: Predictive factor, Performance characteristics, Prostate-specific antigen density, Biopsy core details, Robot-assisted radical prostatectomy

Background

Prostate cancer (PCa) has recently become the most prevalent malignant disease and was categorized as the 6th highest cause of death in Japanese men [1]. In addition, radical prostatectomy is a first-line therapy, and a robot-assisted procedure has become a standard method for patients with localized PCa. Despite the widespread use of prostate-specific antigen (PSA) screening, a saturation biopsy protocol with multiple cores, and progress in diagnostic imaging, contemporary PCa patients still include a highly heterogeneous population of oncological outcomes. The established risk stratification system consisting of PSA, Gleason score (GS), and clinical T stage seem to insufficiently identify patients with unfavorable pathologic features preoperatively, leading to biochemical, local, and systemic recurrence [2]. We previously raised this issue from data that selected Japanese patients with low-risk PCa who still demonstrated advanced-stage ($\geq$ pT3) disease at around 15% [3]. Another Japanese study group compared five established risk stratification systems in their cohort, and found that all stratification systems could not discriminate between low- and intermediate-risk groups in terms of biochemical recurrence-free rate [4]. In view of racial differences, criteria developed from a Western cohort analysis cannot always be applied to Japanese or Asian patients [5].

Detailed information obtained from prostate biopsy has been suggested to include predictors of oncological outcomes since the sextant biopsy era [6], and protocols of multiple core biopsy with greater than 12 cores has enhanced its predictive value [7]. Currently, many urologic surgeons refer to biopsy core details for further risk assessment and decision making, and to determine whether an extended resection and/or lymph node dissection should be performed during radical prostatectomy. Furthermore, pretreatment use of PSA density (PSAD) for further risk stratification has been emphasized, not only for patients with low-risk PCa, but also those with intermediate- and high-risk PCa [8].

This study focused on these preoperative parameters and compared predictive impact on oncological outcomes, including unfavorable pathologic features and biochemical recurrence in Japanese patients with intermediate- and high-risk PCa.

Aims of study

The established risk stratification system is convenient but insufficient to make decisions for patients who need definitive therapy and for a urologic surgeon to decide upon the surgical strategy. On the other hand, prediction nomograms can offer individualized risk of PCa, but several variations exist and an ambiguity remains in the interpretation of the calculated probabilities. Accordingly, we must continue to refine the risk stratification system adapted to the demands of contemporary PCa patients. The aim of this study is to identify potential factors associated with oncological outcomes in the entire cohort and in each risk group, and to clarify the performance characteristics of predictive ability. Finally, we propose an improved risk assessment from the results.

Methods

Inclusion criteria of patients

The study population consisted of 250 consecutive patients that underwent robot-assisted radical prostatectomy between October 2012 and October 2016 at a single Japanese academic hospital with observation periods longer than 6 months. Of these patients, 155 patients were classified as being at intermediate-risk defined as having at least one characteristic among clinical stage T2b-c or GS of 7 or PSA level of 10 to 20 ng/mL, and 95 patients were classified as high-risk defined as having at least one characteristic among clinical stage $\geq$ T3a or GS $\geq$8 or PSA level $\geq$20 ng/mL, according to the National Comprehensive Cancer Network (NCCN) classification [9]. Fourteen patients (14.7%) with either very-high-risk PCa featured by $\geq$5 cores with a Gleason sum of 8 to10, or multiple NCCN high-risk features were not excluded, and were analyzed as a high-risk group in this study. None of the patients received hormonal treatments including antiandrogens, luteinizing hormone-releasing hormone analogues, or 5-alpha reductase inhibitors preoperatively. Robot-assisted radical prostatectomy was carried out using an intraperitoneal anterior approach by six surgeons. Lymph node invasion (LNI) risk was evaluated by using a Briganti nomogram [7], and lymph nodes were dissected in 70% of patients. Patients with a LNI risk $\geq$5% underwent extended dissection, and those with a LNI risk <5% underwent standard dissection or were spared dissection according to the surgeon's decision.

Preoperative clinical data, biopsy, and radiographic findings

We retrospectively reviewed the records of clinical data, findings of multiple core biopsy, and radiographic images. Preoperative patient characteristics are provided in Table 1. PSAD was determined as a pre-biopsy PSA value divided by magnetic resonance imaging (MRI)-estimated prostate volume [10]. Systematic prostate biopsy was performed through a transperineal approach without a MRI-fusion method at our hospital and related facilities. The median number of biopsy cores per procedure was 20 and no patient had fewer than 10 cores. Biopsy specimens were evaluated for GS, number of cores involved with cancer, maximum percentage of cancer extent in each positive core, and percentage of cancer measured by subtracting the intervening benign glands. Gleason scoring of the biopsy specimens was done according to the International Society of Urological Pathology (ISUP) Consensus 2005 [11]. The findings of multiparametric MRI were centrally read by one specialist of urologic radiology, whether there were typical

suspicious lesions for malignancy or not, and we did not use a Prostate Imaging Reporting and Data System (PIR-ADS) preoperatively in this study [12]. We comprehensively determined clinical T stage together with findings from the digital rectal examination.

Evaluation of prostatectomy specimens

Prostatectomy specimens obtained through robot-assisted surgery were processed according to the Stanford protocol [13], were step sectioned transversely at 4 mm intervals, and mounted as half or quarter sections for microscopic evaluation. These were evaluated for GS, extraprostatic extension, surgical margin status, seminal vesicle invasion, and tumor volume. Gleason scoring was also done as recommended in the ISUP Consensus 2005 [11]. One specialist of urologic pathology centrally evaluated the histopathology. Prostate cancer volume was estimated from the three-dimensional measurements of the index tumor, using an ellipsoid formula without correction by a shrinkage factor due to formalin fixation [14]: major diameter × minor diameter × anteroposterior diameter × Pi/6. The anteroposterior diameter was estimated from the number of step sections of 4 mm occupied by cancer.

Table 1 Preoperative patient characteristics

	Number (%) or Median (IQR)		
	Intermediate-risk	High-risk	p-value
Number	155 (100)	95 (100)	
Age (year)	66 (62–69)	67 (63–71)	0.197
PSA (ng/ml)	6.4 (5.0–8.6)	7.8 (5.9–11.8)	**<0.001**
PSA density (ng/ml/cc)	0.184 (0.136–0.259)	0.221 (0.170–0.332)	**<0.001**
Number of biopsy core (n)	20 (14–20)	18 (14–20)	0.127
Number of positive core (n)	3 (2–5)	4 (2–6)	**0.006**
% of positive cores (%)	16.7 (9.3–27.3)	21.4 (14.0–35.0)	**0.001**
% of positive cores dominant side (%)	30.0 (14.3–42.9)	37.5 (20.0–57.1)	**0.001**
% of cancer extent (%)	42.7 (21.4–66.7)	50.0 (28.3–70.0)	0.055
Biopsy Gleason score			
5–7	155 (100)	15 (15.8)	**<0.001**
8–9	0 (0)	80 (84.2)	
DRE T stage			
cT1	118 (76.1)	60 (63.2)	**0.035**
cT2a-c	37 (23.9)	33 (35.6)	
cT3a-b	0 (0)	2 (1.2)	
MRI T stage			
NA	0 (0)	1 (1.1)	**<0.001**
cT1	51 (32.9)	22 (23.2)	
cT2a-c	104 (67.1)	58 (61.1)	
cT3a-b	0 (0)	14 (14.7)	

IQR interquartile range, % cancer extent maximum % of cancer extent in each positive core, DRE digital rectal examination, Bold indicates statistically significant

Statistical analyses

PSAD and biopsy core details, including the percentage of positive cores, the percentage of positive cores from the dominant side, and the maximum percentage of cancer extent in each positive core were analyzed in association with unfavorable pathologic results of prostatectomy specimens, and further with biochemical recurrence. In this study, biochemical recurrence was defined as a PSA level greater than 0.1 ng/mL with subsequent rising PSA. When the PSA level did not decline to less than 0.1 ng/mL after prostatectomy, the date of surgery was defined as that of recurrence (immediate recurrence).

Quantitative data were compared using a Mann–Whitney U test, and qualitative data were compared using a Fisher's exact test. The cut-off values of PSAD, percentage of positive cores, percentage of positive cores from the dominant side, and maximum percentage of cancer extent in each positive core were set to be 0.345 ng/ml/cc, 21.4%, 37.5%, and 55.6%, respectively for the entire cohort; 0.190 ng/ml/cc, 21.4%, 36.4%, and 57.1% respectively for the intermediate-risk group; and 0.345 ng/ml/cc, 35.0%, 40%, and 55.6% respectively for the high-risk group by using receiver-operating characteristic curve analyses for deciding the effective point of judging biochemical recurrence.

Logistic regression and Cox proportional hazards regression models were used for univariate and multivariate analyses, and a stepwise selection procedure was used to elucidate significant factors. Recurrence-free survival was estimated using the Kaplan–Meier method, and differences were compared with the log-rank test. All statistical analyses were performed with EZR, which is a graphical user interface for R (The R Foundation for Statistical Computing, version 2.13.0). All statistical tests were two-sided, with p-values of less than 0.05 considered to be statistically significant.

Results

In the preoperative characteristics indicated in Table 1, significant differences were observed in PSA (6.4 versus 7.8 ng/ml in median value, $p < 0.001$), PSAD (0.184 versus 0.221 ng/ml/cc in median value, $p < 0.001$), the number of positive cores (3 versus 4 in median value, $p = 0.006$), the percentage of positive cores (16.7 versus 21.4% in median value, $p = 0.001$), the percentage of positive cores from the dominant side (30.0 versus 37.5% in median value, $p = 0.001$), and the composition of biopsy GS, T stage by digital rectal examination or MRI ($p < 0.001$, 0.035, <0.001, respectively) between the intermediate- and high-risk groups, but not in the number of biopsy core (20 versus 18 in median value, $p = 0.127$), and the maximum percentage of cancer extent in each positive core (42.7 versus

50.0% in median value, $p = 0.055$). The tumor characteristics of the prostatectomy specimens are provided in Table 2. Significant differences were observed in the pathologic tumor stage (≥pT3: 20.0 versus 40.0%, $p = 0.010$), surgical margin status (positive: 12.3 versus 23.2%, $p = 0.034$), and prostatectomy GS (≥8: 11.6 versus 43.2%, $p < 0.001$) between the intermediate- and high-risk group, but not in index tumor volume (1.18 versus 1.05 cc in median value, $p = 0.776$).

Among those unfavorable pathologic findings, advanced tumor stage ≥ pT3, increased index tumor volume >0.718 ml, and high GS ≥8 showed independent predictive value for biochemical recurrence, but surgical margin status did not show independent value in this study (see Additional file 1: Table S1). During a median follow-up of 24.5 months (interquartile range 14.0–36.0), it was discovered that 19 patients (12.3%) in the intermediate-risk group and 26 patients (27.4%) in the high-risk group developed biochemical recurrence.

The results of the univariate and multivariate analyses for the associations between preoperative factors and unfavorable pathologic results or biochemical recurrence are provided in Tables 3, 4, 5 and 6. In the entire cohort, a higher PSAD, percentage of positive cores, and maximum percentage of cancer extent in each positive core were independently associated with advanced tumor stage ≥ pT3 (odds ratio 4.370, 2.100, and 1.960, respectively) and increased index tumor volume >0.718 ml (odds ratio 2.860, 5.110, and 2.370, respectively). The higher percentage of positive cores from the dominant side showed independent association only with

Table 2 Tumor characteristics of prostatectomy specimens

	Number (%) or Median (IQR)		
	Intermediate-risk	High-risk	p-value
Number	155 (100)	95 (100)	
Pathologic T stage			
pT0	1 (0.6)	2 (2.1)	**0.010**
pT2a-c	123 (79.4)	55 (57.9)	
pT3a-b	31 (20.0)	36 (37.9)	
pT4	0 (0)	2 (2.1)	
Surgical margin			
Negative	136 (87.7)	73 (76.8)	**0.034**
Positive	19 (12.3)	22 (23.2)	
Prostatectomy Gleason score			
≤ 6	4 (2.6)	1 (1.1)	**<0.001**
7	133 (85.8)	53 (55.8)	
≥ 8	17 (11.0)	39 (41.1)	
NA	1 (0.6)	2 (2.1)	
Index tumor volume (cc)	1.18 (0.39–3.37)	1.05 (0.43–2.95)	0.776

IQR interquartile range, *NA* not available due to pT0, Bold indicates statistically significant

Table 3 Factors associated with tumor stage ≥ pT3 in entire cohort and each risk group

| | Entire cohort | | | | | |
| | Univariate analyses | | | Multivariate analyses | | |
	OR	95%CI	p-value	OR	95%CI	p-value
PSAD >0.345 vs ≤0.345 ng/ml/cc	5.850	2.820–12.20	**<0.001**	4.370	2.000–9.540	**<0.001**
% positive cores >21.4 vs ≤21.4%	3.150	1.770–5.630	**<0.001**	2.100	1.110–3.990	**0.028**
% dominant side >37.5 vs ≤37.5%	2.210	1.250–3.910	**0.006**			
% cancer extent >55.6 vs ≤55.6%	2.600	1.450–4.650	**0.001**	1.960	1.030–3.720	**0.041**
NCCN risk high vs intermediate	2.440	1.380–4.320	**0.002**	1.910	1.020–3.580	**0.042**
	Intermediate-risk					
	Univariate analyses			Multivariate analyses		
	OR	95%CI	p-value	OR	95%CI	p-value
PSAD >0.190 vs ≤0.190 ng/ml/cc	1.920	0.864–4.260	0.110			
% positive cores >21.4 vs ≤21.4%	3.260	1.450–7.320	**0.004**	3.260	1.450–7.320	**0.004**
% dominant side >36.4 vs ≤36.4%	2.400	1.070–5.380	**0.033**			
% cancer extent >57.1 vs ≤57.1%	2.180	0.970-4.900	0.059			
	High-risk					
	Univariate analyses			Multivariate analyses		
	OR	95%CI	p-value	OR	95%CI	p-value
PSAD >0.345 vs ≤0.345 ng/ml/cc	4.730	1.680–13.30	**0.003**	4.510	1.580–12.90	**0.004**
% positive cores >35.0 vs ≤35.0%	3.140	1.180–8.390	**0.023**			
% dominant side >40.0 vs ≤40.0%	1.880	0.811–4.360	0.141			
% cancer extent >55.6 vs ≤55.6%	2.810	1.170–6.760	**0.021**			

OR Odds ratio, *95%CI* 95% confidence interval, *% dominant side* % positive cores from dominant side, *% cancer extent* maximum % of cancer extent in each positive core, Bold indicates statistically significant

biochemical recurrence (odds ratio 2.648). NCCN classification showed an association with a tumor stage ≥ pT3 (odds ratio 1.910) and GS ≥8 (odds ratio 5.650), and the attribution of biochemical recurrence was also sustained (odds ratio 2.069). In each risk group of the NCCN classification, these preoperative factors showed various associations with unfavorable pathological results except for a high GS. In the intermediate-risk group, the higher percentage of positive cores and maximum percentage of cancer extent in each positive core showed a predictive value for biochemical recurrence in the univariate analysis, and a higher percentage of positive cores showed independent value in the multivariate analysis (odds ratio 3.910). In the high-risk group, PSAD and all biopsy core details showed predictive value in the univariate analysis, and a higher PSAD remained an independent value in the multivariate analysis (odds ratio 3.103). When analysis included the NCCN sub classification (very high-risk versus high-risk) in the high-risk group, the independent predictive value of PSAD remained unchanged, while the NCCN sub classification lost the independent value in the early stepwise selection procedure. Furthermore, PSAD showed more statistical superiority than PSA in the high-risk group.

Figure 1 shows the Kaplan–Meier event curves for biochemical recurrence-free survivals. The entire cohort was divided into 4 subgroups according to the NCCN risk, percentage of positive cores, and PSAD: subgroup 1 ($n = 100$): intermediate-risk with low percentage of positive cores, subgroup 2 ($n = 55$): intermediate-risk with high percentage of positive cores, subgroup 3 ($n = 74$): high-risk with low PSAD, and subgroup 4 ($n = 21$): high-risk with high PSAD. Pairwise comparisons among groups revealed that subgroup 2 and 3 showed almost the same recurrence curves, and the entire cohort could be stratified into three different risk groups. The frequency of immediate recurrence was significantly higher in subgroup 4 than in the other subgroups (33.3% versus 6.1%, $p < 0.001$).

Discussion

Our study demonstrated that PSAD and biopsy core details had predictive value for unfavorable pathologic results and biochemical recurrence in addition to the NCCN risk classification, and there was a difference in performance characteristics for the prediction of oncologic outcomes in each NCCN risk groups. The most significant predictor for biochemical recurrence was the percentage of positive cores in the intermediate-risk

Table 4 Factors associated with index tumor volume > 0.718 in entire cohort and each risk group

| | Entire cohort | | | | | |
| | Univariate analyses | | | Multivariate analyses | | |
	OR	95%CI	p-value	OR	95%CI	p-value
PSAD >0.345 vs ≤0.345 ng/ml/cc	3.780	1.520–9.440	**0.004**	2.860	1.060–7.680	**0.038**
% positive cores >21.4 vs ≤21.4%	6.640	3.520–12.50	**<0.001**	5.110	2.660–9.840	**<0.001**
% dominant side >37.5 vs ≤37.5%	6.140	3.250–11.60	**<0.001**			
% cancer extent >55.6 vs ≤55.6%	3.240	1.790–5.880	**<0.001**	2.370	1.250–4.520	**0.009**
NCCN risk high vs intermediate	1.220	0.717–2.070	0.465			
	Intermediate-risk					
	Univariate analyses			Multivariate analyses		
	OR	95%CI	p-value	OR	95%CI	p-value
PSAD >0.190 vs ≤0.190 ng/ml/cc	2.330	1.190–4.560	**0.014**			
% positive cores >21.4 vs ≤21.4%	8.050	3.320–19.50	**<0.001**	6.760	2.750–16.70	**<0.001**
% dominant side >36.4 vs ≤36.4%	5.900	2.610–13.40	**<0.001**			
% cancer extent >57.1 vs ≤57.1%	3.460	1.570–7.650	**0.002**	2.370	1.010–5.58	**0.048**
	High-risk					
	Univariate analyses			Multivariate analyses		
	OR	95%CI	p-value	OR	95%CI	p-value
PSAD >0.345 vs ≤0.345 ng/ml/cc	1.950	0.643–5.900	0.239			
% positive cores >35.0 vs ≤35.0%	7.380	1.610–33.90	**0.010**	7.380	1.610–33.90	**0.010**
% dominant side >40.0 vs ≤40.0%	3.560	1.390–9.100	**0.008**			
% cancer extent >55.6 vs ≤55.6%	2.410	0.959–6.050	0.061			

OR Odds ratio, *95%CI* 95% confidence interval, *% dominant side* % positive cores from dominant side, *% cancer extent* maximum % of cancer extent in each positive core, Bold indicates statistically significant

group and PSAD in the high-risk PCa group. To our knowledge, this study was the first attempt to improve a stratification model of intermediate- to high-risk PCa by using the difference in performance characteristics of these preoperative factors, and the entire cohort could be stratified into three distinct risk groups. Moreover, PSAD predicted biochemical recurrence more efficiently than a NCCN sub-classification of very high-risk or high-risk, and immediate recurrence was remarkably frequent in high-risk PCa patients with high PSAD. These results suggest that both PSAD and biopsy core details are important factors for predicting the oncologic outcome of contemporary PCa patients, but those with intermediate- and high-risk PCa, which include a highly heterogeneous population, are not uniformly stratified by a single factor, and a preoperative risk classification system should consider differences in performance characteristics when incorporating these factors.

The percentage of positive cores and percentage of cancer extent in each positive core are representative factors among biopsy core details to assess cancer involvement in the prostate, and these predictive values of oncologic outcome have been investigated since the sextant biopsy era [6]. Egawa, et al. reported that these two factors in conjunction with the three known variables

(PSA, clinical stage, and biopsy GS) improved the predictability of non-organ-confined PCa [15]. Meanwhile, Freeland et al. reported that a combination of PSA, biopsy GS, and percentage of cancer extent defined a preoperative model for predicting PSA recurrence [16], and almost simultaneously, they reported that the percentage of positive cores from the dominant side was a slightly better predictor of PSA recurrence than the total percentage of positive cores [17]. Briganti et al. performed a comprehensive analysis of the importance of the information contained within the variable that codes either the number or the percentage of positive cores; the percentage of cores improved stage predictions, and the number of cores improved mostly biochemical recurrence predictions [18]. The protocols of multiple core biopsy would contribute to enhance the predictive value of the biopsy core details. Briganti et al. later updated their analyses by increasing the number of cores taken from biopsy, and they repeatedly emphasized that the inclusion of the percentage of positive cores should be mandatory in the prediction model for lymph node invasion of PCa [7, 19]. Hinev, et al. demonstrated that Briganti's nomograms showed a higher predictive accuracy for lymph node invasion as compared with the Memorial Sloan-Kettering Cancer Center nomogram,

Table 5 Factors associated with pathological Gleason score ≥ 8 in entire cohort and each risk group

	OR	95%CI	p-value
Entire cohort			
Univariate analyses			
PSAD >0.345 vs ≤0.345 ng/ml/cc	1.510	0.697–3.280	0.296
% positive cores >21.4 vs ≤21.4%	1.350	0.739–2.450	0.331
% dominant side >37.5 vs ≤37.5%	1.440	0.788–2.620	0.237
% cancer extent >55.6 vs ≤55.6%	1.460	0.789–2.710	0.228
NCCN risk high vs intermediate	5.650	2.950–10.80	**<0.001**
Intermediate-risk			
Univariate analyses			
PSAD >0.190 vs ≤0.190 ng/ml/cc	1.860	0.668–5.160	0.236
% positive cores >21.4 vs ≤21.4%	0.733	0.244–2.200	0.580
% dominant side >36.4 vs ≤36.4%	0.696	0.243–1.990	0.500
% cancer extent >57.1 vs ≤57.1%	1.660	0.590–4.650	0.338
High-risk			
Univariate analyses			
PSAD >0.345 vs ≤0.345 ng/ml/cc	1.100	0.412-2.930	0.849
% positive cores >35.0 vs ≤35.0%	1.260	0.483–3.310	0.632
% dominant side >40.0 vs ≤40.0%	2.100	0.912–4.830	0.081
% cancer extent >55.6 vs ≤55.6%	1.020	0.437–2.390	0.959

OR Odds ratio, 95%CI 95% confidence interval, % dominant side % positive cores from dominant side, % cancer extent maximum % of cancer extent in each positive core, Bold indicates statistically significant

which provide predictions without information on biopsy cores [20]. Despite the positive correlation between the percentage of positive cores and the percentage of cancer extent in each positive core, each of the two factors also shows an independent predictive value for the advanced tumor stage and an increased index tumor volume in our entire cohort. Statistical superiority or inferiority between these factors might have arisen from the difference in the composition of patient data set or the saturation degree of biopsy. The relatively large number of biopsy cores might support universality as a prediction tool of these factors, but an advantage of the percentage of positive cores from the dominant side was only observed in prediction of biochemical recurrence in the entire cohort. Currently, many urologic surgeons refer to biopsy core details through prediction nomograms to assess individual risk for lymph node invasion and to make decisions regarding whether an extended resection and/or lymph node dissection should be performed during surgery.

PSAD is a convenient tool to offset the impact of prostate size that contributes to an elevated PSA and intensifies the potential value of PSA. Therefore, PSAD was

initially proposed as a means of distinguishing benign hyperplasia from cancer [21]. PSAD as a predictor for adverse pathologic features or biochemical recurrence has also been debated since the middle 1990s [22]. Some studies demonstrated that PSAD provided greater advantages in predicting oncologic outcome than PSA alone in the entire cohort that underwent definitive therapy [8, 23], but conflicting results were also reported [24, 25]. Because PSAD has been incorporated into the major criteria of clinically insignificant cancer or the protocol of active surveillance for lower-risk cancer, such as Epstein or Prostate Cancer Research International: Active Surveillance (PRIAS) criteria with strict thresholds, clinical interest and discussion of PSAD have shifted toward lower risk cancers [26, 27]. Against these backgrounds, the predictive value of PSAD in risk groups of those who require definitive therapy is not more widely recognized than that of biopsy core details. Similar to our study, Koie et al. analyzed subjects limited to high-risk PCa and revealed that PSAD had independent predictive value for an adverse pathologic stage and biochemical recurrence [28]. More interestingly, Hamada et al. demonstrated that both PSAD and the percentage of cores positive from the dominant side had independent predictive value for biochemical recurrence in high-risk PCa, and they stratified patients into three groups using a statistical formula [29]. Although our study did not show the predictive value of PSAD with any threshold in intermediate-risk PCa, Narita et al. and Kang et al. demonstrated a predictive value, and Kang et al. further proposed incorporating PSAD to identify patients for whom active surveillance would be appropriate [30, 31]. The predictive value of PSAD might become conspicuous when patients are stratified into each risk group, implicitly suggesting that it is important to recognize the difference in the performance characteristics of predictive factors. Because variations in the methods for prostate size measurement may influence PSAD, such that it becomes an unstable factor, our method of estimating prostate size from MRI measurements can be recommended to minimize the fluctuation between examiners [3, 10].

Pretreatment risk stratification or nomograms must be sophisticated to make decisions for patients who need definitive therapy and for a urologic surgeon to decide upon the treatment strategy. Beyond the clinical and pathological factors, non-invasive biomarkers from urine or peripheral blood and genetic panels consisting of multiple gene profiling would help distinguish aggressive cancer from an indolent case and forecast a clinical course of PCa in a pre- and post-treatment setting [32–34]. Thus, clinical and translational research are urgently required to realize future individualized management of PCa patients.

Table 6 Factors associated with biochemical recurrence in entire cohort and each risk group

	Entire cohort					
	Univariate analyses			Multivariate analyses		
	HR	95%CI	*p*-value	HR	95%CI	*p*-value
PSAD >0.345 vs ≤0.345 ng/ml/	3.105	1.669–5.776	**<0.001**			
% positive cores >21.4 vs ≤21.4%	2.490	1.363–4.551	**0.003**			
% dominant side >37.5 vs ≤37.5%	3.793	2.016–7.136	**<0.001**	2.648	1.369–5.121	**0.004**
% cancer extent >55.6 vs ≤55.6%	3.301	1.778–6.130	**<0.001**	2.505	1.324–4.741	**0.005**
NCCN risk high vs intermediate	2.517	1.391–4.555	**0.002**	2.069	1.129–3.791	**0.019**
	Intermediate-risk					
	Univariate analyses			Multivariate analyses		
	HR	95%CI	*p*-value	HR	95%CI	*p*-value
PSAD >0.190 vs ≤0.190 ng/ml/cc	2.040	0.803–5.185	0.134			
% positive cores >21.4 vs ≤21.4%	3.910	1.485–10.29	**0.006**	3.910	1.485–10.29	**0.006**
% dominant side >36.4 vs ≤36.4%	1.111	0.871–1.418	0.398			
% cancer extent >57.1 vs ≤57.1%	3.207	1.288–7.984	**0.012**			
	High-risk					
	Univariate analyses			Multivariate analyses		
	HR	95%CI	*p*-value	HR	95%CI	*p*-value
PSAD >0.345 vs ≤0.345 ng/ml/cc	3.121	1.428–6.824	**0.004**	3.103	1.373–7.012	**0.006**
% positive cores >35.0 vs ≤35.0%	3.005	1.374–6.572	**0.006**			
% dominant side >40.0 vs ≤40.0	2.404	1.089–5.306	**0.030**			
% cancer extent >55.6 vs ≤55.6%	2.788	1.218–6.382	**0.015**			

HR Hazard ratio, *95%CI* 95% confidence interval, *% dominant side* % positive cores from dominant side, *% cancer extent* maximum % of cancer extent in each positive core, Bold indicates statistically significant

The current study has some limitations; it is a retrospective study based on a relatively small population, the median follow-up time was also short to fully determine oncological outcomes, and the results might not apply to patients of other races. The cut-off values of PSAD or biopsy core details used in this study were tentative data used to find the potential predictive impacts, and therefore, we did not intend to draw a conclusion regarding distinct thresholds for these factors. Furthermore, we did not perform lymph node dissection in all patients and the degree of dissection varies, thus we could not address the association between factors and LVI. Simultaneously, this

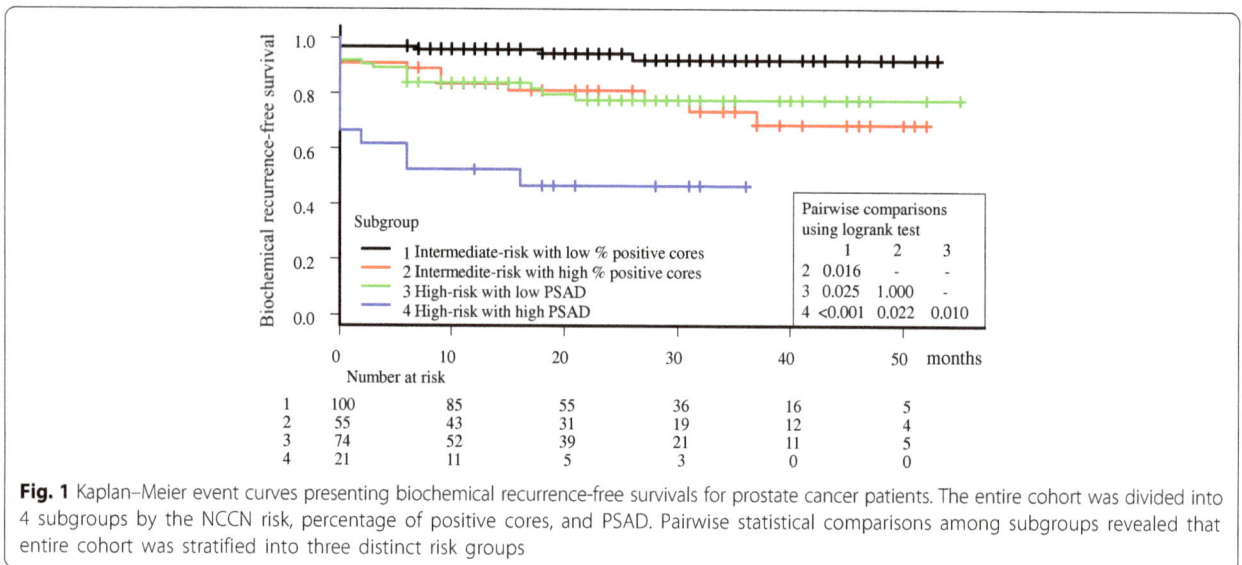

Fig. 1 Kaplan–Meier event curves presenting biochemical recurrence-free survivals for prostate cancer patients. The entire cohort was divided into 4 subgroups by the NCCN risk, percentage of positive cores, and PSAD. Pairwise statistical comparisons among subgroups revealed that entire cohort was stratified into three distinct risk groups

would to a certain extent also affect the interpretation of the results of biochemical recurrence. Nevertheless, both PSAD and biopsy core details are important preoperative predictors in addition to the NCCN classification, and the findings of this study should be validated using a larger, independent dataset.

Conclusions

Contemporary PCa patients who require definitive therapy include a highly heterogeneous population of oncological outcomes, and the established risk stratification system is insufficient to offer individualized management of PCa. PSAD and biopsy core details are important preoperative factors to predict oncologic outcomes, and should be incorporated into risk assessment for intermediate- and high-risk PCa patients. In addition, we must recognize the difference in the performance characteristics of these factors when PCa patients are stratified into each of the NCCN risk groups; where the percentage of positive cores and PSAD are independent predictors for biochemical recurrence in the intermediate- and high-risk groups, respectively.

Abbreviations
GS: Gleason score; ISUP: International Society of Urological Pathology; LNI: Lymph node invasion; MRI: Magnetic resonance imaging; NCCN: National Comprehensive Cancer Network; PCa: Prostate cancer; PSA: Prostate-specific antigen; PSAD: Prostate-specific antigen density

Acknowledgements
The authors are special thanks to Tomoya Mizuno, Director of Urology at Nasu Red Cross Hospital, Tochigi, Japan, for his practical advice and statistical work in conducting this study.

Funding
Not applicable.

Authors' contributions
MY, AN and TaK initiated this study, participated in its design and coordination, carried out the study and drafted the manuscript. YT, KT, IS, KS performed the statistical analysis. MY, HY, TsK, HB, HA, YF and were surgeons of robot-assisted radical prostatectomy and carried out the study. YN and YK were uropathologist and uroradiologist, respectively, and advised the manuscript design. All authors read and approved the final manuscript.

Competing interests
The authors declare that they have no competing interests.

Author details
[1]Department of Urology, Dokkyo Medical University, 880 Kitakobayashi, Mibu, Shimotsuga, Tochigi 321-0293, Japan. [2]Department of Pathology, Dokkyo Medical University, Tochigi, Japan. [3]Department of Radiology, Dokkyo Medical University, Tochigi, Japan.

References
1. Hori M, Matsuda T, Shibata A, Katanoda K, Sobue T, Nishimoto H, et al. Cancer incidence and incidence rates in Japan in 2009: a study of 32 population-based cancer registries for the Monitoring of Cancer Incidence in Japan (MCIJ) project. Jpn J Clin Oncol. 2015;45:884–91.
2. Reese AC, Pierorazio PM, Han M, Partin AW. Contemporary evaluation of the National Comprehensive Cancer Network prostate cancer risk classification system. Urology. 2012;80:1075–9.
3. Yashi M, Mizuno T, Yuki H, Masuda A, Kambara T, Betsunoh H, et al. Prostate volume and biopsy tumor length are significant predictors for classical and redefined insignificant cancer on prostatectomy specimens in Japanese men with favorable pathologic features on biopsy. BMC Urol. 2014;14:43.
4. Koie T, Mitsuzuka K, Narita S, Yoneyama T, Kawamura S, Tsuchiya N, et al. Efficiency of pretreatment risk stratification systems for prostate cancer in a Japanese population treated with radical prostatectomy. Int J Urol. 2015;22:70–3.
5. Lee SE, Kim DS, Lee WK, Park HZ, Lee CJ, Doo SH, et al. Application of the Epstein criteria for prediction of clinically insignificant prostate cancer in Korean men. BJU Int. 2010;105:1526–30.
6. Peller PA, Young DC, Marmaduke DP, Marsh WL, Badalament RA. Sextant prostate biopsies. A histopathologic correlation with radical prostatectomy specimens. Cancer. 1995;75:530–8.
7. Briganti A, Larcher A, Abdollah F, Capitanio U, Gallina A, Suardi N, et al. Updated nomogram predicting lymph node invasion in patients with prostate cancer undergoing extended pelvic lymph node dissection: the essential importance of percentage of positive cores. Eur Urol. 2012;61:480–7.
8. Radwan MH, Yan Y, Luly JR, Figenshau RS, Brandes SB, Bhayani SB, et al. Prostate-specific antigen density predicts adverse pathology and increased risk of biochemical failure. Urology. 2007;69:1121–7.
9. NCCN Clinical Practice Guidelines in Oncology Prostate Cancer Version 2. 2017-February 21, 2017. https://www.nccn.org/professionals/physician_gls/PDF/prostate.pdf Accessed 4 Jun 2017.
10. Karademir I, Shen D, Peng Y, Liao S, Jiang Y, Yousuf A, et al. Prostate volumes derived from MRI and volume-adjusted serum prostate-specific antigen: correlation with Gleason score of prostate cancer. AJR Am J Roentgenol. 2013;201:1041–8.
11. Epstein JI, Allsbrook Jr WC, Amin MB, Egevad LL, Grading Committee ISUP. The 2005 International Society of Urological Pathology (ISUP) Consensus Conference on Gleason Grading of Prostatic Carcinoma. Am J Surg Pathol. 2005;29:1228–42.
12. Vargas HA, Hötker AM, Goldman DA, Moskowitz CS, Gondo T, Matsumoto K, et al. Updated prostate imaging reporting and data system (PIRADS v2) recommendations for the detection of clinically significant prostate cancer using multiparametric MRI: critical evaluation using whole-mount pathology as standard of reference. Eur Radiol. 2016;26:1606–12.
13. McNeal JE, Redwine EA, Freiha FS, Stamey TA. Zonal distribution of prostatic adenocarcinoma. Correlation with histologic pattern and direction of spread. Am J Surg Pathol. 1988;12:897–906.
14. Perera M, Lawrentschuk N, Bolton D, Clouston D. Comparison of contemporary methods for estimating prostate tumour volume in pathological specimen. BJU Int. 2014;113 Suppl 2:29–34.
15. Egawa S, Suyama K, Matsumoto K, Satoh T, Uchida T, Kuwao S, et al. Improved predictability of extracapsular extension and seminal vesicle involvement based on clinical and biopsy findings in prostate cancer in Japanese men. Urology. 1998;52:433–40.
16. Freedland SJ, Aronson WJ, Csathy GS, Kane CJ, Amling CL, Presti Jr JC, et al. Comparison of percentage of total prostate needle biopsy tissue with cancer to percentage of cores with cancer for predicting PSA recurrence after radical prostatectomy: results from the SEARCH database. Urology. 2003;61:742–7.
17. Freedland SJ, Aronson WJ, Terris MK, Kane CJ, Amling CL, Dorey F, et al. The percentage of prostate needle biopsy cores with carcinoma from the more involved side of the biopsy as a predictor of prostate specific antigen recurrence after radical prostatectomy: results from the Shared Equal Access Regional Cancer Hospital (SEARCH) database. Cancer. 2003;98:2344–50.
18. Briganti A, Chun FK, Hutterer GC, Gallina A, Shariat SF, Salonia A, et al. Systematic assessment of the ability of the number and percentage of positive biopsy cores to predict pathologic stage and biochemical recurrence after radical prostatectomy. Eur Urol. 2007;52:733–43.

19. Briganti A, Karakiewicz PI, Chun FK, Gallina A, Salonia A, Zanni G, et al. Percentage of positive biopsy cores can improve the ability to predict lymph node invasion in patients undergoing radical prostatectomy and extended pelvic lymph node dissection. Eur Urol. 2007;51:1573–81.

20. Hinev AI, Anakievski D, Kolev NH, Hadjiev VI. Validation of nomograms predicting lymph node involvement in patients with prostate cancer undergoing extended pelvic lymph node dissection. Urol Int. 2014;92:300–5.

21. Benson MC, Whang IS, Pantuck A, Ring K, Kaplan SA, Olsson CA, et al. Prostate specific antigen density: a means of distinguishing benign prostatic hypertrophy and prostate cancer. J Urol. 1992;147:815–6.

22. Seaman EK, Whang IS, Cooner W, Olsson CA, Benson MC. Predictive value of prostate-specific antigen density for the presence of micrometastatic carcinoma of the prostate. Urology. 1994;43:645–8.

23. Freedland SJ, Wieder JA, Jack GS, Dorey F, deKernion JB, Aronson WJ. Improved risk stratification for biochemical recurrence after radical prostatectomy using a novel risk group system based on prostate specific antigen density and biopsy Gleason score. J Urol. 2002;168:110–5.

24. Ingenito AC, Ennis RD, Hsu IC, Begg MD, Benson MC, Schiff PB. Re-examining the role of prostate-specific antigen density in predicting outcome for clinically localized prostate cancer. Urology. 1997;50:73–8.

25. Brassell SA, Kao TC, Sun L, Moul JW. Prostate-specific antigen versus prostate-specific antigen density as predictor of tumor volume, margin status, pathologic stage, and biochemical recurrence of prostate cancer. Urology. 2005;66:1229–33.

26. Bastian PJ, Mangold LA, Epstein JI, Partin AW. Characteristics of insignificant clinical T1c prostate tumors. A contemporary analysis. Cancer. 2004;101:2001–5.

27. Bul M, Zhu X, Valdagni R, Pickles T, Kakehi Y, Rannikko A, et al. Active surveillance for low-risk prostate cancer worldwide: the PRIAS study. Eur Urol. 2013;63:597–603.

28. Koie T, Mitsuzuka K, Yoneyama T, Narita S, Kawamura S, Kaiho Y, et al. Prostate-specific antigen density predicts extracapsular extension and increased risk of biochemical recurrence in patients with high-risk prostate cancer who underwent radical prostatectomy. Int J Clin Oncol. 2015;20:176–81.

29. Hamada R, Nakashima J, Ohori M, Ohno Y, Komori O, Yoshioka K, et al. Preoperative predictive factors and further risk stratification of biochemical recurrence in clinically localized high-risk prostate cancer. Int J Clin Oncol. 2016;21:595–600.

30. Narita S, Mitsuzuka K, Tsuchiya N, Koie T, Kawamura S, Ohyama C, et al. Reassessment of the risk factors for biochemical recurrence in D'Amico intermediate-risk prostate cancer treated using radical prostatectomy. Int J Urol. 2015;22:1029–35.

31. Kang HW, Jung HD, Lee JY, Kwon JK, Jeh SU, Cho KS, et al. Prostate-specific antigen density predicts favorable pathology and biochemical recurrence in patients with intermediate-risk prostate cancer. Asian J Androl. 2016;18:480–4.

32. Sharma P, Zargar-Shoshtari K, Pow-Sang JM. Biomarkers for prostate cancer: present challenges and future opportunities. Future Sci OA. 2015;2(1):FSO72.

33. Behesnilian AS, Reiter RE. Risk stratification of prostate cancer in the modern era. Curr Opin Urol. 2015;25:246–51.

34. Ross AE, Johnson MH, Yousefi K, Davicioni E, Netto GJ, Marchionni L, et al. Tissue-based Genomics Augments Post-prostatectomy Risk Stratification in a Natural History Cohort of Intermediate- and High-Risk Men. Eur Urol. 2016;69:157–65.

Permissions

The contributors of this book come from diverse backgrounds, making this book a truly international effort. This book will bring forth new frontiers with its revolutionizing research information and detailed analysis of the nascent developments around the world.

We would like to thank all the contributing authors for lending their expertise to make the book truly unique. They have played a crucial role in the development of this book. Without their invaluable contributions this book wouldn't have been possible. They have made vital efforts to compile up to date information on the varied aspects of this subject to make this book a valuable addition to the collection of many professionals and students.

This book was conceptualized with the vision of imparting up-to-date information and advanced data in this field. To ensure the same, a matchless editorial board was set up. Every individual on the board went through rigorous rounds of assessment to prove their worth. After which they invested a large part of their time researching and compiling the most relevant data for our readers.

The editorial board has been involved in producing this book since its inception. They have spent rigorous hours researching and exploring the diverse topics which have resulted in the successful publishing of this book. They have passed on their knowledge of decades through this book. To expedite this challenging task, the publisher supported the team at every step. A small team of assistant editors was also appointed to further simplify the editing procedure and attain best results for the readers.

Apart from the editorial board, the designing team has also invested a significant amount of their time in understanding the subject and creating the most relevant covers. They scrutinized every image to scout for the most suitable representation of the subject and create an appropriate cover for the book.

The publishing team has been an ardent support to the editorial, designing and production team. Their endless efforts to recruit the best for this project, has resulted in the accomplishment of this book. They are a veteran in the field of academics and their pool of knowledge is as vast as their experience in printing. Their expertise and guidance has proved useful at every step. Their uncompromising quality standards have made this book an exceptional effort. Their encouragement from time to time has been an inspiration for everyone.

The publisher and the editorial board hope that this book will prove to be a valuable piece of knowledge for researchers, students, practitioners and scholars across the globe.

List of Contributors

Peng Zhang, Bohan Fan, Biao Wang, Xiaodong Zhang, Hu Han and Yue Xu
Urology department, Beijing Chaoyang hospital, Capital Medical University, 8 Gongren Tiyuchang Nanlu, Chaoyang District, Beijing 100020, China

S. De Luca, C. Fiori, R. M. Scarpa and F. Porpiglia
Division of Urology, San Luigi Gonzaga Hospital and University of Torino, Orbassano, Italy

R. Passera
Division of Nuclear Medicine, San Giovanni Battista Hospital and University of Torino, Corso AM Dogliotti 14, 10126 Torino, Italy

A. Sottile
Division of Laboratory Medicine, Candiolo Cancer Institute, Candiolo, Italy

Dechao Wei, Yili Han, Mingchuan Li, Yongxing Wang, Yatong Chen, Yong Luo and Yongguang Jiang
Department of Urology, Beijing Anzhen Hospital, Capital Medical University, Beijing 100029, People's Republic of China

Demisew Anemu Sori, Ahadu Workineh Azale and Desta Hiko Gemeda
Jimma University College of Public Health and Medical Sciences, Jimma, Ethiopia

Bianjiang Liu, Gong Cheng, Ninghong Song, Min Gu and Zengjun Wang
Department of Urology, The First Affiliated Hospital of Nanjing Medical University, Nanjing 210029, China

Quan Li
Department of Urology, Suzhou Municipal Hospital, Suzhou 215000, China

Ulf Lützen, Marlies Marx, Yi Zhao, Michael Jüptner and Maaz Zuhayra
Department of Nuclear medicine, Molecular Imaging Diagnostics and Therapy, University Hospital Schleswig Holstein, Campus Kiel, Kiel, Germany

Carsten Maik Naumann, Daniar Osmonov, Katrin Bothe and Klaus-Peter Jünemann
Department of Urology and Pediatric Urology, University Hospital Schleswig Holstein, Campus Kiel, Kiel, Germany

Jens Dischinger
Northern German Seminar for Radiation Protection gGmbH at the Christian-Albrechts-University Kiel, Kiel, Germany

René Baumann
Department of Radio Oncology, University Hospital Schleswig Holstein, Campus Kiel, Kiel, Germany

Jean-Baptiste Beauval, Mathieu Roumiguié, Thibaut Benoit, Bernard Malavaud and Michel Soulié
Department of Urology, Andrology and Renal Transplantation, CHU Rangueil, 1, av J Pouilhès, 31059 Toulouse, France

Thomas Filleron
Institut Claudius Regaud, IUCT-O, Toulouse F-31059, France

Alexandre de la Taille and Laurent Salomon
Department of Urology, Andrology and Renal Transplantation, CHU Mondor, Créteil, France

Guillaume Ploussard
Department of Urology, Clinique St Jean du Languedoc, Toulouse, France

Stephanie C. Knüpfer, Mareike M. Averhoff, Carsten M. Naumann and Moritz F. Hamann
Department of Urology and Pediatric Urology, University Medical Centre Schleswig-Holstein, Arnold-Heller-Strasse 3, Campus Kiel 24105, Germany

Susanne A. Schneider and Günther Deuschl
Department of Neurology, University Medical Centre Schleswig-Holstein, Campus Kiel, Germany

Serge P. Marinkovic, Scott Hughes, Donghua Xie, Lisa M. Gillen and Christina M. Marinkovic
Department of Urology, Detroit Medical Center, Harper/Hutzel Hospital, Detroit, MI 48202, USA

Hai Huang, Ren Jizhong, Lei Yin, Danfeng Xu and Yi Hong
Department of Urinary Surgery of Changzheng Hospital, Second Military Medical University, No. 415, Fengyang Road, Huangpu District, Shanghai 200003, China

Yi Huang
Department of Urinary Surgery of Changzheng Hospital, Second Military Medical University, No. 415, Fengyang Road, Huangpu District, Shanghai 200003, China
Department of Urinary Surgery of Navy Hospital of Xiamen, No. 23, Zhenhai Road, Siming District, Xiamen 361000, China

Xiuwu Pan and Lin Li
Department of Urinary Surgery of Changzheng Hospital, Second Military Medical University, No. 415, Fengyang Road, Huangpu District, Shanghai 200003, China
Department of Urinary Surgery of Third Affiliated Hospital, Second Military Medical University, No. 700, Moyu Road, Jiading District, Shanghai 201805, China

Xingang Cui
Department of Urinary Surgery of Third Affiliated Hospital, Second Military Medical University, No. 700, Moyu Road, Jiading District, Shanghai 201805, China

Qiwei Zhou
Department of Urinary Surgery of No. 313 Hospital of PLA, No. 50, Haibinnan Road, Longgang District, Huludao City, Liaoning 125000, China

Guodong Wang
Department of Stomatology of Changzheng Hospital, Second Military Medical University, Shanghai, China

Kenneth R. MacKenzie and Jonathan Aning
Department of Urology, The Newcastle upon Tyne Hospitals NHS Foundation Trust, Freeman Hospital, Newcastle-Upon-Tyne NE7 7DN, UK

Keishiro Fukumoto, Eiji Kikuchi, Akira Miyajima and Mototsugu Oya
Department of Urology, Keio University School of Medicine, 35 Shinanomachi, Shinjuku-ku, Tokyo 160-0016, Japan

Shuji Mikami
Division of Diagnostic Pathology, Keio University School of Medicine, Tokyo, Japan

Bishoy A. Gayed, Ramy Youssef, Oussama Darwish, Aditya Bagrodia, Ganesh Raj, Arthur Sagalowsky and Vitaly Margulis
Department of Urology, University of Texas Southwestern Medical Center, 5323 Harry Hines Blvd., Dallas, TX 75390-9110, USA

Payal Kapur
Departments of Pathology, University of Texas Southwestern Medical Center, Dallas, TX, USA

James Brugarolas
Departments of Medicine and Developmental Biology, University of Texas Southwestern Medical Center, Dallas, TX, USA

J. Michael Di Maio
Departments of Cardiothoracic Surgery, University of Texas Southwestern Medical Center, Dallas, TX, USA

Abeni Oitchayomi, Arnaud Doerfler, Sophie Le Gal, Charles Chawhan and Xavier Tillou
Urology and Transplantation Department, University Hospital of Caen, CHU Cote de Nacre, Avenue de Cote de Nacre, 14033 Caen, France

Jianrong Huang, Leming Song, Xiaolin Deng, Min Hu, Zuofeng Peng, Tairong Liu, Chuance Du, Lei Yao, Shengfeng Liu, Shulin Guo and Jiuqing Zhong
Department of Urology, The Affiliated Ganzhou Hospital of Nanchang University, 17 Hongqi Avenue, Ganzhou, Jiangxi 341000, China

Donghua Xie
Department of Urology, The Affiliated Ganzhou Hospital of Nanchang University, 17 Hongqi Avenue, Ganzhou, Jiangxi 341000, China
Department of Urology, Detroit Medical Center, Detroit, MI 48201, USA

Monong Li
Department of Urology, The affiliated Qingdao Municipal Hospital of Medical College of Qingdao University, Qingdao, Shandong 266021, China

Xinying Li, Ping Wang, Yili Liu and Chunlai Liu
Department of Urology, The Fourth Hospital of China Medical University, 4 Chongshan Road, Shenyang 110032, China

Musa Kayondo and Joseph Njagi
Faculty of Medicine, Mbarara University of Science and Technology, Mbarara, Uganda
Department of Obstetrics and Gynecology, Mbarara Regional Referral Hospital, Mbarara, Uganda

Peter Kivuniike Mukasa
United Nation Fund for Population Activities, Kampala, Uganda

Tom Margolis
Department of Obstetrics and Gynecology, University of California, Los Angeles, USA
Medled Medical Missions, Burlingame, California, USA

Andrea Mogorovich and Cesare Selli
Urology Unit University of Pisa, Pisa, Italy

Francesco Francesca and Giorgio Pomara
Urology Unit AOUP, Pisa, Italy

Riccardo Bartoletti
Urology Unit University of Pisa, Pisa, Italy
Urology University Unit, Cisanello Hospital, Via Paradisa 2, 56124 Pisa, Italy

Z. Talat, B. Onal, B. Cetinel, C. Demirdag, S. Citgez and C. Dogan
Department of Urology, Istanbul University-Cerrahpasa, Cerrahpasa Medical Faculty, Fatih, 34098 Istanbul, Turkey

Yunjin Bai, Xiaoming Wang, Yubo Yang, Ping Han and Jia Wang
Department of Urology, Institute of Urology, West China Hospital, Sichuan University, Chengdu, China

Jeong Woo Lee
Department of Urology, Dongguk University Ilsan Hospital, Dongguk University College of Medicine, 27, Dongguk-ro, Ilsandong-gu, Goyang-si, Gyeonggi-do 410-773, Republic of Korea

Min Gu Park
Department of Urology, Seoul Paik Hospital, Inje University College of Medicine, 9, Mareunnae-ro, Jung-gu, Seoul 100-032, Republic of Korea

Sung Yong Cho
Department of Urology, Seoul Metropolitan Government-Seoul National University Boramae Medical Center, Seoul National University College of Medicine, 20, Boramae-ro 5-Gil, Dongjak-gu, Seoul 156-707, Republic of Korea

R. M. Kumar
Division of Urology, Department of Surgery, The Ottawa Hospital, University of Ottawa, Ottawa, ON, Canada

M. Horrigan, S. Cnossen, R. Mallick, M. Fung-Kee-Fung, K. Witiuk and D. A. Fergusson
Ottawa Hospital Research Institute, Ottawa, ON, Canada

R. H. Breau, L. T. Lavallee, I. Cagiannos and C. Morash
Division of Urology, Department of Surgery, The Ottawa Hospital, University of Ottawa, Ottawa, ON, Canada
Ottawa Hospital Research Institute, Ottawa, ON, Canada

D. Stacey
Ottawa Hospital Research Institute, Ottawa, ON, Canada
Faculty of Health Sciences, University of Ottawa, Ottawa, ON, Canada

R. Morash and J. Smylie
The Ottawa Hospital Cancer Program, Ottawa, Canada

Yongquan Tang
Department of Pediatric Surgery, West China Hospital, Sichuan University, No. 37 of Guoxue Xiang, Chengdu 610041, China

Zhihong Liu, Jiayu Liang, Kan Wu, Chuan Zhou, Fuxun Zhang and Yiping Lu
Department of Urology, Institute of Urology, West China Hospital, Sichuan University, Chengdu, China

Ruochen Zhang
Department of Urology, Fujian Provincial Hospital, Fuzhou, China

Zijun Zou
Department of Urology, the Third Affiliated Hospital, Sun Yat-sen University, Guangzhou, China

Yajie Yu, Chao Liang and Pengfei Shao
Department of Urology, The First Affiliated Hospital of Nanjing Medical University, Nanjing 210029, China

Meiling Bao
Department of Pathology, The First Affiliated Hospital of Nanjing Medical University, Nanjing 210029, China

Nici Markus Dreger, Stephan Roth, Alexander Sascha Brandt and Stephan Degener
Department of Urology, Helios Medical Center Wuppertal, Helios University Hospital Wuppertal, University of Witten/Herdecke, Heusnerstraße 40, Wuppertal 42283, Germany

Friedrich Carl von Rundstedt
Scott Department of Urology, Baylor College of Medicine Medical Center, 7200 Cambridge, Houston, TX, USA
Department of Urology, Jena Medical Center, Friedrich-Schiller University, Bachstraße 18, Jena 07743, Germany

Meng-Yi Yan, Jesun Lin and Pao-Hwa Chen
From the Division of Urology, Department of Surgery, Changhua Christian Hospital, 135, Nanxiao St., Changhua City, Changhua County 500, Taiwan

Yao-Li Chen
From the Transplant Medicine and Surgery Research Center, Changhua Christian Hospital, Changhua, Taiwan
School of Medicine, Kaohsiung Medical University, Kaohsiung, Taiwan

Heng-Chieh Chiang
From the Division of Urology, Department of Surgery, Changhua Christian Hospital, 135, Nanxiao St., Changhua City, Changhua County 500, Taiwan
School of Medicine, Kaohsiung Medical University, Kaohsiung, Taiwan

Hai-bin Wei, Xiao-long Qi, Feng Liu, Qi Zhang, En-hui Li, Xuan-yu Chen and Da-hong Zhang
Department of Urology, Zhejiang Provincial People's Hospital, No. 158, Shangtang Road, Xiacheng District, Hangzhou, Zhejiang 310014, China

Jie Wang
Department of Nephrology, Sir Run Run Shaw Hospital, No. 3, East Qingchun Road, Jianggan District, Hangzhou, Zhejiang 310076, China

Xiao-feng Ni
Department of general surgery, Central Hospital of Huzhou, No. 198, Hongqi Road, Wuxing District, Huzhou, Zhejiang 313003, China

Ken Fukushi, Shingo Hatakeyama, Hayato Yamamoto, Yuki Tobisawa, Osamu Soma, Teppei Matsumoto, Itsuto Hamano, Takuma Narita, Atsushi Imai, Takahiro Yoneyama and Takuya Koie
Department of Urology, Hirosaki University Graduate School of Medicine, 5 Zaifu-chou, Hirosaki 036-8562, Japan

Tohru Yoneyama and Yasuhiro Hashimoto
Department of Advanced Transplant and Regenerative Medicine, Hirosaki University Graduate School of Medicine, Hirosaki, Japan

Chikara Ohyama
Department of Urology, Hirosaki University Graduate School of Medicine, 5 Zaifu-chou, Hirosaki 036-8562, Japan
Department of Advanced Transplant and Regenerative Medicine, Hirosaki University Graduate School of Medicine, Hirosaki, Japan

Yuriko Terayama and Tomihisa Funyu
Department of Urology, Oyokyo Kidney Research Institute, Hirosaki, Japan

Christophe K. Mannaerts and Arnoud W. Postema
Department of Urology, Amsterdam University Medical Centers, University of Amsterdam, Amsterdam, The Netherlands

Rogier R. Wildeboer and Massimo Mischi
Department of Electrical Engineering, Eindhoven University of Technology, Eindhoven, The Netherlands

Hessel Wijkstra
Department of Urology, Amsterdam University Medical Centers, University of Amsterdam, Amsterdam, The Netherlands
Department of Electrical Engineering, Eindhoven University of Technology, Eindhoven, The Netherlands

Johanna Hagemann, Lars Budäus, Derya Tilki and Georg Salomon
Martini Clinic, Prostate Cancer Center, University Hospital Hamburg-Eppendorf, Hamburg, Germany

Masahiro Yashi, Akinori Nukui, Yuumi Tokura, Kohei Takei, Issei Suzuki, Kazumasa Sakamoto, Hideo Yuki, Tsunehito Kambara, Hironori Betsunoh, Hideyuki Abe, Yoshitatsu Fukabori and Takao Kamai
Department of Urology, Dokkyo Medical University, 880 Kitakobayashi, Mibu, Shimotsuga, Tochigi 321-0293, Japan

Yoshimasa Nakazato
Department of Pathology, Dokkyo Medical University, Tochigi, Japan

Yasushi Kaji
Department of Radiology, Dokkyo Medical University, Tochigi, Japan

Index